The Epidemiological Transition

POLICY AND PLANNING IMPLICATIONS FOR DEVELOPING COUNTRIES

WORKSHOP
PROCEEDINGS

James N. Gribble and Samuel H. Preston, Editors

Committee on Population
Commission on Behavioral and Social Sciences and Education
National Research Council

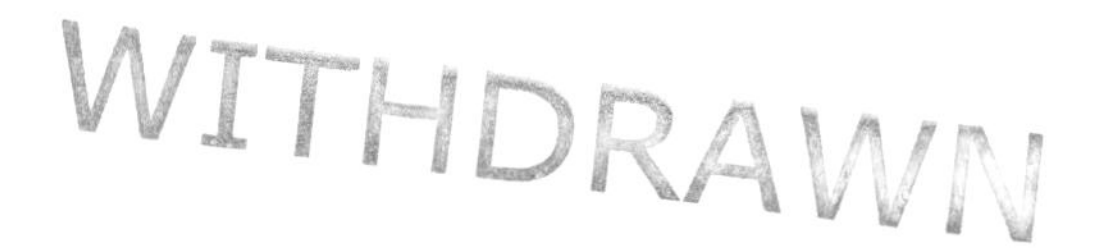

NATIONAL ACADEMY PRESS
Washington, D.C. 1993

National Academy Press • 2101 Constitution Avenue, N.W. • Washington, D.C. 20418

NOTICE: The project that is the subject of this report was approved by the Governing Board of the National Research Council, whose members are drawn from the councils of the National Academy of Sciences, the National Academy of Engineering, and the Institute of Medicine. The members of the committee responsible for the report were chosen for their special competences and with regard for appropriate balance.

This report has been reviewed by a group other than the authors according to procedures approved by a Report Review Committee consisting of members of the National Academy of Sciences, the National Academy of Engineering, and the Institute of Medicine.

The National Academy of Sciences is a private, nonprofit, self-perpetuating society of distinguished scholars engaged in scientific and engineering research, dedicated to the furtherance of science and technology and to their use for the general welfare. Upon the authority of the charter granted to it by the Congress in 1863, the Academy has a mandate that requires it to advise the federal government on scientific and technical matters. Dr. Bruce Alberts is president of the National Academy of Sciences.

The National Academy of Engineering was established in 1964, under the charter of the National Academy of Sciences, as a parallel organization of outstanding engineers. It is autonomous in its administration and in the selection of its members, sharing with the National Academy of Sciences the responsibility for advising the federal government. The National Academy of Engineering also sponsors engineering programs aimed at meeting national needs, encourages education and research, and recognizes the superior achievements of engineers. Dr. Robert M. White is president of the National Academy of Engineering.

The Institute of Medicine was established in 1970 by the National Academy of Sciences to secure the services of eminent members of appropriate professions in the examination of policy matters pertaining to the health of the public. The Institute acts under the responsibility given to the National Academy of Sciences by its congressional charter to be an adviser to the federal government and, upon its own initiative, to identify issues of medical care, research, and education. Dr. Kenneth I. Shine is president of the Institute of Medicine.

The National Research Council was organized by the National Academy of Sciences in 1916 to associate the broad community of science and technology with the Academy's purposes of furthering knowledge and advising the federal government. Functioning in accordance with general policies determined by the Academy, the Council has become the principal operating agency of both the National Academy of Sciences and the National Academy of Engineering in providing services to the government, the public, and the scientific and engineering communities. The Council is administered jointly by both Academies and the Institute of Medicine. Dr. Bruce Alberts and Dr. Robert M. White are chairman and vice chairman, respectively, of the National Research Council.

Support for the meeting that is the subject of this report was provided by the Office of Health of the U.S. Agency for International Development.

Library of Congress Catalog Card No. 93-84592
International Standard Book Number 0-309-04830-7

Additional copies of this report are available from: National Academy Press, 2101 Constitution Avenue, N.W., Box 285, Washington, D.C. 20055 Call 800-624-6242 or 202-334-3313 (in the Washington Metropolitan Area).

B060

Printed in the United States of America

WORKSHOP ON THE POLICY AND PLANNING IMPLICATIONS OF THE EPIDEMIOLOGICAL TRANSITION IN DEVELOPING COUNTRIES

November 20-22, 1991

Participant List

Presenters

NANCY BIRDSALL, World Bank
ROBERT BLUM, University of Minnesota
JAMES BLUMSTEIN, Vanderbilt University
JOSE LUIS BOBADILLA, World Bank
RODOLFO BULATAO, World Bank
JOHN CALDWELL, Australian National University
PAT CALDWELL, Australian National University
CHANPEN CHOPRAPAWAN, National Epidemiology Board of Thailand
RICHARD FEACHEM, London School of Hygiene and Tropical Medicine
LARRY HELIGMAN, United Nations Population Division
CLYDE HERTZMAN, University of British Columbia
DEAN JAMISON, University of California, Los Angeles
RUTH LEVINE, The Urban Institute
DAVID MECHANIC, Rutgers University
W. HENRY MOSLEY, Johns Hopkins University
PHILIP MUSGROVE, World Bank
ANNE R. PEBLEY, Princeton University
SAMUEL H. PRESTON, University of Pennsylvania
ANTHONY ROBBINS, Boston University
ERIC STALLARD, Duke University
JULIA WALSH, Harvard University

Guests

SUE ANTHONY, Office of Nutrition, U.S. Agency for International Development
PETER BERMAN, Harvard University
ROBERT BERNSTEIN, Office of Health, U.S. Agency for International Development
RICHARD BISSELL, Bureau for Research and Development, U.S. Agency for International Development
MARTIN BROCKERHOFF, Office of Population, U.S. Agency for International Development

ROBERT CLAY, Office of Health, U.S. Agency for International Development
ROBIN ESPENSCHADE, Office of Health, U.S. Agency for International Development
JOHN FARRAR, International Clinical Epidemiology Network
HOLLY FLUTY, Office of Health, U.S. Agency for International Development
DIAA HAMMAMY, International Science and Technology Institute
PAMELA JOHNSON, Office of Health, U.S. Agency for International Development
KEVIN KINSELLA, Center for International Research, Bureau of the Census
JAMES KOCHER, Center for Development Policy, Research Triangle Institute
SUE KOLODIN, Office of Health, U.S. Agency for International Development
TERRY LUCAS, Near East Bureau, U.S. Agency for International Development
MIKE MALISON, International Health Program Office, Centers for Disease Control
MELANIE MARLETT, Directorate for Policy, U.S. Agency for International Development
ROY MILLER, International Science and Technology Institute
ELLYN OGDEN, Statistica, Inc.
MARGUERITE PAPPAIOANOU, Epidemiology Program Office, Centers for Disease Control
TOM PARK, Latin America Bureau, U.S. Agency for International Development
CRISTINA POSSAS, Takemi Fellow, Harvard University
PETRA REYES, Office of Health, U.S. Agency for International Development
RICHARD SUZMAN, Office of Demography of Aging, National Institute on Aging
JOHN TOMARO, Office of Health, U.S. Agency for International Development
BARBARA BOYLE TORREY, Center for International Research, Bureau of the Census
DAVID WILLIS, Office of Demography of Aging, National Institute on Aging
OLEH WOLOWYNA, Center for Development Policy, Research Triangle Institute
JUN ZHU, Office of Population Research, Princeton University

Committee on Population Staff

LINDA G. MARTIN, *Director*
CAROLE L. JOLLY, *Program Officer*
JAMES N. GRIBBLE, *Program Officer*
DOMINIQUE A. MEEKERS, *Research Associate*
DIANE L. GOLDMAN, *Administrative Assistant*
JOAN MONTGOMERY HALFORD, *Project Assistant*

Division on International Health Staff

POLLY HARRISON, *Director*
CAROLYN HALL, *Program Associate*
DANA HOTRA, *Research Associate*
CHRISTOPHER HOWSON, *Deputy Director*
VIOLAINE MITCHELL, *Study Director*
NALINI PHILIPOSE, *Research Assistant*
SHARON SCOTT-BROWN, *Administrative Assistant*
DELORES SUTTON, *Project Assistant*

COMMITTEE ON POPULATION

INSTITUTE OF MEDICINE
BOARD ON INTERNATIONAL HEALTH

Contents

Preface

In November 1991, with support from the Office of Health of the U.S. Agency for International Development, the Committee on Population, in collaboration with the Board on International Health of the Institute of Medicine, organized a workshop to discuss the changing demographic and epidemiologic profiles of developing countries and responses from the health sector to these changes. The Workshop on the Policy and Planning Implications of the Epidemiological Transition in Developing Countries was held November 20-22, 1991, at the National Academy of Sciences' Georgetown facility in Washington, D.C. This report includes ten of the papers presented during the workshop.

The workshop covered three broad topics related to the epidemiological transition. First, participants considered the issue of projecting realistic scenarios of the populations and cause-of-death structures of developing countries, as well as discussed health over the life course. Second, the workshop turned to the mechanisms used to establish priorities in the allocation of health resources in response to the changing demographic and epidemiologic profiles. Particular attention was given to the appropriate use of data in establishing priorities. The third topic was the role of government, private medicine, and families in providing health services.

The committee wishes to thank the Office of Health of the U.S. Agency for International Development for supporting this workshop. A planning meeting, at which the foundation for the workshop was developed, was attended by Julio Frenk, Charles Griffin, Connie Carino, Gerald Rosenthal, Davidson Gwatkin, Marguerite Pappaioanou, and Pamela Johnson, as well as others mentioned below. The workshop participants were responsible for the commissioned papers, presentations, and discussion that took place. Anne Pebley and Dean Jamison facilitated the discussion by chairing parts of the workshop.

The committee is grateful to Linda Martin, Director of the Committee on Population, Polly Harrison, Director of the Division on International Health, and Petra Reyes, Deputy Director of the Applied Research Division, Office of Health, U.S. Agency for International Development, for their time and effort in developing the workshop. The committee also wishes to thank James Gribble who coordinated the workshop activities. Joan Montgomery Halford provided the logistical and administrative work for the workshop. Florence Poillon copy edited this volume, and Paula Melville and Elaine McGarraugh assisted in its publication.

SAMUEL H. PRESTON, *Chair*
Committee on Population

The Epidemiological Transition

POLICY AND PLANNING IMPLICATIONS FOR DEVELOPING COUNTRIES

Introduction

As child survival programs continue to achieve their goals of reducing infant and child mortality, the age structure and overall health status of the populations of most developing countries are changing. A decline in fertility in many parts of the world has resulted in a shift toward an older population. With an increasing proportion of the population falling into the adult and elderly age groups, the epidemiological profiles of developing countries increasingly reflect the diseases and health problems of adults rather than of children. In particular, chronic and degenerative diseases, and accidents and injuries, are becoming more important causes of death. In most countries, this process has been accelerated by a more rapid reduction in infant and child mortality rates than those of adults. This shift in demographic and disease profiles, often referred to as the epidemiological transition, is currently under way in most developing countries. The transition occurs at different paces in different places, depending on the rate of fertility changes, the distribution of risk factors that contribute to the incidence of disease, and the health system's ability to respond to the changing epidemiological profile.

Although scientists are beginning to understand better some of the trends in the changing disease and mortality patterns, policymakers need to know how to use this information to make decisions about the priorities for the health sector. To emphasize the importance of using demographic and epidemiologic data in decision making, a workshop was convened by the National Academy of Sciences' Committee on Population and the Institute on Medicine's Board on International Health, with support from the Office of Health of the U.S. Agency for International Development. The workshop was designed to bring together medical experts, epidemiologists, demographers, and other social scientists involved in research on the epidemiological transition and to foster discussion on specific topics. This volume contains papers presented at the meeting that served as a basis for discussion. The papers deal with the quantitative dimension of demographic and epidemiological changes, the processes used in establishing priorities in the health sector, and the roles of governments and families in providing health services.

TRANSITIONS IN MORTALITY AND EPIDEMIOLOGIC PATTERNS

Changes in mortality structure are the principal outcome indicator by which the epidemiological transition is assessed. Heligman and colleagues (see Heligman et al., Table 8, in this volume) show that whereas 27.3 percent of deaths in less developed regions occurred at ages 50 and above in 1960-1965, 41.9 percent were in that age range in 1980-1985 and 63.0 percent are projected for these ages in 2010-2015.

Changing mortality patterns are the product not only of changes in age structure but also of changes in the distribution of risk factors and in age-specific incidence and case-fatality rates of various diseases. In some cases, mortality rates may be declining faster than morbidity and disability rates because better treatments for diseases have reduced their case-fatality rates. Oral rehydration therapy, for example, has not reduced the incidence of diarrheal disease, but has contributed to a reduction in the number of fatalities per case.

The populations of developing countries are gradually shifting from environments with greater exposure to infectious diseases (poor water and food quality, unhygienic sanitation practices) to areas with a higher prevalence of risk factors for noncommunicable diseases, such as motor vehicles, unsafe workplaces, and air pollution (Smith, 1990). At the same time, personal behaviors are often changing in ways that increase the chances of developing a chronic disease. The presence of a risk factor does not necessarily imply that a disease will be observed at the level expected on the basis of relationships in developed countries. Nevertheless, epidemiological studies indicate that smoking, hypertension, dietary fat, motor vehicles, occupational hazards, and poverty are among the leading risk factors for death from noncommunicable diseases in developing and developed countries alike.

Smoking, for example, although known to be responsible for a number of diseases, has grown in popularity. The increase between 1970 and 1985 in tobacco consumption per adult amounted to 41.6 percent in Africa, 24.0

percent in Latin America and the Caribbean, and 22.1 percent in Asia (Masironi and Rothwell, 1988).

Increasing numbers of motor vehicles and unsafe workplaces are risk factors for accidents and injuries. In Brazil, for example, traffic accident death rates are not dissimilar from rates observed in the United States, but they are much higher on both a per-vehicle basis and a per-mile-driven basis than in developed countries (Baker, 1984). Injuries in the workplace tend to be much more common and severe in developing countries (Stansfield et al., 1993). The death rate for factory workers in India was about 50 percent higher than in the United States (Mohan, 1982). Agricultural injury death rates are estimated to be three to eight times higher in developing countries than in developed ones (International Labour Organization, 1988).

DATA DEFICIENCIES

A number of factors prevent a precise understanding of the epidemiological transition and impede policy formulation. Paramount among these is the absence of good data on mortality. Cause-of-death data either do not exist or are unreliable for most developing countries. Although a number of Latin American countries have high-quality data, no African and very few Asian countries have data on death registration or cause of death. In the absence of reliable data, the cause structure can be estimated from data on the overall level of mortality, by using a model based on the relationship between mortality level and cause-of-death structure in populations with good data (see Bulatao, in this volume). However, this approach raises concern about the relevance of mortality patterns of advanced developing countries or the historical experience of developed countries to the current experience of the world's poorest countries. As a result, much of the analysis on cause-of-death structure and cause-specific death rates is limited to a few developing countries or subnational populations with reliable data.

Another difficulty in studying the epidemiological transition in many countries is that the existing data are not representative of the whole population, but rather often come from a more privileged segment of the population. Urban-based or hospital-based studies may represent one segment of the population, but results from such studies are not readily generalizable. The poorer subpopulations of developing countries are often thought to suffer more from infectious and parasitic diseases, and the wealthier segments are thought to suffer more often from noncommunicable diseases. However, the poor have greater exposure to many of the risk factors associated with communicable and noncommunicable diseases alike. Studies in Brazil, for example, indicate that the highest levels of hypertension, smoking, alcohol use, lack of exercise, and obesity are to be found among those with the lowest educational level (Briscoe, 1990). Cause-specific death rates for cancer, cardiovascular disease, respiratory disease, and external causes were higher among poor men than wealthy men in Porto Alegre, Brazil (Briscoe, 1990). National-level figures illustrate large-scale changes; to understand the variation that occurs within a country, the population needs to be disaggregated, and the changes taking place within the major subpopulations must be examined.

ORGANIZATION OF THIS VOLUME

Demographic and Epidemiologic Data

Policy and planning implications of the epidemiological transition are based in part on an understanding of how population and mortality structures are likely to change. Larry Heligman, Nancy Chen, and Ozer Babakol provide a projection of changes in population structure over the next 25 years in Latin America, Africa, and developing areas of Asia and Oceania. They describe changes in the number of people, growth, and age structures of populations residing in rural and urban areas, and they examine life-table mortality patterns, numbers dying, and the age structure of deaths in these areas, as well as potential consequences of AIDS on mortality in Africa.

A projection of the mortality structure is also useful in planning for the specific types of services that will be needed. Rodolfo Bulatao estimates and projects the cause-of-death pattern for six age groups (0, 1 to 4, 5 to 14, 15 to 44, 45 to 64, and 65 and older), by sex for four calendar years (1970, 1985, 2000, 2015) and by six country groupings (industrial market economies, industrial nonmarket economies, Latin America and the Caribbean, sub-Saharan Africa, the Middle East and North Africa, and Asia and the Pacific). This exercise clearly demonstrates an impending decline in mortality from communicable diseases and the relative emergence of noncommunicable causes. These first two papers provide a quantitative background for subsequent discussions.

The projections that achieve worldwide coverage are necessarily rather mechanical exercises in which epidemiologic issues are suppressed. The next two papers introduce additional epidemiological considerations into the analysis of mortality patterns. Henry Mosley and Ronald Gray examine childhood precursors of adult morbidity and mortality, drawing attention to the fact that health insults as early as gestation can influence one's health status as an adolescent or adult. In developed countries, about 6 to 10 percent of adults die between ages 15 and 60; in developing countries, it is often the case that 25 to 35 percent die during this age interval. The authors suggest that as many as one-third of the preventable deaths in developing countries are the consequences of infection and other conditions acquired during infancy and childhood. These life-cycle connections must be taken into account in assessing the relative value of health programs directed at children and adults.

The shift toward an aging population and the resulting changes in the epidemiological profile call for a better understanding of the complexity of chronic and degenerative diseases. Kenneth Manton and Eric Stallard consider the issues related to projecting morbidity and mortality during the reproductive and postreproductive years by developing a dynamic model based on risk factor regressions and multivariate hazard functions. Combining data sources to produce longitudinal data that include the levels of risk factors in developing countries yields more accurate forecasts than using the generally available data from developed countries. Using examples of active life expectancy and an intervention to reduce risk factors for cardiovascular diseases, the authors illustrate how the model can be employed to project morbidity, mortality, and their associated costs.

Setting Priorities in a Changing Epidemiological Environment

In determining whether the focus of health investments should be on childhood or adult diseases, a number of indices have been developed that assess the different outcomes based on the types of inputs used. A commonly used index is the healthy years of life saved by specific interventions. Samuel Preston critically examines this index, identifying circumstances in which it yields reliable and unreliable information. A distinction is drawn between interventions that occur over only one year and those that extend into the future. He also discusses whether and how the index accounts for the benefits accrued by those who are not yet born when the intervention is initiated. He argues that population projections can often provide a better vehicle for assessing the consequences of interventions and incorporating other dimensions such as total gain in production or changes in per capita income.

José Luis Bobadilla and Cristina Possas examine health policy issues arising from the epidemiological transition in Mexico, Brazil, and Colombia. They develop a framework for health policy decisions based jointly on population dynamics, which provides an idea of the magnitude of the health needs, and on the available health system, which describes the configuration of services available to meet the current level of need. Although it is not possible to formulate a homogeneous health policy agenda for developing countries because each country's transition is different, the authors offer a set of issues that will help each health system to be more responsive to its population's needs: redistribute welfare through providing health services, reform the health care model, improve the efficiency and quality of care, and build a national capacity for strategic health planning.

The World Summit for Children in 1990 drew attention again to the continuing high levels of mortality and morbidity among infants and children in developing countries. At that meeting, policy statements were put forward that set goals for reducing mortality, morbidity, and the prevalence of risk factors. Anne Pebley examines these goals, focusing on their demographic plausibility and the potential consequences of achieving them. She raises the issue of whether pursuing numerical goals will draw attention away from the need to focus on durable programs that will have sustained effects on children's health. The changing health environment raises questions of whether the "child survival" strategy is the best approach for improving children's health in the 1990s and whether some of the goals can be achieved without improving health care infrastructure.

As noted earlier, the demographic and epidemiologic changes that are taking place in developing countries are often aggregated into national-level numbers, but within each population are groups, in widely differing circumstances. The wealthy and poor typically follow different epidemiologic and demographic trajectories. In examining the distributional implications of alternative policy strategies focused on children and adult health, Davidson Gwatkin compares the least healthy segment of the population with the healthiest segment. The comparison is made both for high- and low-mortality scenarios. He demonstrates that paying greater attention to the health problems of adults and the elderly may often exacerbate social inequalities in mortality. Similarly, he shows that the least healthy are likely to benefit more from a reduction in mortality from communicable diseases, whereas a decline in noncommunicable diseases would differentially benefit the healthier segment of the population. Perhaps surprisingly, he shows that a health policy tilt toward adult noncommunicable diseases would be likely to increase inequalities more in low-mortality than in high-mortality developing countries.

Providers of Services: Roles of Government, Private Sector, and Families

Moving from the debate over whether priority should shift toward adult health, the workshop turned its attention to who should provide services, considering the roles of government, private medicine, and the informal sector. Nancy Birdsall and Estelle James state the case for shifting more of the provision of services to the private sector because of the inefficiencies and inequities associated with government spending. They suggest that informational programs and basic services that cannot be supported in a private, competitive market, such as maternal and child health programs in rural areas, receive public funding. However, services such as hospitals, which presently represent a large percentage of health budgets and serve only a small portion of the health needs of the population, may warrant privatization, with fees covered by mandated health insurance.

Regardless of whether the public or the private sector finances and provides the majority of health services, the informal sector will continue to play a vital role in caregiving. John and Pat Caldwell examine the roles of women, families, and communities in preventing illness and providing health services. They observe that in many parts of the world, mothers are constrained in their ability to care for sick children because of social and economic impediments. Societies that are relatively unaffected by cultural and technological imports often have health beliefs that promote incautious behavior. In some cases, women view child care as a community activity and may be less attentive to their children's survival because family systems can induce a sense of being powerless to influence events. In some societies, the mother must submit to her mother-in-law or husband regarding the type of care a sick child will receive. In more modern, transitional societies, some women are educated and may take advantage of the health care system. The less educated women are often alienated from the system and, because of their traditional health beliefs, do not use the system as effectively as they could. The authors cite women's groups and female health visitors as ways of empowering young mothers to care better for themselves and for their children.

CONCLUSION

Although this volume covers a range of issues related to changing disease profiles in developing countries, it is clearly not an exhaustive account of how societies should adapt to these changes. The papers do not form a cohesive set of policy recommendations; rather they address a set of issues that health planners in developing countries will have to consider as the epidemiological profile of their populations change. In a sense, the adaptation-to-change paradigm is itself rather arbitrary because government policy will play a central role in the pace and direction of future changes. Nevertheless, the widespread declines in fertility and child mortality, both of which contribute to the shifting age structures of developing countries, are not likely to be reversed and have imposed significant changes in the context for thinking about health policy.

The demographic changes discussed here will have far-reaching consequences in the social and economic sectors of developing countries. In this report a number of issues related to the health sector's response are raised. As populations move toward an older age structure, how much emphasis on child survival will be needed? What mechanisms will be used to allocate resources into different health programs? Who will be responsible for providing health care services?

The formulation of health initiatives in this new context involves many considerations, including assessments of the likely cost and effectiveness of specific programs. But there are dangers in prematurely narrowing discussion to technical issues of cost and effectiveness. How governments and families actually behave, how interventions affect various social groups, what long-term effects programs may have on the cohorts that experience them, and even how program effects should be measured and modeled, are questions that need to be addressed before cost-effectiveness calculations can be confidently invoked. This volume represents a contribution to the discussion of these broader issues.

REFERENCES

Baker, S.P.
1984 *The Injury Fact Book.* Washington, D.C.: Heath and Company.

Briscoe, J.
1990 *Brazil: The New Challenge of Adult Health.* Washington, D.C.: World Bank.

International Labour Organization
1988 *Yearbook on Labor Statistics*, 48th Issue. Geneva: International Labor Organization.

Masironi, R., and K. Rothwell
1988 Tendances et effets du tabagisme dans le monde. *World Health Statistics Quarterly* 41:228-241.

Mohan, D.
1982 Accidental death and disability in India—A case of criminal neglect. *Industrial Safety Chronicle* (April-June):24-43.

Smith, K.R.
1990 The risk transition. *International Environmental Affairs* 2(3):227-251.

Stansfield, S.K., G.S. Smith, and W.P. McGreevey
1993 Injury and poisoning. In D.T. Jamison and W.H. Mosley, eds., *Disease Control Priorities in Developing Countries.* New York: Oxford University Press for the World Bank.

Shifts in the Structure of Population and Deaths in Less Developed Regions

Larry Heligman, Nancy Chen, and Ozer Babakol

INTRODUCTION

During the process of the demographic transition, the age structure of a population changes toward one that is older. The age structure of deaths also changes toward one in which greater proportions of deaths take place at the oldest ages; this shift in the structure of deaths is a consequence of the greater share of population that has reached the older ages, and interrelatedly, the low probabilities of dying in all but the oldest age groups.

In general, countries exhibit relatively similar demographic structures at the beginnings and the ends of their demographic transitions, although the movement from here to there is neither smooth nor uniform. Many of the same factors underlie the mortality and fertility changes that comprise the demographic transition; nevertheless the two components move at different paces both within and among countries. In particular the transition process has differed in Africa, Asia, and Latin America. As the United Nations (1991a:12) described:

> During the period 1950-1955, the earliest data for which the United Nations provides demographic estimates on a regular basis, population growth rates ranged from 2.7 percent per year in Latin America to 2.2 percent in Africa and 1.9 percent in Asia. The high Latin American population growth rate is primarily explained by the region's earlier start of mortality reduction. Life expectancy at birth in the major area was 10 years greater than

L. Heligman and N. Chen are with Population Division, United Nations, New York; O. Babakol is with Statistics Division, United Nations, New York. The views expressed in this paper are those of the authors and do not necessarily reflect the views of the United Nations.

in Africa and Asia and the crude death rate about 10 deaths per 1,000 lower. Africa and Asia exhibited similar life expectancies at birth and similar crude death rates but African women, on average, exhibited about 0.7 more births per woman than their Asian counterparts; the African population growth rate was hence higher.

A temporary convergence in growth rates occurred during the period 1965-1970. Africa, Asia and Latin America had similar growth rates, varying only from 2.4 to 2.6 percent per year. The population growth rate had risen sharply from the earlier period in Africa and Asia owing to falling mortality rates and little or moderate fertility change. The Latin American population growth rate held steady, as crude birth and death rates fell by similar amounts. Currently, population growth rates have diverged again. The African population growth rate has risen to 3 percent per year owing to falling mortality and little fertility change; whereas, Asian and Latin American population growth rates fell to 1.9 percent and 2.1 percent respectively.

This paper focuses on describing the changes in certain population characteristics projected to take place during the next quarter-century in Africa, developing regions of Asia and Oceania, and Latin America. To put these projected changes into a context, changes during the past 25 years are also described. In particular, we describe past and projected changes in (1) the number of people, growth, and age structures of population residing in the total, urban, and rural sectors of these major areas; and (2) life-table mortality patterns, numbers dying, and the age structure of deaths for these regions, including the potential implications of the AIDS pandemic in Africa. Because Africa exhibits very high mortality and there is greater uncertainty with respect to future trends, a special section is included on African mortality.

The analysis in this paper is carried out at the level of major area: that is, Africa, developing regions of Asia and Oceania (i.e., excluding Japan, Australia, and New Zealand), and Latin America. From here on, "Asia" is used to refer to the developing regions of Asia and Oceania. The tables present data for India and China separately because of their particularly large population sizes. Eight age groups are considered.

The major sources of data considered for this paper are the 1990 revisions of the official United Nations total, urban, and rural population projections for countries of the world (United Nations, 1991a-c). We have also made new and consistent estimates and projections of the age distribution of urban and rural populations, of age patterns of mortality, and of the potential number of deaths due to the AIDS epidemic in some African countries.

POPULATION GROWTH AND AGE STRUCTURES

In 1990, approximately 4.1 billion persons resided in the less developed regions (LDRs) of the world (Table 1). Of these, 73 percent reside in Asia,

TABLE 1 Total Population and Percentage of Population in Less Developed Regions, 1965, 1990, and 2015

Region	1965			1990			2015		
	Both	Male	Female	Both	Male	Female	Both	Male	Female
	Population (thousands)								
Total	2333400	1186835	1146565	4085638	2078534	2007104	6332461	3205134	3127327
Africa	317056	157039	160017	642111	319381	322731	1301371	649645	651726
Latin America	250843	125665	125178	448076	223523	224553	673172	334458	338714
Developing regions of Asia and Oceania	1765501	904131	861370	2995451	1535630	1459820	4357918	2221031	2136887
China	729191	375124	354067	1139060	586189	552871	1435683	732233	703450
India	495196	255886	239270	853094	440888	412206	1304001	668729	635272
	Distribution (%)								
Total	100.0	100.0	100.0	100.0	100.0	100.0	100.0	100.0	100.0
Africa	13.6	13.2	14.0	15.7	15.4	16.1	20.6	20.3	20.8
Latin America	10.8	10.6	10.9	11.0	10.8	11.2	10.6	10.4	10.8
Developing Regions of Asia and Oceania	75.7	76.2	75.1	73.3	73.9	72.7	68.8	69.3	68.3
China	41.3	41.5	41.1	38.0	38.2	37.9	32.9	33.0	32.9
India	28.0	28.3	27.8	28.5	28.7	28.2	29.9	30.1	29.7

16 percent in Africa, and 11 percent in Latin America. During the next 25 years, the population of the LDRs is projected to increase more than half, to 6.3 billion. The fastest growth is projected for Africa, which will increase more than twice, from 642 million persons to 1.3 billion, and will contain 20 percent of the total LDR population in 2015. Asia and Latin America are projected to increase 45 and 50 percent, respectively, from 3.0 billion to 4.4 billion in the case of Asia, and from 448 million to 673 million for Latin America.

As fertility and mortality have declined, the age structures of the populations of the LDRs have aged. For example, in 1965, 42 percent of the LDR population was under age 15, whereas 36 percent is now—an increase from 977 million in 1965 to 1.45 billion. Simultaneously, the population aged 15-64 has risen from 54 to 60 percent, and that aged 65 and over from 3.7 to 4.5 percent (Tables 2 and 3).

With projected fertility and mortality declines, these trends will continue during the next 25 years. By 2015, the population under age 15 will have declined to 29 percent, and the share in the age group 15-64 and age 65 and over will have risen to 65 and 6 percent, respectively. Nonetheless, even among those ages, which will exhibit declines in their relative shares, large absolute and percentage increases in numbers of people will occur between 1990 and 2015. The numbers of persons aged 0-4 and 5-14 are projected to rise by 15 and 33 percent, respectively (Table 4). The population in the reproductive ages (15-49) will rise by 60 percent, and those aged 50 and over will more than double in size. In fact, the population aged 80 and over in the LDRs is projected to rise by 170 percent, from 21.4 million to 58.1 million.

Child Population Aged 0-14

In 1990 there were about 544 million children under the age of 5 and 909 million aged 5-14. Representing respectively 13 and 22 percent of the LDR population, these preschool and early school-age children make up well over one-third of the LDR population. The 1990-2015 average annual growth rates for these age groups are projected to be only 1.38 and 0.54 percent annually, respectively. Nonetheless, significant absolute increments will occur because of the large population bases. Nearly 80 million children (15 percent increase) aged 0-4 and nearly 300 million children (33 percent increase) aged 5-14 will be added to the populations during the next 25 years.

Reproductive Age Population Aged 15-49

The less developed regions were home to 2.1 billion persons in 1990 in the reproductive ages of 15-49, representing slightly more than one-half of

TABLE 2 Total, Urban, and Rural Population and Percentage Urban in Less Developed Regions, 1965, 1990, and 2015

Age	Total Population (thousands)			Urban Population (thousands)			Rural Population (thousands)			Percentage Urban		
	1965	1990	2015	1965	1990	2015	1965	1990	2015	1965	1990	2015
Less Developed Regions												
0-4	384656	543767	622983	82716	183713	318002	301941	360054	304981	21.5	33.8	51.0
5-14	592277	909253	206081	123438	302865	606637	468840	606389	599443	20.8	33.3	50.3
15-49	1067037	2081612	3328506	275082	834421	1926834	791956	1247191	1401672	26.0	40.1	57.9
15-24	407221	832733	1159758	105828	333756	671542	301393	498977	488216	25.8	40.1	57.9
50-64	202385	368987	787823	45988	131147	429546	156397	237840	358276	22.7	35.5	54.5
65+	87044	182018	387068	19054	62554	203437	67990	119464	183632	21.9	34.4	52.6
65-79	78963	160572	328989									
80+	8081	21446	58079									
Total	2333400	4085638	6332461	546278	1514701	3484458	1787122	2570938	2848002	23.4	37.1	55.0
Africa												
0-4	57787	115751	189646	10505	35062	88626	47282	80690	101020	18.2	30.3	46.7
5-14	83439	173478	335541	15983	54384	158759	67455	119094	176782	19.2	31.3	47.3
15-49	143020	289335	633647	32444	108673	345836	110575	180660	287809	22.8	38.0	55.1
15-24	58183	122136	262387	13257	46389	144500	44925	75746	117887	22.7	37.6	54.6
50-64	23240	44200	98891	4609	13858	47448	18631	30342	51444	19.8	31.4	48.0
65+	9571	19346	43646	1789	5462	18708	7782	13884	24939	18.7	28.2	42.9
65-79	8713	17387	38512									
80+	858	1959	5134									
Total	317056	642111	1301371	65331	217440	659378	251725	424671	641993	20.6	33.9	50.7

continued

TABLE 2 *Continued*

Age	Total Population (thousands)			Urban Population (thousands)			Rural Population (thousands)			Percentage Urban		
	1965	1990	2015	1965	1990	2015	1965	1990	2015	1965	1990	2015
Latin America												
0-4	42461	57413	64482	20480	38243	49816	21981	19170	14667	48.2	66.6	77.3
5-14	65596	103261	123914	32292	69917	96841	33305	33344	27073	49.2	67.7	78.2
15-49	112806	227589	353154	64219	168588	293052	48585	59000	60102	56.0	73.4	82.6
15-24	45086	89468	117125	25235	65639	96794	19851	23828	20330	56.9	74.1	83.0
50-64	20620	38380	86226	11633	28113	71235	8988	10268	14990	56.4	73.2	82.6
65+	9362	21434	45396	5191	15631	37383	4169	5802	8013	55.5	72.9	82.3
65-79	8313	18163	37559									
80+	1049	3271	7837									
Total	250843	448076	673172	133816	320493	548327	117028	127583	124845	53.3	71.5	81.5
Developing Regions of Asia and Oceania												
0-4	284408	370603	368855	51731	110408	179560	232678	260194	189294	18.2	29.8	48.7
5-14	443242	632514	746626	75163	178564	351037	368080	453951	395588	17.0	28.2	47.0
15-49	811211	1564688	2341705	178419	557160	1287946	632796	1007531	1053761	22.0	35.6	55.0
15-24	303952	621129	780246	67336	221728	430248	236617	399403	349999	22.2	35.7	55.1
50-64	158525	286407	602706	29746	89176	310863	128778	197230	291842	18.8	31.1	51.6
65+	68111	141238	298026	12074	41461	147346	56039	99778	150680	17.7	29.4	49.4
65-79	61937	125022	252918									
80+	6174	16216	45108									
Total	1765501	2995451	4357918	347131	976768	2276753	1418369	2018684	2081164	19.7	32.6	52.2

China												
0-4	112275	112328	89803	16711	30642	46712	95564	81686	43090	14.9	27.3	52.0
5-14	180719	189144	182401	26149	50359	93403	154569	138784	88997	14.5	26.6	51.2
15-49	333339	647436	773358	70803	237785	487116	262537	409651	286241	21.2	36.7	63.0
15-24	121005	252808	231621	24708	90891	142959	96298	161918	88661	20.4	36.0	61.7
50-64	70800	123868	258307	13566	41688	153491	57233	82180	104816	19.2	33.7	59.4
65+	32058	66284	131814	5480	20329	74008	26577	45955	57806	17.1	30.7	56.1
65-79	28944	58255	110305									
80+	3114	8029	21509									
Total	729191	1139060	1435683	132711	380803	854731	596480	758257	580952	18.2	33.4	59.5
India												
0-4	78964	114364	117060	13504	28253	47335	65460	86110	69724	17.1	24.7	40.4
5-14	121137	196961	245969	20986	49247	100581	100150	147714	145388	17.3	25.0	40.9
15-49	233924	422266	698267	48625	124629	322369	185300	297638	375896	20.8	29.5	46.2
15-24	87825	165174	244012	19095	50674	116685	68730	114501	127327	21.7	30.7	47.8
50-64	43613	81099	159533	7262	19490	63145	36350	61609	96389	16.7	24.0	39.6
65+	17518	36403	83173	2707	8649	31250	14811	29753	51922	15.5	22.5	37.6
65-79	16267	34743	71861									
80+	1251	3660	11312									

TABLE 3 Distribution of Total, Urban, and Rural Population in Less Developed Regions, 1965, 1990, and 2015

	Total Population (%)			Urban Population (%)			Rural Population (%)		
Age	1965	1990	2015	1965	1990	2015	1965	1990	2015
Less Developed Regions									
0-4	16.48	13.31	9.84	15.14	12.13	9.13	16.90	14.00	10.71
5-14	25.38	22.25	19.05	22.60	20.00	17.41	26.23	23.59	21.05
15-49	45.73	50.95	52.56	50.36	55.09	55.30	44.31	48.51	49.22
15-24	17.45	20.38	18.31	19.37	22.03	19.27	16.86	19.41	17.14
50-64	8.67	9.03	12.44	8.42	8.66	12.33	8.75	9.25	12.58
65+	3.73	4.46	6.11	3.49	4.13	5.84	3.80	4.65	6.45
65-79	3.38	3.93	5.20						
80+	0.35	0.52	0.92						
Total	100.00	100.00	100.00	100.00	100.00	100.00	100.00	100.00	100.00
Africa									
0-4	18.23	18.03	14.57	16.08	16.12	13.44	18.78	19.00	15.74
5-14	26.32	27.02	25.78	24.47	25.01	24.08	26.80	28.04	27.54
15-49	45.11	45.06	48.69	49.66	49.98	52.45	43.93	42.54	44.83
15-24	18.35	19.02	20.16	20.29	21.33	21.91	17.85	17.84	18.36
50-64	7.33	6.88	7.60	7.05	6.37	7.20	7.40	7.14	8.01
65+	3.02	3.01	3.35	2.74	2.51	2.84	3.09	3.27	3.88
65-79	2.75	2.71	2.96						
80+	0.27	0.31	0.39						
Total	100.00	100.00	100.00	100.00	100.00	100.00	100.00	100.00	100.00
Latin America									
0-4	16.93	12.81	9.58	15.30	11.93	9.09	18.78	15.03	11.75
5-14	26.15	23.05	18.41	24.13	21.82	17.66	28.46	26.13	21.69
15-49	44.97	50.79	52.46	47.99	52.60	53.44	41.52	46.24	48.14
15-24	17.97	19.97	17.40	18.86	20.48	17.65	16.96	18.68	16.28

50-64	8.22	8.57	12.81	8.69	8.77	12.99	7.68	8.05	12.01
65+	3.73	4.78	6.74	3.88	4.88	6.82	3.56	4.55	6.42
65-79	3.31	4.05	5.58						
80+	0.42	0.73	1.16						
Total	100.00	100.00	100.00	100.00	100.00	100.00	100.00	100.00	100.00
Developing Regions of Asia and Oceania									
0-4	16.11	12.37	8.46	14.90	11.30	7.89	16.40	12.89	9.10
5-14	25.11	21.12	17.13	21.65	18.28	15.42	25.95	22.49	19.01
15-49	45.95	52.24	53.73	51.40	57.04	56.57	44.61	49.91	50.63
15-24	17.22	20.74	17.90	19.40	22.70	18.90	16.68	19.79	16.82
50-64	8.98	9.56	13.83	8.57	9.13	13.65	9.08	9.77	14.02
65+	3.86	4.72	6.84	3.48	4.24	6.47	3.95	4.94	7.24
65-79	3.51	4.17	5.80						
80+	0.35	0.54	1.04						
Total	100.00	100.00	100.00	100.00	100.00	100.00	100.00	100.00	100.00
China									
0-4	15.4	9.9	6.3	12.6	8.0	5.5	16.0	10.8	7.4
5-14	24.8	16.6	12.7	19.7	13.2	10.9	25.9	18.3	15.3
15-49	45.7	56.8	53.9	53.4	62.4	57.0	44.0	54.0	49.3
15-24	16.6	22.2	16.1	18.6	23.9	16.7	16.1	21.4	15.3
50-64	9.7	10.9	18.0	10.2	10.9	18.0	9.6	10.8	18.0
65+	4.4	5.8	9.2	4.1	5.3	8.7	4.5	6.1	10.0
65-79	4.0	5.1	7.7						
80+	0.4	0.7	1.5						
Total	100.00	100.00	100.00	100.00	100.00	100.00	100.00	100.00	100.00

continued

TABLE 3 *Continued*

Age	Total Population (%)			Urban Population (%)			Rural Population (%)		
	1965	1990	2015	1965	1990	2015	1965	1990	2015
India									
0-4	16.0	13.4	9.0	14.5	12.3	8.4	16.3	13.8	9.4
5-14	24.5	23.1	18.9	22.5	21.4	17.8	24.9	23.7	19.7
15-49	47.2	49.5	53.6	52.2	54.1	57.1	46.1	47.8	50.8
15-24	17.7	19.4	18.7	20.5	22.0	20.7	17.1	18.4	17.2
50-64	8.8	9.5	12.2	7.8	8.5	11.2	9.0	9.9	13.0
65+	3.5	4.5	6.4	2.9	3.8	5.5	3.7	4.8	7.0
65-79	3.3	4.1	5.5						
80+	0.2	0.4	0.9						
Total	100.00	100.00	100.00	100.00	100.00	100.00	100.00	100.00	100.00

the total population (Table 5). Of these, 1.02 billion persons are women. About one of every four persons in the developing world is a woman of reproductive age.

The number of people in this age group doubled from 1.07 billion in 1965 to 2.09 billion in 1990 and is projected to increase another 60 percent during the next quarter century, adding 1.2 billion persons. By 2015, 53 percent of all persons in less developed regions will be between the ages of 15 and 49.

Currently about 40 percent of persons aged 15-49 are adolescents in the 15-24 age group. The number of adolescents will grow by about 40 percent by 2015; they are making up a declining share of the reproductive age populations of the developing world.

Postreproductive Age Population: Those 50 and Older

The most rapid population growth is projected to occur among the older population. The population aged 50 and over is projected to increase at an average annual rate of 3 percent per year, so that this population will double by 2015, from 551 million to 1.2 billion. As a result, this age group will rise from 13 to 19 percent of the total population (Table 3).

About 182 million people were age 65 and over in 1990, and the population of this group is also expected to double during the next 25 years. Particularly rapid growth, however, is projected among the old old (i.e., those aged 80 and over), whose number may increase at 4 percent per year, rising from 21 million to 58 million. Among persons aged 65 and over, those over age 80 rose from 9 percent in 1965 to 12 percent in 1990 and are projected to rise further to 15 percent in 2015.

Up to about age 65, one can safely make the generalization that "half the population are men and half are women." However, due to greater longevity, women make up greater shares in older age groups. At ages 50-64, women comprised 50 percent of the population in 1990, but the female share rose to 53 percent for ages 65-79 and nearly 60 percent for ages 80 and over.

Urban-Rural Makeup

Thirty-seven percent of the LDR population lived in urban areas in 1990 (Table 2). Age differences in the percent urban population range from about one-third under age 15 and over age 50, to about 40 percent between ages 15 and 49. The result is a noticeably younger population in rural areas, where 38 percent is under age 15 compared to 32 percent in urban areas. The trade-off comes at ages 15-49: 55 percent of the urban population is between these ages, compared to 49 percent of the rural population.

TABLE 4 Change (percent) and Average Annual Rate of Change of Population, by Age, in Less Developed Regions, 1965-1990 and 1990-2015

	Total Population				Urban Population				Rural Population			
	Change (%)		Rate of Change		Change (%)		Rate of Change		Change (%)		Rate of Change	
Age	1965-1990	1990-2015	1965-1990	1990-2015	1965-1990	1990-2015	1965-1990	1990-2015	1965-1990	1990-2015	1965-1990	1990-2015
Less Developed Regions												
0–4	41.4	14.6	1.38	0.54	122.1	73.1	3.19	2.19	19.2	–15.3	0.70	–0.66
5–14	53.5	32.6	1.71	1.13	145.4	100.3	3.59	2.78	29.3	–1.1	1.03	–0.05
15–49	95.1	59.9	2.67	1.88	203.3	130.9	4.44	3.35	57.5	12.4	1.82	0.47
15–24	104.5	39.3	2.86	1.33	215.4	101.2	4.59	2.80	65.6	–2.2	2.02	–0.09
50–64	82.3	113.5	2.40	3.03	185.2	227.5	4.19	4.75	52.1	50.6	1.68	1.64
65+	109.1	112.7	2.95	3.02	228.3	225.2	4.76	4.72	75.7	53.7	2.25	1.72
65–79	103.4	104.9	2.84	2.87								
80+	165.4	170.8	3.90	3.99								
Total	75.1	55.0	2.24	1.75	177.3	130.0	4.08	3.33	43.9	10.8	1.45	0.41
Africa												
0–4	100.3	63.8	2.78	1.97	233.8	152.8	4.82	3.71	70.7	25.2	2.14	0.9
05–14	107.9	93.4	2.93	2.64	240.3	191.9	4.90	4.29	76.6	48.4	2.27	1.58
15–49	102.3	119.0	2.82	3.14	235.0	218.2	4.84	4.63	63.4	59.3	1.96	1.86
15–24	109.9	114.8	2.97	3.06	249.9	211.5	5.01	4.54	68.6	55.6	2.09	1.77
50–64	90.2	123.7	2.57	3.22	200.7	242.4	4.40	4.92	62.9	69.5	1.95	2.11
65+	102.1	125.6	2.81	3.25	205.3	242.5	4.46	4.92	78.4	79.6	2.32	2.34
65–79	99.6	121.5	2.76	3.18								
80+	128.3	162.1	3.30	3.85								
Total	102.5	102.7	2.82	2.83	232.8	203.2	4.81	4.44	68.7	51.2	2.09	1.65

0–4	35.2	12.3	1.21	0.46	86.7	30.3	2.5	1.06	–0.1	–23.5	–0.55	–1.07
5–14	57.4	20.0	1.81	0.73	116.5	38.5	3.09	1.30	0.1	–18.8	0.00	–0.83
15–49	101.8	55.2	2.81	1.76	162.5	73.8	3.86	2.21	21.4	1.9	0.78	0.07
15–24	98.4	30.9	2.74	1.08	160.1	47.5	3.82	1.55	20.0	–14.7	0.73	–0.64
50–64	86.1	124.7	2.49	3.24	141.7	153.4	3.53	3.72	14.2	46.0	0.53	1.51
65+	128.9	111.8	3.31	3.00	201.1	139.2	4.41	3.49	39.2	38.1	1.32	1.29
65–79	118.5	106.8	3.13	2.91								
80+	211.8	139.6	4.55	3.50								
Total	78.6	50.2	2.32	1.63	139.5	71.1	3.49	2.15	9.0	–2.1	0.35	–0.09
Developing Regions of Asia and Oceania												
0–4	30.3	–0.5	1.06	–0.02	113.4	62.6	3.03	1.95	11.8	–27.2	0.45	–1.27
5–14	42.7	18.0	1.42	0.66	137.6	96.6	3.46	2.70	23.3	–12.9	0.84	–0.55
15–49	92.9	49.7	2.63	1.61	212.3	131.2	4.55	3.35	59.2	4.6	1.86	0.18
15–24	104.4	25.6	2.86	0.91	229.3	94.0	4.77	2.65	68.8	–12.4	2.09	–0.53
50–64	80.7	110.4	2.37	2.98	199.8	248.6	4.39	4.99	53.2	48.0	1.71	1.57
65+	107.4	111.0	2.92	2.99	243.4	255.4	4.93	5.07	78.1	51.0	2.31	1.65
65–79	101.9	102.3	2.81	2.82								
80+	162.6	178.2	3.86	4.09								
Total	69.7	45.5	2.11	1.5	181.4	133.1	4.14	3.39	42.3	3.1	1.41	0.12
China												
0–4	0.0	–20.1	0.00	–0.90	83.4	52.4	2.43	1.69	–14.5	–47.2	–0.63	–2.56
5–14	4.7	–3.6	0.18	–0.15	92.6	85.5	2.62	2.47	–10.2	–35.9	–0.43	–1.78
15–49	94.2	19.4	2.66	0.71	235.8	104.9	4.85	2.87	56.0	–30.1	1.78	–1.43
15–24	108.9	–8.4	2.95	–0.35	267.9	57.3	5.21	1.81	68.1	–45.2	2.08	–2.41
50–64	75.0	108.5	2.24	2.94	207.3	268.2	4.49	5.21	43.6	27.5	1.45	0.97
65+	106.8	98.9	2.91	2.75	271.0	264.1	5.24	5.17	72.9	25.8	2.19	0.92
65–79	101.3	89.3	2.80	2.55								
80+	157.8	167.9	3.79	3.94								
Total	56.2	26.0	1.78	0.93	186.9	124.5	4.22	3.23	27.1	–23.4	0.96	–1.07

continued

TABLE 4 *Continued*

Age	Total Population				Urban Population				Rural Population			
	Change (%)		Rate of Change		Change (%)		Rate of Change		Change (%)		Rate of Change	
	1965-1990	1990-2015	1965-1990	1990-2015	1965-1990	1990-2015	1965-1990	1990-2015	1965-1990	1990-2015	1965-1990	1990-2015
India												
0–4	44.8	2.4	1.48	0.09	109.2	67.5	2.95	2.06	31.5	–19.0	1.10	–0.84
5–14	62.6	24.9	1.94	0.89	134.7	104.2	3.41	2.86	47.5	–1.6	1.55	–0.06
15–49	80.5	65.4	2.36	2.01	156.3	158.7	3.76	3.80	60.6	26.3	1.90	0.93
15–24	88.1	47.7	2.53	1.56	165.4	130.3	3.90	3.34	66.6	11.2	2.04	0.42
50–64	86.0	96.7	2.48	2.71	168.4	224.0	3.95	4.70	69.5	56.5	2.11	1.79
65+	107.8	128.5	2.93	3.31	219.5	261.3	4.65	5.14	100.9	74.5	2.79	2.23
65–79	113.6	106.8	3.04	2.91								
80+	192.6	209.1	4.29	4.51								
Total	72.3	52.9	2.18	1.70	147.4	145.2	3.62	3.59	54.9	18.7	1.75	0.69

The share of population of ages 50-64 and 65 and over is about the same in the two areas: about 9 percent aged 50-64 and 6 percent aged 65+.

Both urban and rural areas contain more males than females; males exceed females by 6 percent in urban areas and 2 percent in rural areas. Urban areas exhibit higher sex ratios than do rural areas at every age group except 5-14 and 65 and over. Particularly, urban areas exhibit a large "male excess" at ages 15-49, where males exceed females by 9 percent. The female population significantly exceeds the number of males only at the older ages: for ages 65 and over, by 21 percent in urban areas and 11 percent in rural areas (Table 6).

The percentage of urban residents is projected to rise to 55 by 2015, with differentials among age groups ranging between only from 50 to 58 percent. The urban population is projected to grow by a factor of 2.3 between 1990 and 2015 (whereas the rural population will increase by only 11 percent). Urban growth is projected to be particularly rapid among those aged 50 and over (more than 4.7 percent per year) so that the share of urban population at these older ages will rise to 18 percent (from the current 13 percent). Nonetheless, the urban population will also be doubling at younger ages, from 485 million to 925 million at ages 0-14 and from 834 million to 1.9 billion at ages 15-49.

The rural population is also projected to age during the next 25 years, with a decline in the preschool population from 360 million to 305 million, and a stabilization in the size of the population aged 5-24 at about 1.1 billion persons. However, the number of persons aged 50 and over will probably increase by 50 percent to 542 million. As a result, the percentage of the rural population aged 0-14 is projected to decline from 38 to 32 percent. The percentage aged 50 and over will rise from 14 percent to 19 percent, similar to that in urban areas.

Africa is expected to add 659 million people during the next 25 years. Of these, 442 million (67 percent) will be in urban areas, and 217 million (33 percent) will be rural dwellers. Rural growth rates are projected to average only 1.65 percent per year during the next quarter of a century; urban growth is projected to average 4.44 percent (Table 4).

Africa's age distribution in urban areas is characterized by smaller population shares under age 15 than their rural counterparts. Among urban populations, 50 percent is between ages 15 and 49, 41 percent under age 15, and 9 percent age 50 and over; among rural populations, the corresponding shares are 43 percent age 15-49, 47 percent under age 15, and 10 percent age 50 and over. Both areas will exhibit rises during the next 25 years in population share aged 15-49 (from 50 to 52 percent in urban areas, and 43 to 45 percent in rural areas). Of similar size, but in the opposite direction, declines of relative share are expected among the preschool and child population: from 41 to 38 percent in urban areas, and 47 to 43 percent in rural areas.

TABLE 5 Total Population by Sex and Age in Less Developed Regions, 1965, 1990, and 2015

	1965			1990			2015		
Age	Males	Females	Sex Ratio	Males	Females	Sex Ratio	Males	Females	Sex Ratio
Less Developed Regions									
0-4	196253	188403	1.04	277886	265881	1.05	317586	305397	1.04
5-14	302683	289594	1.05	465445	443808	1.05	614883	591198	1.04
15-49	546706	520331	1.05	1064569	1017043	1.05	1697318	1631188	1.04
15-24	208513	198708	1.05	426861	405872	1.05	591621	568137	1.04
50-64	100687	101698	0.99	185718	183269	1.01	395399	392424	1.01
65+	40505	46539	0.87	84916	97102	0.87	179949	207119	0.87
65-79	37141	41822	0.89	76159	84413	0.90	155806	173183	0.90
80+	3364	4717	0.71	8757	12689	0.69	24143	33936	0.71
Total	1186835	1146565	1.04	2078534	2007104	1.04	3205134	3127327	1.02
Africa									
0-4	29067	28720	1.01	58341	57410	1.02	95808	93838	1.02
5-14	41873	41566	1.01	87369	86109	1.01	169123	166418	1.02
15-49	70762	72258	0.98	143995	145340	0.99	317056	316591	1.00
15-24	28948	29235	0.99	61304	60832	1.01	131858	130529	1.01
50-64	11108	12132	0.92	21034	23165	0.91	48043	50848	0.94
65+	4230	5341	0.79	8640	10706	0.81	19614	24032	0.82
65-79	3885	4828	0.80	7854	9533	0.82	17520	20992	0.83
80+	345	513	0.67	786	1173	0.67	2094	3040	0.69
Total	157039	160017	0.98	319381	322731	0.99	649645	651726	1.00
Latin America									
0-4	21531	20930	1.03	29158	28255	1.03	32824	31658	1.04
5-14	33150	32446	1.02	52266	50995	1.02	62933	60981	1.03
15-49	56479	56327	1.00	113712	113877	1.00	177020	176134	1.01
15-24	22705	22381	1.01	45082	44386	1.02	59265	57860	1.02
[illegible]	[illegible]	[illegible]	[illegible]	[illegible]	[illegible]	[illegible]	[illegible]	[illegible]	[illegible]

65-79	3926	4387	0.89	8379	9784	0.86	16956	20603	0.82
80+	455	594	0.77	1389	1882	0.74	3119	4718	0.66
Total	125665	125178	1.00	223523	224553	1.00	334458	338714	0.99
Developing Regions of Asia and Oceania									
0-4	145655	138753	1.05	190387	180216	1.06	188954	179901	1.05
5-14	227660	215582	1.06	325810	306704	1.06	382827	363799	1.05
15-49	419465	391746	1.07	806862	757826	1.06	1203242	1138463	1.06
15-24	156860	147092	1.07	320475	300654	1.07	400498	379748	1.05
50-64	79455	79070	1.00	146065	140343	1.04	305749	296957	1.03
65+	31894	36217	0.88	66508	74730	0.89	140260	157766	0.89
65-79	29330	32607	0.90	59926	65096	0.92	121330	131588	0.92
80+	2564	3610	0.71	6582	9634	0.68	18930	26178	0.72
Total	904131	861370	1.05	1535630	1459820	1.05	2221031	2136887	1.04
China									
0-4	57709	54566	1.06	57946	54382	1.07	46162	43641	1.06
5-14	92791	87928	1.06	97651	91493	1.07	93781	88620	1.06
15-49	175922	157417	1.12	335427	312009	1.08	397921	375437	1.06
15-24	63881	57124	1.12	130227	122581	1.06	119162	112459	1.06
50-64	34340	36460	0.94	64827	59041	1.10	131878	126429	1.04
65+	14361	17697	0.81	30338	35946	0.84	62490	69324	0.90
65-79	13137	15807	0.83	27465	30790	0.89	53794	56511	0.95
80+	1224	1890	0.65	2873	5156	0.56	8696	12813	0.68
Total	375124	354067	1.06	586189	552871	1.06	732233	703450	1.04

continued

TABLE 5 *Continued*

Age	1965			1990			2015		
	Males	Females	Sex Ratio	Males	Females	Sex Ratio	Males	Females	Sex Ratio
India									
0-4	40744	38220	1.07	58837	55527	1.06	59916	57144	1.05
5-14	63142	57995	1.09	101988	94973	1.07	126199	119700	1.05
15-49	120378	113546	1.06	219947	202319	1.09	360868	337399	1.07
15-24	44902	42923	1.05	86178	78996	1.09	125559	118453	1.06
50-64	22782	20831	1.09	41007	40092	1.02	82133	77400	1.06
65+	8840	8678	1.02	19110	19293	0.99	39613	43560	0.91
65-79	8304	7963	1.04	17323	17420	0.99	34548	37313	0.93
80+	536	715	0.75	1787	1873	0.95	5065	6247	0.81
Total	255886	239270	1.07	440888	412206	1.07	668729	635272	1.05

TABLE 6 Age-Specific Sex Ratios of Urban and Rural Populations of Less Developed Regions, 1965, 1990, and 2015

	1965		1990		2015	
Age	Urban	Rural	Urban	Rural	Urban	Rural
Less Developed Regions						
0-4	1.05	1.04	1.05	1.04	1.05	1.03
5-14	1.03	1.05	1.03	1.06	1.03	1.05
15-49	1.09	1.04	1.09	1.02	1.09	0.98
15-24	1.07	1.04	1.08	1.04	1.07	1.00
50-64	1.01	0.98	1.04	1.00	1.04	0.97
65+	0.81	0.89	0.82	0.90	0.84	0.90
Total	1.05	1.03	1.06	1.02	1.05	1.00
Africa						
0-4	1.03	1.01	1.03	1.01	1.03	1.02
5-14	0.98	1.01	0.98	1.03	0.98	1.05
15-49	1.10	0.95	1.11	0.92	1.10	0.90
15-24	1.06	0.97	1.08	0.96	1.07	0.95
50-64	1.01	0.89	0.98	0.88	1.01	0.89
65+	0.79	0.79	0.78	0.82	0.78	0.84
Total	1.04	0.97	1.05	0.96	1.04	0.95
Latin America						
0-4	1.05	1.01	1.04	1.01	1.04	1.02
5-14	1.00	1.04	1.01	1.06	1.02	1.07
15-49	0.94	1.09	0.96	1.11	0.98	1.13
15-24	0.95	1.10	0.98	1.13	1.00	1.16
50-64	0.87	1.09	0.89	1.12	0.90	1.13
65+	0.75	1.06	0.75	1.11	0.74	1.08
Total	0.96	1.06	0.96	1.08	0.96	1.10
Developing Regions of Asia and Oceania						
0-4	1.06	1.05	1.06	1.05	1.06	1.05
5-14	1.06	1.06	1.06	1.06	1.05	1.05
15-49	1.14	1.05	1.13	1.03	1.11	1.00
15-24	1.11	1.05	1.10	1.05	1.09	1.01
50-64	1.07	0.99	1.11	1.01	1.08	0.98
65+	0.83	0.89	0.86	0.90	0.87	0.91
Total	1.09	1.04	1.09	1.03	1.07	1.00
China						
0-4	1.06	1.06	1.06	1.07	1.06	1.06
5-14	1.06	1.05	1.07	1.06	1.06	1.05
15-49	1.17	1.10	1.09	1.05	1.08	1.02
15-24	1.16	1.11	1.08	1.05	1.08	1.03
50-64	1.05	0.92	1.10	1.05	1.10	0.97
65+	0.82	0.81	0.77	0.84	0.91	0.90
Total	1.11	1.05	1.07	1.04	1.07	1.00

continued

TABLE 6 *Continued*

	1965		1990		2015	
Age	Urban	Rural	Urban	Rural	Urban	Rural
India						
0-4	1.07	1.06	1.06	1.06	1.05	1.05
5-14	1.08	1.09	1.07	1.08	1.05	1.06
15-49	1.19	1.03	1.21	1.04	1.16	1.00
15-24	1.13	1.02	1.17	1.06	1.12	1.01
50-64	1.19	1.08	1.10	1.00	1.13	1.02
65+	0.97	1.03	0.95	1.00	0.88	0.93
Total	1.14	1.05	1.14	1.05	1.11	1.01

During the past 25 years, the Latin American urban population increased at an average annual rate of 3.5 percent and the rural population less than 0.4 percent. During the next 25 years, the urban population is projected to increase at 2.2 percent, and the rural population is projected to decline slightly in size.

The population residing in urban areas in Latin American is therefore projected to rise from 71.5 percent in 1990 to 81.5 percent in 2015 (Table 2). The percentage urban is notably higher for ages 15 and over than for younger ages both in 1990 (73 and 68 percent, respectively) and, as projected, in 2015 (83 and 78 percent, respectively). The urban population is hence older than the rural population. In 1990, 34 percent of the urban population was under age 15, compared to 41 percent of the rural population. Correspondingly, 53 percent of the urban population and 46 percent of the rural population are between ages 15 and 49.

Asia is much less urban than Latin America; only 33 percent of Asians resided in urban areas in 1990. However, the urban population is projected to grow by 3.4 percent per year during the next 25 years (compared to 0.1 percent for rural areas) and the urban population will increase to 52 percent of the total.

The share of population aged 15-49 is more pronounced in Asia and Oceania than in Latin America, for both urban and rural areas. In urban areas, 57 percent is currently age 15-49 (compared to 53 percent in Latin America); in rural areas, 50 percent is age 15-49 (compared to 46 percent in Latin America).

DISTRIBUTION OF DEATHS BY SEX AND AGE

Africa, Latin America, and Asia vary not only according to mortality level but also according to the age and sex patterns of mortality. Different mortality patterns, along with variant sex and age patterns of population at risk, lead to very different distributions of deaths across regions.

The effect of mortality level can be indicated with just a few figures. Although 16 percent of the LDR population in 1990 was African, the continent contributed 23 percent of deaths during 1985-1990 (Table 7). Developing Asia and Oceania comprise 73 percent of the LDR population, but 69 percent of deaths. Latin America makes up the remaining 11 percent of population and 8 percent of deaths.

Different age and sex patterns lead to other interesting variations. For example, during 1985-1990, 48 percent of deaths in Africa occurred to preschool children (Table 8). For developing Asia and Oceania the corresponding percentage is 32, and for Latin America, 26 percent deaths occur under age 5. At the other end of the age spectrum, the share of deaths to those 65 and over varies from 15 percent in Africa, to 33 percent in developing Asia, to 36 percent in Latin America. The male to female sex ratio of total deaths is 1.10 for Africa and 1.09 for Asia and Oceania, but 1.26 for Latin America. Sex ratios are less than unity among the elderly in Africa and Latin America, but slightly more than unity in developing Asia. (Detailed tables on deaths by sex are not included here, in the interest of space, but the most salient gender differences are discussed in the text.)

In general, the age distribution of deaths is youngest in Africa and oldest in Latin America. As a result, although 23 percent of total deaths in the LDRs are among Africans, 31 percent of preschool deaths and 38 percent of early-school-age deaths are. Correspondingly, only 12 percent of LDR deaths at ages 65 and over are African. Latin America contributes 8 percent toward LDR deaths, 6 percent of deaths at ages 0-4, 5 percent of 5- to 14-year-old deaths, and 10 percent of deaths among those 65 and over. Asia and Oceania comprise 69 percent of total deaths in LDRs, 62 percent of preschool deaths, 57 percent of 5- to 14-year-old deaths, and 78 percent of deaths at age 65 and older.

Age Patterns of Mortality

Figure 1 and Table 9 present age- and sex-specific mortality rates (${}_nm_x$) for each of the three major areas for the period 1985-1990. These age-specific mortality rates are calculated from aggregations of country-specific population and deaths. They are aggregations of heterogeneous experiences and do not necessarily represent a typical country experience.

The country-specific life tables on which the data in Figure 1 and Table 9 are from diverse sources. Some (particularly for Africa) are based on model life tables because of the absence of reliable data. Others are based on the application of indirect techniques to census or survey tabulations such as child survival and parental orphanhood. As many as possible are

TABLE 7 Total Deaths and Percentage of Deaths in Less Developed Regions, 1960-1965, 1985-1990, and 2010-2015

	1960-1965			1985-1990			2010-2015		
Region	Both	Male	Female	Both	Male	Female	Both	Male	Female
				Deaths (thousands)					
Total	201578	103746	97832	189991	99604	90387	219494	118361	101133
Africa	34160	17758	16402	43970	23005	20965	52194	27648	24546
Latin America	14245	7673	6572	15752	8782	6971	21187	11758	9429
Developing Regions of Asia and Oceania	153173	78315	74858	130269	67818	62452	146113	78954	67159
China	59281	30779	28502	36707	19397	17310	50421	27710	22711
India	45530	22710	22821	45804	23481	22323	44255	23846	20409
				Distribution (%)					
Total	100.0	100.0	100.0	100.0	100.0	100.0	100.0	100.0	100.0
Africa	17.0	17.1	16.8	23.1	23.1	23.2	23.8	23.4	24.3
Latin America	7.1	7.4	6.7	8.3	8.8	7.7	9.6	9.9	9.3
Developing Regions of Asia and Oceania	76.0	75.5	76.5	68.6	68.1	69.1	66.6	66.7	66.4
China	38.7	39.3	38.1	28.2	28.6	27.7	34.5	35.1	33.8
India	29.7	30.0	30.5	35.2	34.6	35.7	30.3	30.2	30.4

TABLE 8 Distribution of Deaths by Age in Less Developed Regions, 1960-1965, 1985-1990, and 2010-2015

	1960-1965		1985-1990		2010-2015	
Age	Number	Percentage	Number	Percentage	Number	Percentage
Less Developed Regions						
0-4	91611	45.45	65782	34.62	40872	18.62
5-14	19658	9.75	14040	7.39	9366	4.27
15-24	9251	4.59	8139	4.28	6669	3.04
15-49	35341	17.53	30487	16.05	30975	14.11
50-64	21180	10.51	24946	13.13	35390	16.12
65-74	17870	8.86	24847	13.08	38274	17.44
65+	33788	16.76	54737	28.81	102892	46.88
75+	15918	7.90	29890	15.73	64618	29.44
Total	201578	100.00	189991	100.00	219494	100.00
Africa						
0-4	17291	50.62	20599	46.85	18076	34.63
5-14	4316	12.63	5306	12.07	5255	10.07
15-24	1770	5.18	2383	5.42	3204	6.14
15-49	5934	17.37	7682	17.47	10513	20.14
50-64	2723	7.97	3787	8.61	5867	11.24
65-74	2086	6.11	3218	7.32	5407	10.36
65+	3897	11.41	6595	15.00	12483	23.92
75+	1811	5.30	3377	7.68	7076	13.56
Total	34160	100.00	43970	100.00	52194	100.00
Latin America						
0-4	6367	44.70	4151	26.35	2515	11.87
5-14	1097	7.70	752	4.77	490	2.31
15-24	573	4.02	687	4.36	537	2.53
15-49	2409	16.91	2980	18.91	3403	16.06
50-64	1634	11.47	2266	14.38	3859	18.22
65-74	1314	9.22	2180	13.84	3728	17.60
65+	2738	19.22	5605	35.58	10920	51.54
75+	1425	10.00	3425	21.74	7192	33.95
Total	14245	100.00	15752	100.00	21187	100.00
Developing Regions of Asia and Oceania						
0-4	67953	44.36	41032	31.50	20282	13.88
5-14	14246	9.30	7982	6.13	3621	2.48
15-24	6928	4.51	5070	3.89	2928	2.00
15-49	26998	17.63	19825	15.22	17059	11.68
50-64	16824	10.98	18893	14.50	25663	17.56
65-74	14770	9.45	19449	14.93	29139	19.94
65+	27152	17.73	42537	32.65	79488	54.40
75+	12683	8.28	23088	17.72	50349	34.46
Total	153173	100.00	130269	100.00	146113	100.00

continued

TABLE 8 *Continued*

Age	1960-1965		1985-1990		2010-2015	
	Number	Percentage	Number	Percentage	Number	Percentage
China						
0-4	22593	38.1	4750	12.9	1439	2.9
5-14	4909	8.3	1011	2.8	337	0.7
15-24	2600	4.4	1159	3.2	482	1.0
15-49	11057	18.7	5009	13.6	3995	7.9
50-64	7526	12.7	7136	19.4	9788	19.4
65-74	6915	11.7	8322	22.7	12023	23.9
65+	13197	22.3	18801	51.2	34862	69.1
75+	6282	10.6	10479	28.6	22839	45.3
Total	59281	100.00	36707	100.0	50421	100.0
India						
0-4	22316	49.0	17607	38.4	8644	19.5
5-14	4584	10.1	3241	7.1	1222	2.8
15-24	2154	4.7	1912	4.2	982	2.2
15-49	7655	16.8	7174	15.7	5399	12.2
50-64	4267	9.4	5601	12.2	6742	15.2
65-74	3709	8.2	5772	12.6	8156	18.4
65+	6707	14.7	12182	26.6	22247	50.3
75+	2998	6.6	6411	14.0	14091	31.8
Total	45530	100.0	45804	100.0	44255	100.0

based on recorded deaths and population by age and sex (from censuses, surveys, or civil registration), adjusted when necessary for incompleteness.

Life expectancy at birth for the less developed regions averaged 61.4 years for this period (60.1 years for males and 62.8 for females). Africa exhibits the lowest life expectancy, 52 years, compared to 66.7 years for Latin America and 62.3 years for Asia. Latin America's life expectancy exceeds that of Asia by 4.4 years, but male-female differences are large. Among males, Latin American life expectancy exceeds that of Asia by 2.6 years, but among females the difference is 6.3 years. For both males and females, African death rates are the highest among the three areas at all ages.

Female death rates for Latin America are lower than those for Asia at all ages, but differences are small after age 40 and are negligible between ages 40 and 60. Latin American and Asian death rates exhibit a crossover among males at age 55-60. Latin American male death rates are lower prior to age 15 and again after age 55, but are much higher between ages 15 and 55.

Dechter and Preston (1992) have illustrated that the low Latin Ameri-

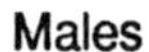

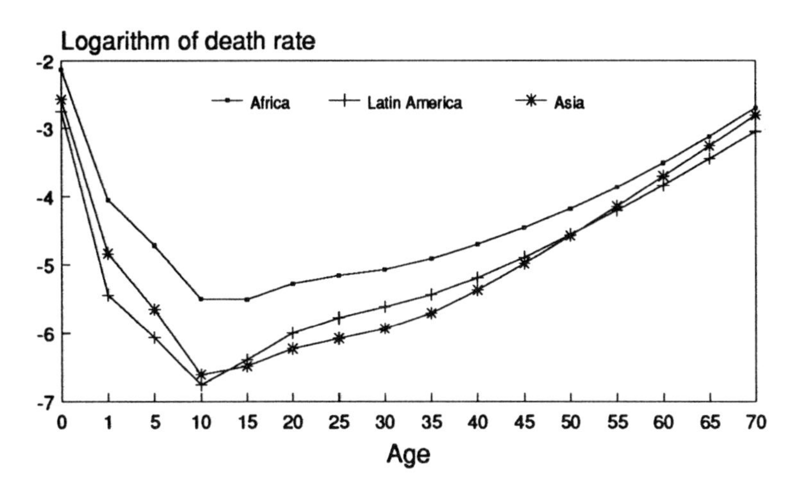

Females

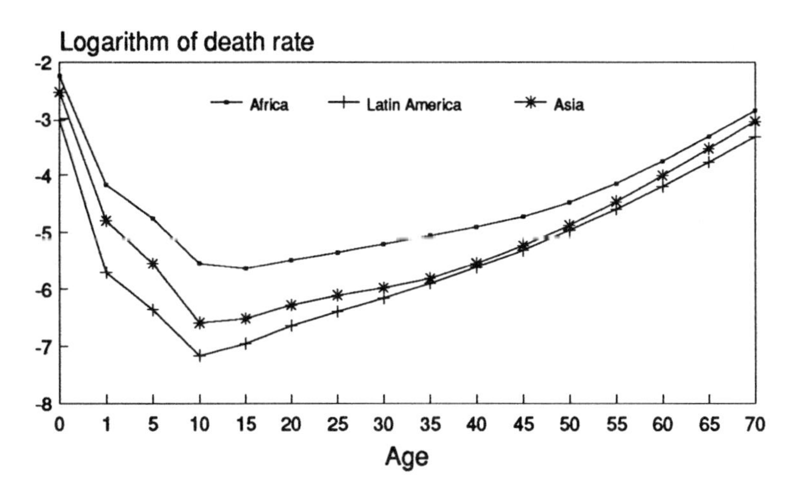

FIGURE 1 Age-specific mortality rates, males and females, 1985-1990.

TABLE 9 Age-Specific Mortality Rates ($_nm_x$) in Less Developed Regions, 1985-1990

Age	Less Developed Regions	Africa	Latin America	Asia
Males				
0-1	.08392	.11822	.06370	.07606
1-4	.00941	.01730	.00435	.00794
5-9	.00440	.00894	.00226	.00352
10-14	.00178	.00410	.00116	.00135
15-19	.00192	.00408	.00168	.00153
20-24	.00246	.00512	.00249	.00198
25-29	.00286	.00578	.00311	.00230
30-34	.00324	.00629	.00365	.00266
35-39	.00395	.00735	.00437	.00333
40-44	.00533	.00908	.00558	.00467
45-49	.00752	.01157	.00751	.00686
50-54	.01087	.01523	.01043	.01028
55-59	.01625	.02088	.01486	.01578
60-64	.02480	.02976	.02152	.02455
65-69	.03824	.04413	.03175	.03831
70-74	.05954	.06734	.04737	.06024
Life expectancy at birth	60.1	50.3	64.0	61.4
Females				
0-1	.08195	.10548	.04856	.07931
1-4	.00919	.01544	.00331	.00827
5-9	.00455	.00860	.00172	.00388
10-14	.00174	.00390	.00077	.00137
15-19	.00173	.00355	.00095	.00147
20-24	.00213	.00412	.00130	.00187
25-29	.00252	.00477	.00167	.00222
30-34	.00289	.00547	.00212	.00253
35-39	.00343	.00637	.00274	.00300
40-44	.00436	.00744	.00364	.00390
45-49	.00578	.00887	.00499	.00534
50-54	.00805	.01137	.00702	.00763
55-59	.01191	.01582	.01012	.01152
60-64	.01846	.02345	.01503	.01816
65-69	.02941	.03641	.02304	.02927
70-74	.04726	.05749	.03594	.04746
Life expectancy at birth	62.8	53.6	69.5	63.2

can death rates at older ages may be partially a function of a common Latin American pattern of age misreporting. In Costa Rica, it is found that correction for age misreporting leads to an age pattern of mortality consistent with the West region of the Coale and Demeny (1983) model life-table system. To see the effects of such age misreporting on the population projections presented here, we prepared a special projection for Latin America, assuming that age-specific death rates followed the West region pattern from ages 45 onward, rather than those exhibited in Table 9. The new life tables exhibit for 1985-1990 a life expectancy at birth 1.8 years below the United Nations estimate.

However, the 2015 age distribution in this new projection (which uses the adjusted life table and assumes that life expectancy improves at the same pace as the United Nations projection, but at the lower level of life expectancy) is altered to only a small degree. With the adjusted life table, the percentages of population in age groups 0-14, 15-49, 50-64, and 65+ are 28.3, 52.9, 12.7, and 6.1, compared with 28.0, 52.5, 12.8, and 6.7 from the United Nations projections (see Table 3 above).

African Distribution of Deaths

Of the 190 million deaths in the less developed regions during 1985-1990, 44 million occurred in Africa; hence, this major area requires a more detailed description of the future evolution of mortality. Slightly more than 52 percent of the deaths are to males, a percentage that has remained nearly unchanged during the past 25 years. However, males make up the majority of deaths only up to age 65: deaths are 53 percent male at ages 0-4, 51 percent male at ages 5-14, and 54 percent male for ages 15-64. From age 65, females make up a majority of deaths: 50.2 percent of all deaths at ages 65-74, and 56 percent of deaths at age 75 and over.

During 1985-1990, 47 percent of African deaths occurred at ages under 5 and another 12 percent between ages 5 and 14. As previously indicated, with 59 percent of deaths under age 15, Africa exhibits a very young death distribution, when compared with 42 percent of deaths occurring under age 15 for the LDRs as a whole. Due to the age pattern of mortality decline during the past 25 years, as well as the fertility decline that has occurred, the number of deaths in Africa has increased more at the older ages. Comparing deaths during the period 1960-1965 with those during 1985-1990, one finds a direct relationship between age and percent increase in number of deaths, as shown in Table 10.

The pattern is very similar if one considers males and females separately, although the percentage increase for male deaths was greater than that for females at all ages. As a result the percentage of deaths occurring under age 14 has fallen during the past 25 years, from 63 to 59 percent; the

TABLE 10 Increase in Africa's Deaths from 1960-1965 to 1985-1990

Age Group	Deaths 1985-1990 (thousands)	Percentage Increase 1960-1965 to 1985-1990
0-4	20599	19.1
5-14	5306	23.0
15-49	7682	29.5
50-64	3787	39.1
65-74	3218	54.2
75+	3377	86.5

percentage at ages 15-49 has remained at 17 percent; at ages 50-64, the share of deaths has risen from 8 to 9 percent; and at age 65 and over, the share has increased from 11 to 15 percent (Table 8).

Changes in Deaths Over the Next 25 Years Without the AIDS Pandemic

The 1990 revision of population estimates and projections by the United Nations projects a continuation of the above trends for the next 25 years, although at a faster pace due to an assumed more rapid decline in fertility. However, the 1990 revision was undertaken before the extent of the AIDS pandemic was known and before even rough estimates could be made of its potential demographic effects. This section therefore describes how the number and distribution of deaths in Africa would evolve if the AIDS pandemic had not occurred, or if it plays itself out with minimal impact on future mortality. The next section presents some preliminary indications of what the effect of AIDS may be on deaths during the next 25 years.

In the absence of AIDS, 52.2 million deaths in Africa are expected during the 2010-2015 period, 19 percent more than occurred during 1985-1990. All of the increase in numbers of deaths will take place among the adult population. In fact, it is projected that the number of deaths under age 5 will be 12 percent below the 1985-1990 level, and the number at ages 5-14 will be 1 percent below. Increases in the number of deaths at age 15 and over are expected to be much greater than they were during the last 25 years. In comparison to 1985-1990, deaths during 2010-2015 will be 37 percent greater at ages 15-49, 55 percent greater at ages 50-64, 68 percent greater at ages 65-74, and 110 percent greater at age 75 and over.

The total number of deaths that would occur in Africa during 2010-2015 is projected to be 24 percent of the deaths that occur in the LDRs in total—only slightly higher than the 23 percent calculated for 1985-1990. However, below age 25 the proportion of LDR deaths that are located in

Africa will continue to rise rapidly. Under age 5, 44 percent of all LDR deaths in 2010-2015 will be African (compared to 19 percent in 1960-1965 and 31 percent in 1985-1990); at ages 5-14, 56 percent of deaths will be African (compared to 22 percent in 1960-1965 and 38 percent in 1985-1990); at ages 15-24, 48 percent of deaths are projected to be African (compared to 19 percent in 1960-1965 and 29 percent in 1985-1990).

Potential Effect of the AIDS Pandemic on the Number and Distribution of African Deaths

However, AIDS exists, and at least in Africa, it will lead to large numbers of additional deaths during the next 25 years. For the 15 countries with the estimated highest current level of human immunodeficiency virus (HIV) prevalence (Malawi, Rwanda, Uganda, Zambia, Zimbabwe, Burundi, Central African Republic, Congo, Tanzania, Zaire, Benin, Burkina Faso, Côte d'Ivoire, Kenya, and Mozambique), potential deaths during the next 25 years due to the AIDS pandemic have been calculated based on the World Health Organization's (WHO) latest estimates of HIV prevalence and the WHO epidemiological model for projecting future infections and resultant AIDS cases and deaths. The application of the model here is conservative in that it assumes no new adult infections after 2005.

Preliminary estimates from this model indicate that these 15 countries will provide in aggregate about 18 million AIDS-related deaths during the next 25 years. (Additional deaths due to AIDS will add up to 13 million persons since many would die from other causes anyway). AIDS deaths will occur predominantly to young children and those in the prime working ages. About one-fourth of projected AIDS deaths will occur to children under age 5, and slightly more than one-half will occur to those aged 15-49. About 23 percent of deaths will be to those aged 50 and over, and less than 1 percent to those between ages 5 and 14.

Figure 2 presents the projected aggregate age-specific mortality rates for the 1990-2015 period, with and without AIDS, for these 15 African countries. Table 11 shows the percentage increase in expected mortality rates due to AIDS. The mortality rates in the absence of AIDS are calculated from the United Nations 1990 Revision.

The death rate under age 5 will be 13 percent higher than originally expected, but the largest rises in age-specific death rates can be expected to occur in the middle age groups. The death rate will rise by at least 20 percent between ages 20 and 65, by about 50 percent or more between ages 25 and 60, and by 100 percent between ages 35 and 45.

As a result, the age distribution of deaths in these countries during the next 25 years will be greatly altered. The percentage of expected deaths between ages 15 and 49 is projected to be 25 rather than 19 percent, and the

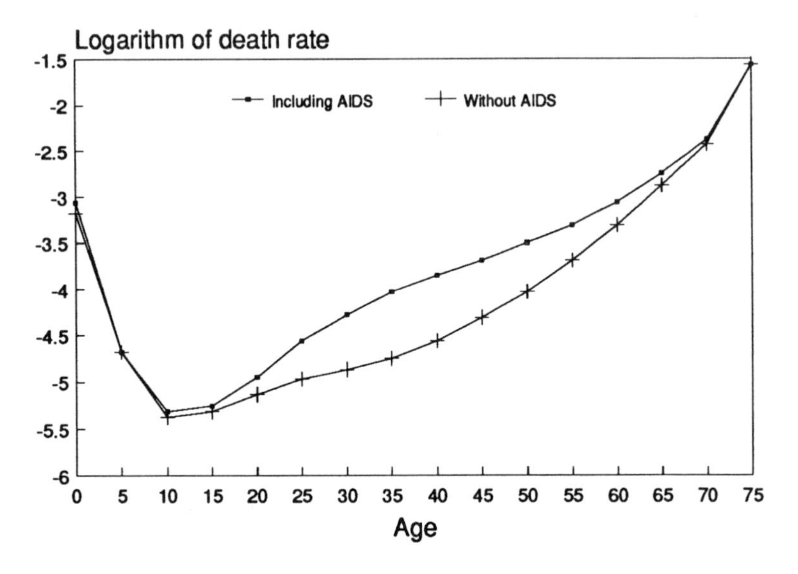

FIGURE 2 Projected aggregate age-specific mortality rates for 15 African countries with and without AIDS, 1990-2015.

TABLE 11 Increase in Mortality Rates Due to AIDS, 1990-2015; 15 Highest-Prevalence African Countries[a]

Age Group	Percentage Increase Due to AIDS
0-4	12.8
5-9	0.1
10-14	3.8
15-19	7.9
20-24	22.6
25-29	49.2
30-34	80.0
35-39	103.1
40-44	105.6
45-49	91.7
50-54	70.0
55-59	48.4
60-64	27.7
65-69	15.3
70-74	8.1
75+	2.2

[a]Countries include: Malawi, Rwanda, Uganda, Zambia, Zimbabwe, Burundi, Central African Republic, Congo, Tanzania, Zaire, Benin, Burkina Faso, Côte d'Ivoire, Kenya, and Mozambique.

TABLE 12 Distribution of Deaths for 15 African Countries With and Without AIDS, 1990-2015[a]

	Percentage	
Age Group	Without AIDS	With AIDS
0-4	43.3	39.7
5-14	11.9	9.8
15-49	19.2	25.3
50-64	8.8	10.5
65+	16.8	14.6
Total	100.0	100.0

[a]Countries include: Malawi, Rwanda, Uganda, Zambia, Zimbabwe, Burundi, Central African Republic, Congo, Tanzania, Zaire, Benin, Burkina Faso, Côte d'Ivoire, Kenya, and Mozambique.

share between ages 50 and 64 will be 11 rather than 9 percent. AIDS mortality will lead to lower shares of deaths at other ages: 40 percent of deaths will be among those 0-4, rather than 43 percent (in spite of an anticipated 13 percent increase in deaths at these ages); 10 percent at ages 5-14 instead of 12 percent; and 15 percent at ages 65 and over instead of 17 percent (Table 12).

It can be expected that these 15 countries will account for the vast majority of all AIDS deaths in Africa, but even if one assumed that no AIDS-related deaths occurred outside these 15 countries, the 1990-2015 total death rate for Africa would be 7 percent higher than otherwise projected. In fact, total expected deaths for Africa will increase by more than 20 percent at ages 30-54, and by at least 10 percent at ages 25-59.

SUMMARY

Currently 4.1 billion persons live in the less developed regions of the world: 642 million in Africa, 448 million in Latin America, and 3.0 billion in the developing regions of Asia and Oceania. During the next 25 years, an average annual population growth rate of 2.8 percent is projected for Africa, compared to 1.6 percent for Latin America and 1.5 percent for Asia. Thus, by 2015, of the 6.3 billion population projected for the less developed regions, 1.3 billion will be African, 673 million Latin American, and 4.4 billion Asian. At mid-1990, 37 percent of the population of the less developed regions lived in urban areas (1.5 billion persons). By 2015, 55 percent of the population of the developing countries is projected to be urban.

The age distribution of population varies significantly across these three major areas. The population share aged 0-4 ranges from 12 and 13 percent in Latin America and Asia, to 18 percent in Africa. The percentage of the population aged 65 and over varies from 3.0 percent in Africa, to 4.7 percent in Asia, to 4.8 percent in Latin America. The population age distribution will be much older by 2015, as the percentage aged 65 and over rises to 3.4 in Africa, 6.7 in Latin America, and 6.8 in Asia.

Africa, Latin America, and Asia vary according to mortality level, and to age and sex patterns of death. Although 16 percent of the LDR population in 1990 is African, the continent contributed 23 percent of the deaths during 1985-1990. Developing Asia and Oceania comprised 73 percent of the LDR population, but 69 percent of deaths, whereas Latin America made up the remaining 11 percent of the population and 8 percent of deaths.

In general, the age distribution of deaths is youngest in Africa. During 1985-1990, 48 percent of deaths in Africa occurred to preschool children, compared to 26 percent in Latin America and 32 percent in Asia. Deaths to those aged 65 and over contribute 15 percent to African deaths, 33 percent to Asian deaths, and 36 percent to Latin American deaths.

Although mortality levels are projected to exhibit substantial declines during the next quarter century, the absolute number of deaths in the less developed regions will be greater in 2010-2015 than during the five years prior to 1990. The age distribution of deaths will, however, be much older, with nearly one-half of all deaths expected to take place at age 65 and over, and less than 20 percent under age 5. For some countries, particularly in Africa, the potential effects of the AIDS pandemic may alter the future course and age patterns of mortality. Preliminary estimates indicate that the 15 African countries with the highest current level of HIV prevalence may experience 18 million additional deaths during the next 25 years due to the AIDS pandemic. These AIDS-related deaths are expected to occur predominantly to young children and to those in the prime working ages. About one-fourth of the projected AIDS deaths during the next 25 years in these countries will occur to children under age 5, and slightly more than one-half will occur to those aged 15-49.

REFERENCES

Coale, A.J., and P. Demeny
1983 *Regional Model Life Tables and Stable Populations*, 2nd ed. New York: Academic Press.

Dechter, A.R., and S.H. Preston
1992 Age misreporting and its effects on adult mortality estimates in Latin America. *Population Bulletin of the United Nations*. No. 31/32. New York: United Nations.

United Nations
1991a *World Population Prospects 1990*. Population Studies No. 120. New York: United Nations.

1991b *The Sex and Age Distributions of Population, The 1990 Revision.* Population Studies No. 122. New York: United Nations.

1991c *World Urbanization Prospects 1990, Estimates and Projections of Urban and Rural Populations and Urban Agglomerations.* Population Studies No. 120. New York: United Nations.

Mortality by Cause, 1970 to 2015

Rodolfo A. Bulatao

BACKGROUND

National data on causes of death provide a view of the overall health status of a population. They suggest what diseases and conditions should be of major concern and where a country stands in relation to others and in relation to the epidemiological transition (Omran, 1971). They can provide guidance on health priorities and feedback on the effects of interventions. As mortality falls worldwide, health conditions increasingly deviate from a simple unilinear trend (Frenk et al., 1989). Consequently, policymakers need to pay close attention to trends in causes of death in order to understand the health needs of changing populations.

Because of the many deficiencies of cause-of-death data, particularly in areas of high mortality, even a simple classification of deaths is difficult to achieve. Country reports to the World Health Organization (WHO) of causes of death are supplemented with regression estimates for the many nonreporting countries. The regression approach, initiated by Preston (1976) and continued by Hakulinen et al. (1986a,b), estimates mortality rates for different

---

Rodolfo A. Bulatao is with the World Bank. The author wishes to thank Alan D. Lopez for data, insights, and suggestions, and Patience W. Stephens for research assistance. Thanks also to David Dunlop, Richard Feachem, E. Robert Greenberg, Scott B. Halstead, Dean T. Jamison, Bernhard Liese, Jose Martinez, Alberto Torres, and Patrick Vaughan, as well as participants in meetings for the World Bank health sector priorities review, for their comments and suggestions.

causes as functions of overall mortality levels. This approach has also been applied to specific causes, such as cancer deaths (Parkin et al., 1988).

The equations developed by Hakulinen et al. for different age-sex groups are applied here. Besides updating their estimates (from 1980 to 1985), this paper incorporates new data not available to them, attempts a more detailed classification based on seven major causes, and provides perspectives on possible future trends.

Estimates were made by sex and age (for six age groups: 0, 1–4, 5–14, 15–44, 45–64, and 65 and older) for four years (1970, 1985, 2000, and 2015) and six regions or country groups (industrial market economies, industrial nonmarket economies, Latin America and the Caribbean, sub-Saharan Africa, the Middle East and North Africa, and Asia and the Pacific).

METHOD

Grouping Causes of Death

The seven major causes of death considered here are infectious and parasitic diseases, neoplasms, circulatory system and certain degenerative diseases, complications of pregnancy, certain perinatal conditions, injury and poisoning, and other causes. These categories are identical to those used by Hakulinen et al. to permit the application of their equations. Categories correspond to specific codes in the International Statistical Classification of Diseases, Injuries, and Causes of Death, eighth and ninth revisions (ICD–8 and ICD–9: World Health Organization, 1977; see Bulatao and Stephens, 1992: Table 1 for the correspondence).

Two categories require some explanation. The infectious and parasitic diseases include bronchitis, emphysema, and asthma because of the important infectious bronchitis component, which was not separable from the others. Circulatory system and certain degenerative diseases include diabetes, nephritis, cirrhosis of the liver, and ulcers of the stomach and duodenum, not because of any presumed similarity in etiology or pathogenesis but to keep the number of categories manageable by combining the degenerative diseases other than cancer.

Three of these major causes were further subdivided into 21 specific causes of death, as shown in Table 1. These specific causes were chosen mainly for substantive interest. One of them—diarrhea—corresponds to a subcategory used by Hakulinen.

Among these specific causes, not all could be defined with precision. For example, the codes selected from ICD–9 for micronutrient disorders were those for disorders of the thyroid gland, anemias, and avitaminosis. This group of causes may be both too broad and too narrow in different ways, but further specification was not possible.

TABLE 1 Major and Specific Causes of Death

Infectious and Parasitic Diseases	Circulatory System and Certain Degenerative Diseases	Other Causes
Diarrhea	Ischemic heart disease	Mental disorders
Tuberculosis	Cerebrovascular disease	Oral health diseases
Acute respiratory infection	Other cardiovascular diseases	Micronutrient disorders
Measles	Diabetes	Malnutrition
Chronic obstructive pulmonary disease (COPD)	Certain degenerative diseases (nephritis, cirrhosis, ulcers)	Unspecified other causes
Polio		
Yellow fever, dengue, and encephalitis		
Malaria		
Schistosomiasis and filariasis		
Intestinal parasites		
Other infectious and parasitic diseases		

Data on Causes of Death

Although data on causes of death can be problematic, these data are used largely as reported by WHO, without attempting such corrections as regrouping codes or reallocating undefined causes. (WHO has procedures for scrutinizing the data before including them in its reports.) The limitations that remain are discussed, and the data for three countries require specific comment.

Reports on causes of death for around 1970 and 1985 cover a limited number of countries, and their reliability is a matter of concern. About 70 countries or territories annually provide WHO with statistics on causes of death by sex and age, using the ICD. For about 40 of these countries, most of them developed, the data can be considered reliable. The remaining 30 countries' reports may cover as little as half of the population (though some cover everyone) and usually include 5–20 percent of deaths ascribed to ill-defined conditions. (Bulatao and Stephens, 1992:Tables A1 and A2, list the countries and give data coverage and quality.)

Data quality depends critically on medical certification of causes of death. In remote areas with few or no physicians, diagnosis is uncertain and many deaths are coded to symptoms and ill-defined conditions. In addition, incomplete coverage by the vital registration system will likely bias the picture toward the chronic disease pattern more common in urban areas. Furthermore, despite the common set of procedures defined by ICD–

9 for coding and certifying the cause of death, data across countries are still affected by variations in diagnostic preferences, cultural factors, medical training, the availability of diagnostic aids, and other factors.

The data provide underlying causes of death; associated or contributory conditions are not reported. It is difficult to predict how the importance of associated causes will change as countries progress through the epidemiological transition. Certainly under the regime of infectious diseases, malnutrition will frequently underlie many deaths from diarrheal diseases or acute respiratory infections. On the other hand, as death is increasingly postponed to older ages, multiple pathologies at or near the time of death become relatively common. Given the complications and the lack of data, this paper discusses only underlying causes.

Of the countries reporting to WHO, China, India, and the former USSR have data with special characteristics. The Chinese data are from a survey covering 57 million urban residents and 42 million rural residents spread over the eastern part of the country. The 580,000 deaths recorded, though only 7 percent of estimated annual Chinese deaths, should be reasonably indicative of the mortality pattern for 70–80 percent of the population.

The Indian data are from a 1986 cause-of-death survey of 1,200 rural primary health care centers spread throughout India, and covered 10,075 male and 8,187 female deaths (0.2 percent of estimated Indian deaths). Coding was idiosyncratic, but the major causes and some of the specific causes were still distinguishable.

For the former USSR (which was still a single country in 1985 and is treated as such in this paper), the data reported to WHO permitted identification of deaths due to diarrhea, most circulatory system diseases (excluding cirrhosis of the liver), and measles. Regression estimates were used to fill in the other causes.

For most other countries reporting to WHO, data were available on each cause of death. The major exceptions were the Latin American and Caribbean countries, for which 1970 but not 1985 data were available on other causes and four specific causes (chronic obstructive pulmonary disease, polio, mental disorders, and micronutrient disorders). Again, regression estimates filled in for the missing data.

Estimating and Projecting Mortality

Before estimating deaths by cause, overall mortality was estimated and projected. This was done country by country, for 187 countries, territories, or groups of small countries or territories covering the entire world (only aggregate results are reported). Life expectancy and infant mortality estimates for the 1985–1990 quinquennium were obtained from the best available sources; adjustments were made as needed for agreement with other demographic parameters; and both forward and backward population projections were made.

Each country's experience with mortality change is used to project its mortality over the period 1990–2005. Each country is assumed to revert to the average mortality trend for the world as a whole for the projection of 2005-2015. This average trend involves slower improvements as life expectancy rises. The procedure involves separate projections of life expectancy and infant mortality and the choice of "split" life tables from the Coale-Demeny (1983) set to match both parameters. Further description of the procedures is provided in Bulatao and Bos (1989).

The mortality trends are applied to the standard World Bank projections (see Bulatao et al., 1990). Two types of alternative projections were also run: "fixed mortality" projections, in which age-specific mortality rates (for five-year age groups) are taken as fixed at 1985–1990 levels throughout the projection period; and "fixed distribution" projections, in which mortality changes as in the standard projections, but the distribution of deaths by cause within each of the six larger age groups does not change from 1985. These alternative projections allow some decomposition of projected changes in the cause-of-death structure.

Estimating Mortality Rates by Major Cause

Mortality rates by major cause were obtained from actual data and from previously estimated regression equations. Data reported to WHO were used wherever possible for the years 1970 and 1985. These data were adjusted proportionally where necessary to produce the mortality levels separately estimated.

The regression equations for major causes of death, obtained from Hakulinen et al. (1986a), predict mortality rates by cause for age-sex groups as linear functions of mortality rates for all causes. To take into account differences in age structure within broad age groups, separate equations (generally only slightly different) were estimated for each of 24 world regions. This was not necessary for the first two age groups, 0 and 1–4, which are narrower than the other groups and for which only world and not regional equations are available.

Essentially these regression equations indicate that mortality rates for most causes, except neoplasms, increase with overall mortality. The increases are greatest for infectious and parasitic diseases (slopes around 0.5, meaning that half of the increase in deaths is attributable to this major cause), followed by other causes (slopes around 0.25) and perinatal conditions (slope of 0.22, for age group 0 only). Slopes vary considerably by age group: for infectious and parasitic diseases, they vary from 0.7 for those 1–4 years old to 0.4 for those 65 and older. Slopes also vary by sex: for neoplasms among those 65 and older, the slope for males is –0.13 and for females –0.04. Nevertheless, the trend across age groups is similar for males and females. In contrast, slopes hardly vary across regions, with the largest gap between regions for a given cause and sex and age group being around 0.04. The equations for lower-mortality, more developed regions do appear to diverge more often from the norm, though only minimally. When the number of regions and the rarity of even small differences in the equations are considered, the case for distinct cause-of-death structures across regions is weak.

Where reported data were not available, results from the equations specific to each of the 24 regions were used. For 2000 and 2015, the same region-specific equations were applied for the industrial market economies. Other countries were allowed to switch to the equations for developed countries as a group if their mortality levels had declined to a standardized death rate (by using the 1985 age structure for the world) below 6. (The industrial market economies as a group have a standardized crude death rate of 5.8 for 1985, as contrasted, for example, with 9.0 for Latin America and the Caribbean.)

Estimating Cause-Specific Mortality Rates

New regression equations were estimated for mortality rates from 21 specific causes by using the rate for the major cause under which each falls as the predictor. The data, the specifications, and the results of the regressions are described.

Data for 1970 and 1985 were pooled; 1970 data were used for 65 countries (34 of them developing, mostly Latin American) and 1985 data for 69 countries (38 developing). China was included, but India and the former USSR were omitted because of the number of causes for which estimates could not be produced. Although data quality varies for the countries included, imposing a more rigorous standard would bias the sample strongly toward developed countries.

For each country, mortality rates by cause were first adjusted to correspond to the separately determined overall mortality levels. Rates based on fewer than 10,000 people in the age-sex group were excluded. Three equations were then estimated for each disease in each age-sex group: a quadratic specification, where the rate for the specific cause depended on the rate for the major cause and the square of this rate, as well as on a dummy variable for data year; a corresponding linear specification; and a specification in which the rate for the specific cause depended only on two dummy variables, for developing country status and data year.

If the quadratic term achieved a 5 percent level of significance, the quadratic equation was chosen; if not, and the linear term achieved a 5 percent level of significance, the linear equation was chosen; in all remaining cases, the dummy variable equation was chosen. Of the 264 final equations, half were quadratic, one-third linear, and the remainder dummy variable equations. The dummy variable for data year had a significant effect in 20 percent of the equations chosen.

Some cause-specific mortality rates were predicted better than others. R^2 varied much more by cause than by age-sex group, permitting the grouping of equations by cause:

(1) mean R^2 greater than .70: diarrhea, acute respiratory infection, other cardiovascular diseases, and unspecified causes;

(2) mean R^2 between .35 and .60: tuberculosis, measles, chronic obstructive pulmonary disease, other infectious and parasitic diseases, cerebrovascular disease, nephritis/cirrhosis/ulcers, micronutrient disorders, and malnutrition;

(3) mean R^2 between .20 and .25: intestinal parasites, ischemic heart disease, and diabetes; and

(4) mean R^2 below .20: polio, malaria, yellow fever/dengue/encephalitis, schistosomiasis/filariasis, mental disorders, and oral health diseases.

The last group also accounted for almost all the dummy variable equations, meaning that developed or developing country averages were essentially applied for these causes.

RESULTS

Demographic Background

Demographic factors affect the cause-of-death structure. From 1985 to 2015, world population is expected to increase by 75 percent, but the population of sub-Saharan Africa will increase by 150 percent. Changes in mortality are implicit in these projections, with much lower overall rates and changes in age-, sex-, and cause-specific rates.

For instance, the population age 45 and over in developing countries is projected to more than double between 1985 and 2015, rising from 17 to 24 percent of the total. Causes of death, which are closely related to age at death, will change accordingly. For developing countries, infant mortality is projected to fall from 78 per thousand in 1985 to 43 per thousand in 2015, and life expectancy at birth to rise by five years. Such mortality trends imply changes in causes of death, which differ by mortality level.

In each region, life expectancy is expected to rise, but starting at different levels and failing to converge by 2015. Life expectancy in industrial market economies will rise from 76.2 years in 1985 to 77.9 years in 2015. Life expectancy in sub-Saharan Africa will rise from 51.3 years in 1985 to

61.3 years in 2015. The other four regions will follow intermediate paths, none of them crossing. Even with projected improvements across the board, regional differentiation will remain sharp: by 2015, life expectancy in sub-Saharan Africa will have barely caught up with 1985 life expectancy in the Middle East and North Africa, and will not have caught up with 1985 life expectancy in any other region.

On the other hand, crude death rates will converge. Regional rates vary as one would expect, being clearly highest in sub-Saharan Africa and lowest in Latin America and the Caribbean. The latter region has more young people than the developed country regions, which accounts for its lower risk of death. With the projected improvements in life expectancy, the crude death rate is not expected to fall monotonically. Rates level off at 5 to 10 per thousand, after which they increase slightly as the numbers of elderly increase. Given these trends, variability across regions in crude death rates is projected to diminish considerably by 2000 and 2015.

Current Causes of Death

Estimated mortality rates by major cause are shown in Table 2 by sex, region, and year, but without age breakdowns, and numbers of deaths by cause and region are shown in Table 3. Patterns for 1970 and 1985 are considered first. The leading causes of death for the world as whole for both 1970 and 1985 were infectious and parasitic diseases and circulatory system diseases. Parasitic and infectious diseases were more important in developing countries, and circulatory system diseases were more important in developed countries. Like infectious and parasitic diseases, death rates from certain perinatal conditions were much more important for developing countries, but for the world as a whole, deaths from certain perinatal conditions accounted for only one-fourth or one-fifth as many deaths as infectious diseases in 1985 (3,321 compared to 14,764). Like circulatory system diseases, neoplasms were more important in developed than in developing countries, but over all countries accounted for only one-third the number of deaths (4,903 compared to 13,208). The category of other causes and injury and poisoning provide weak contrasts between developed and developing countries, and complications of pregnancy account for only a small proportion of deaths.

Figure 1 compares these results with estimates that Hakulinen et al. (1986a) made for 1980. Although the equations were the same, Hakulinen incorporated earlier reported data for fewer countries. Nevertheless, results are generally consistent, with their estimated rates for 1980 usually falling between the 1970 and 1985 estimates. Comparisons for specific regions (not shown), despite being complicated by differences in country groupings, also show general agreement. For sub-Saharan Africa, Hakulinen et al.

TABLE 2 Estimated and Projected Mortality Rates (per 100,000), by Major Cause, Sex, and Region, 1970–2015

	1970		1985		2000		2015	
Region and Cause	Male	Female	Male	Female	Male	Female	Male	Female
World								
All causes	1293	1281	1064	1004	863	802	880	776
Infections	449	449	318	294	176	179	140	133
Neoplasms	95	96	108	96	108	98	128	114
Circulatory	297	324	262	286	292	283	339	314
Pregnancy	0	13	0	9	0	9	0	7
Perinatal	86	70	79	59	48	36	37	27
Injury	93	40	97	56	78	31	79	32
Other	273	289	201	204	161	167	157	150
Developed Countries								
All causes	1054	1069	1047	1013	997	963	1161	1059
Infections	146	112	109	74	78	59	90	63
Neoplasms	167	163	203	172	182	170	213	188
Circulatory	463	552	473	563	486	536	575	597
Pregnancy	0	2	0	1	0	1	0	1
Perinatal	26	10	15	10	13	9	13	7
Injury	99	51	87	40	77	37	80	39
Other	153	180	161	154	160	152	191	163
Developing Countries								
All causes	1383	1373	1070	1001	830	759	823	714
Infections	564	595	382	368	200	211	150	148
Neoplasms	68	68	78	70	90	79	111	98
Circulatory	234	225	198	192	244	216	291	252
Pregnancy	0	18	0	12	0	11	0	9
Perinatal	109	96	98	75	56	43	42	31
Injury	91	35	100	62	78	29	79	30
Other	318	336	213	221	162	171	150	147
Industrial Market								
All causes	1036	1021	986	950	1007	943	1173	1045
Infections	106	85	82	66	64	47	68	38
Neoplasms	186	169	240	192	196	171	236	200
Circulatory	500	567	461	518	513	551	615	639
Pregnancy	0	0	0	0	0	0	0	0
Perinatal	21	7	8	5	10	6	10	5
Injury	98	58	74	40	70	36	74	40
Other	125	135	120	128	154	131	171	123
Nonmarket								
All causes	1089	1155	1162	1126	980	1000	1139	1082
Infections	224	159	158	88	103	79	128	106
Neoplasms	129	152	136	135	158	169	173	168

TABLE 2 *Continued*

	1970		1985		2000		2015	
Region and Cause	Male	Female	Male	Female	Male	Female	Male	Female
Nonmarket—*cont'd*								
Circulatory	392	524	495	644	437	509	505	526
Pregnancy	0	4	0	3	0	2	0	2
Perinatal	37	15	28	17	20	13	19	11
Injury	100	40	109	39	90	38	90	37
Other	209	260	237	200	172	189	225	231
Latin America and Caribbean								
All causes	1097	903	883	706	677	557	722	594
Infections	366	301	211	177	100	86	67	55
Neoplasms	79	76	76	70	94	86	122	109
Circulatory	238	214	228	196	242	215	306	275
Pregnancy	0	12	0	6	0	4	0	3
Perinatal	61	42	65	44	40	28	30	20
Injury	98	31	90	29	76	28	78	29
Other	255	227	213	184	124	111	119	102
Sub-Saharan Africa								
All causes	2163	1882	1727	1448	1196	1024	947	785
Infections	1070	937	817	683	498	430	346	286
Neoplasms	52	57	52	55	54	55	60	60
Circulatory	243	226	209	191	182	169	180	162
Pregnancy	0	27	0	21	0	17	0	14
Perinatal	200	157	167	129	119	90	82	61
Injury	108	39	96	34	86	30	82	28
Other	491	438	386	334	258	233	196	174
Middle East and North Africa								
All causes	1563	1520	1184	1121	775	733	691	624
Infections	624	653	459	473	209	237	142	164
Neoplasms	60	56	65	60	69	62	81	70
Circulatory	250	224	200	183	191	171	209	176
Pregnancy	0	21	0	13	0	12	0	10
Perinatal	140	126	120	97	73	57	52	39
Injury	90	37	80	32	75	28	76	28
Other	400	404	260	263	157	166	131	137
Asia								
All causes	1280	1342	963	946	784	736	833	734
Infections	506	577	319	323	149	176	110	119
Neoplasms	70	70	85	74	101	87	130	113
Circulatory	230	227	191	194	268	235	338	292
Pregnancy	0	17	0	11	0	10	0	8
Perinatal	98	91	88	67	42	32	30	22
Injury	87	34	105	78	77	29	79	31

TABLE 3 Deaths by Major and Specific Cause (in thousands), by Region, 1985

Cause	World	Developed	Developing	Industrial	Nonmarket	LAC	SSA	MENA	Asia
All causes	49899	12047	37852	7313	4735	3183	7203	4314	23151
Infectious, parasitic	14764	1061	13704	558	503	778	3403	1743	7780
Diarrhea	2997	20	2977	5	15	201	1158	507	1111
Tuberculosis	844	39	805	13	25	48	119	76	562
Acute respiratory	5549	422	5127	271	151	286	1407	741	2693
Measles	421	1	420	0	1	16	196	87	121
COPD	1943	334	1608	248	87	113	226	160	1110
Polio	25	1	25	0	0	2	3	2	18
Yellow fever	8	0	8	0	0	0	2	1	5
Malaria	146	0	146	0	0	6	20	16	105
Schistosomiasis	12	0	12	0	0	0	0	1	10
Intestinal parasites	133	3	130	0	2	7	41	18	65
Other infectious	2686	240	2446	20	221	99	230	135	1981
Neoplasms	4903	2190	2714	1629	560	294	242	235	1943
Circulatory	13208	6075	7133	3704	2371	848	909	715	4661
Ischemic heart	3948	2426	1522	1407	1019	213	216	190	904
Cerebrovascular	3813	1547	2266	873	674	176	193	158	1738
Other cardiovascular	3705	1603	2103	1075	527	302	347	254	1199
Diabetes	507	159	348	129	30	62	55	42	189
Certain degenerative	1235	340	895	220	120	96	97	70	631
Pregnancy	225	8	218	0	7	12	48	23	134
Perinatal	3321	143	3178	51	92	218	672	408	1880
Injury, poisoning	3694	729	2965	429	299	239	294	212	2220
Other	9784	1842	7941	941	902	795	1635	978	4534
Mental disorders	95	46	50	36	10	5	4	3	38
Oral health diseases	3	1	2	0	0	1	0	0	1
Micronutrient	252	42	210	20	23	23	45	27	115
Malnutrition	372	26	346	6	20	24	67	37	218
Unspecified	9061	1728	7333	879	849	742	1519	911	4162

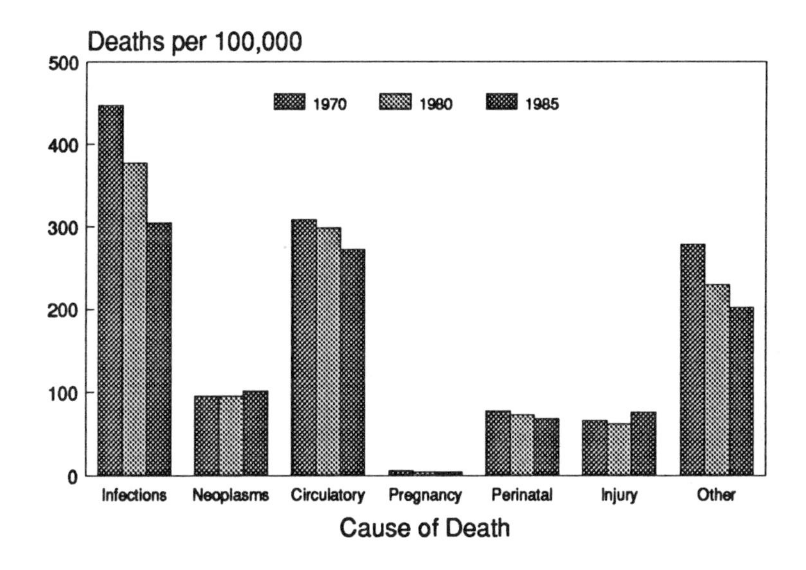

FIGURE 1 Mortality by cause, world, 1970-1985.

assumed slightly higher overall mortality levels than those used here, but their distribution of deaths across causes is still similar.

The estimates suggest that substantial change can take place in a short period. For developing countries, the mortality rate for infectious and parasitic diseases is estimated to have declined 17 percent from 1970 to 1980 and an exceptional 22 percent in the next five years, from 1980 to 1985.

Breakdowns for 1985 of the three largest categories of major causes are summarized in Table 3, which gives numbers of deaths for both major and specific causes. Table 4 provides mortality rates standardized by using the 1985 world age structure.

Among infectious and parasitic diseases, four specific causes are the most important, accounting for at least nine out of ten deaths in each region: acute respiratory infections (pneumonia, influenza, acute bronchitis, whooping cough, and diphtheria, but not measles, which has been separated); diarrhea; other infectious and parasitic diseases; and chronic obstructive pulmonary disease. (The last, as noted earlier, is not infectious but is included here for convenience.) Tuberculosis and measles account for a few percent more, and the remaining categories are relatively rare.

Among the four dominant causes, the distribution varies considerably across regions. A major contrast is the greater relative importance of chronic obstructive pulmonary disease in developed (industrial and nonmarket) regions and the greater relative importance of diarrhea in developing regions. Acute respiratory infections, being important in both developed and developing regions, are responsible for a larger share of deaths than either of these two other causes. The predominance of these four specific causes in the estimates accurately reflects the data reported to WHO. For instance, among reporting Latin American countries, acute respiratory infections account for one-quarter to one-half of all deaths due to infectious diseases in each age-sex group, and acute respiratory infections and diarrhea combined account for three-fourths of deaths under 5 years of age.

Among circulatory system diseases, ischemic heart disease, cerebrovascular disease, and other cardiovascular diseases are nearly equal in importance for the world as a whole. Regionally, ischemic heart disease is responsible for the largest share of circulatory system disease deaths in developed regions; cerebrovascular disease has the largest share in Asia; and other cardiovascular diseases have the largest share in the remaining developing regions. All of these categories are important everywhere, and each always accounts for one-fifth or more of the deaths under the major category. Diabetes is of lesser importance in these estimates, with less than 5 percent of deaths under the major category, and nephritis, cirrhosis of the liver, and ulcers of the stomach and duodenum account for roughly twice this proportion.

For the category of other causes, an attempt was made to distinguish mental disorders, oral health diseases, micronutrient deficiencies, and malnutrition. Combined, these accounted for less than 10 percent of other causes, however, leaving a large remainder unspecified.

The estimates from the regressions were compared with estimates compiled by Walsh (1988) and experts working on the World Bank health sector priorities review. In all major categories except one, the Walsh estimates were higher than the regression and experts' estimates. The comparisons illustrate the difficulty in determining the correct mortality structure of developing countries with limited data. In principle, the expert estimates could be attained if substantial numbers of deaths classified as due to ill-defined causes were in fact caused by these specific diseases.

Trends in Major Causes of Death

Given uncertainties in figures for specific causes, only the major causes are projected into the future. Figures 2 and 3 show how the actual numbers of deaths are expected to change for developed and developing countries, and Figure 4 shows the proportional mortality trends. The two most important major causes show opposite trends, infectious diseases declining from causing 35 percent of deaths in 1970 to 16 percent of deaths in 2015, whereas diseases of the circulatory system rise, from causing 24 percent of

Cause	World	Developed	Developing	Industrial	Nonmarket	LAC	SSA	MENA	Asia
All causes	1046	692	1147	578	894	901	1621	1243	1077
Infectious, parasitic	308	77	386	43	126	199	658	422	350
Diarrhea	62	2	78	1	5	48	221	114	47
Tuberculosis	18	3	25	1	5	14	33	24	25
Acute respiratory	116	29	141	20	40	72	258	173	120
Measles	9	0	10	0	0	4	31	17	5
COPD	41	18	54	18	16	33	54	49	56
Polio	1	0	1	0	0	0	0	0	1
Yellow fever	0	0	0	0	0	0	0	0	0
Malaria	3	0	4	0	0	1	3	4	5
Schistosomiasis	0	0	0	0	0	0	0	0	0
Intestinal parasites	3	0	3	0	1	2	7	4	3
Other infectious	56	24	69	3	59	26	50	35	88
Neoplasms	103	117	92	125	97	91	86	92	93
Circulatory	280	298	255	260	381	272	328	297	237
Ischemic heart	84	119	55	99	164	69	85	82	46
Cerebrovascular	81	74	84	59	106	57	74	68	91
Other cardiovascular	78	78	73	75	86	97	119	103	59
Diabetes	11	8	12	9	5	20	20	18	10
Certain degenerative	26	19	30	17	21	29	30	26	30
Pregnancy	5	1	6	0	2	3	11	7	5
Perinatal	69	20	77	12	32	48	89	76	79
Injury, poisoning	77	56	83	51	67	64	71	61	94
Other	205	123	248	87	189	223	377	288	219
Mental disorders	2	2	2	2	2	2	2	1	2
Oral health diseases	0	0	0	0	0	0	0	0	0
Micronutrient	5	3	6	2	4	7	12	9	5
Malnutrition	8	3	9	0	6	6	11	8	9
Unspecified	190	115	231	83	177	209	352	269	202

NOTE: Rates are standardized by using the 1985 world age structure; COPD, chronic obstructive pulmonary disease; LAC, Latin America and the Caribbean; SSA, Sub-Saharan Africa; MENA, Middle East and North Africa.

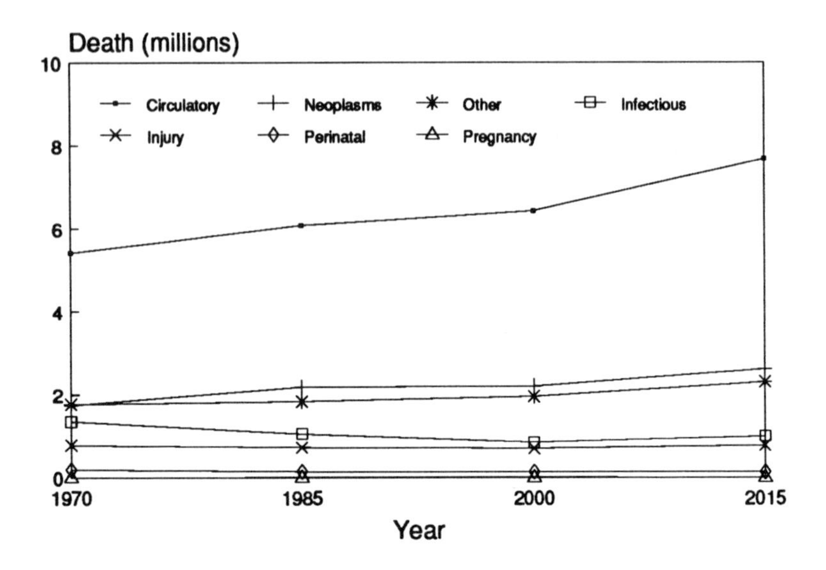

FIGURE 2 Annual deaths by cause, more developed countries, 1970-2015.

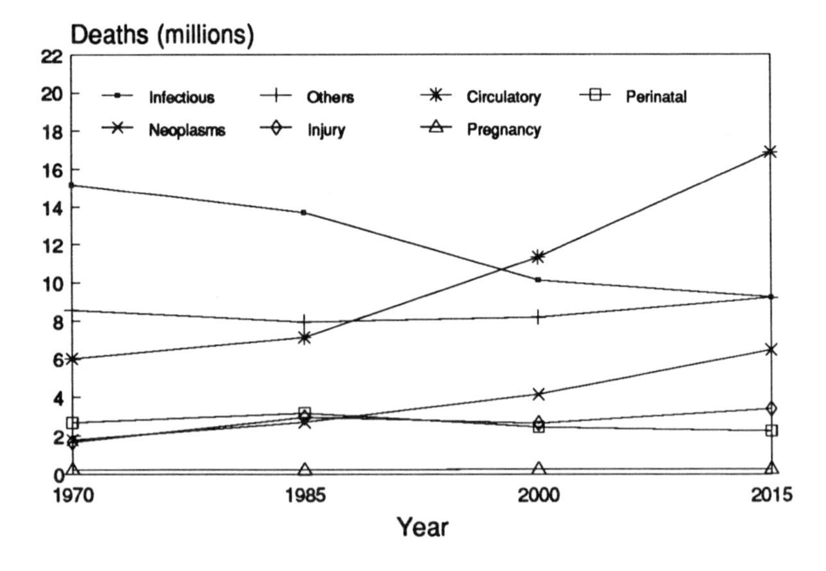

FIGURE 3 Annual deaths by cause, less developed countries, 1970-2015.

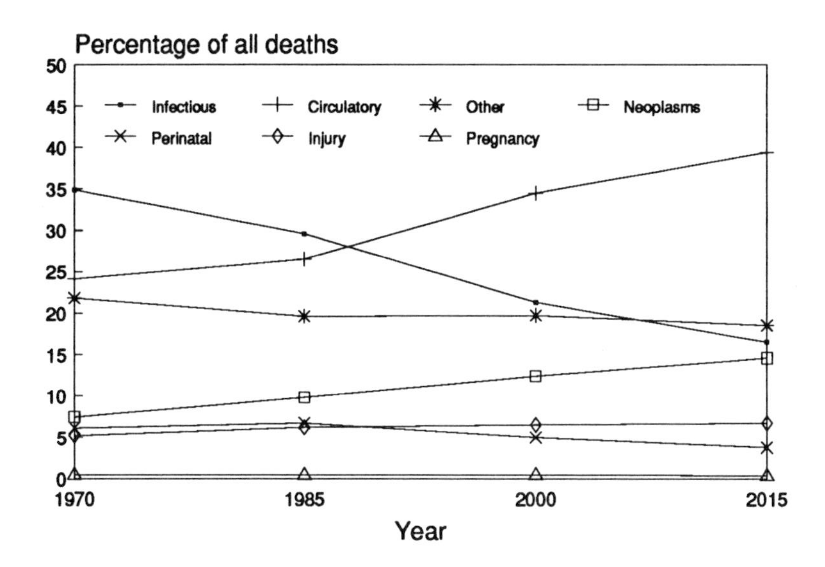

FIGURE 4 Percentage of deaths due to each major cause, world, 1970-2015.

deaths in 1970 to 39 percent in 2015. The infectious disease trend is due mainly to lower mortality from this cause in developing countries, whereas the circulatory disease trend is due to higher mortality from this cause in both developed and developing countries.

Deaths from certain perinatal conditions show a decline parallel to that for infectious and parasitic diseases. Neoplasms show an increase parallel to that for circulatory system diseases. The category of other causes is responsible for more deaths than either of these causes and is expected to decline, but somewhat gradually, and possibly because of better reporting rather than actual change. Injury and poisoning, accounting for 5 to 10 percent of deaths, and complications of pregnancy, accounting for less than 1 percent of deaths, show no clear trend.

All regions exhibit the same basic trends, the differences among them having to do mainly with being more or less advanced in the process of epidemiological transition. Mortality patterns and trends for Asia, the region with the largest population, are closest to those for the world as a whole, as shown in Table 4, with Latin America and the Caribbean, industrial nonmarket economies, and industrial market economies successively more advanced, on the one hand, and the Middle East and North Africa, and sub-Saharan Africa, successively less advanced, on the other. A convenient index for summarizing these regional contrasts, as well as the manner in which they change over time, is the ratio of deaths from circulatory system

TABLE 5 Ratio of Deaths from Circulatory System Diseases to Deaths from Infectious and Parasitic Diseases, by Region, 1970–2015

Region	1970	1985	2000	2015
World	0.69	0.89	1.62	2.39
Developed countries	3.98	5.73	7.52	7.69
Developing countries	0.40	0.52	1.12	1.82
Industrial market	5.63	6.64	9.61	11.88
Industrial nonmarket	2.44	4.72	5.24	4.41
Latin America and Caribbean	0.68	1.09	2.46	4.74
Sub-Saharan Africa	0.23	0.27	0.38	0.54
Middle East and North Africa	0.37	0.41	0.81	1.26
Asia	0.42	0.60	1.55	2.75
India	0.40	0.29	1.01	1.64
China	0.53	1.19	3.52	8.37
Other Asia	0.32	0.56	1.04	1.69

diseases to deaths from infectious and parasitic diseases, as shown in Table 5. For the world as a whole, this ratio is estimated at 0.7 for 1970, 0.9 for 1985, 1.6 for 2000, and 2.4 for 2015.

The greatest numbers of deaths will continue to be in Asia, where almost half of all deaths in the world take place. This proportion is not projected to change from the pattern shown in Table 3. For all causes combined, in fact, each region will contribute about the same proportion of deaths in 2015 as in 1985. For particular causes, some changes are projected, however, with Asia contributing smaller proportions of deaths from infectious and parasitic diseases and perinatal conditions, and larger proportions of deaths from circulatory system diseases and neoplasms. Sub-Saharan African deaths will increase in proportion for the first two of these causes, and industrial market economy deaths will decrease in proportion for the last two of these causes.

The projections of mortality by cause are not straightforward extrapolations from past experience, but involve a combination of population projections with predictive equations for mortality rates by cause. An alternative, much simpler, procedure would have been to take the change in percentage of deaths due to a given cause from 1970 to 1985 and extrapolate this linearly into the future. This alternative procedure would have given quite different results: for the world as a whole by 2000, a larger share of deaths due to infectious and parasitic diseases (24 instead of 21 percent), a correspondingly smaller share due to circulatory system diseases (29 instead of 35 percent), and smaller variations for other causes. For specific regions, the differences would have been greater: for the Middle East and North Africa by 2015, for instance, a linear extrapolation would give 39 percent of deaths due to infectious and parasitic diseases, whereas the regression-based procedures give only 23 percent.

Some insight into why the calculations come out as they do can be obtained by decomposing future changes in the distribution of deaths. Such changes may be related to changes in the age-sex structure of the population, changes in mortality levels from all causes within age-sex groups, or changes in the distribution of deaths by cause within age-sex groups. Projections with fixed mortality or fixed distributions of deaths by cause can help distinguish these components of change, if one accepts the necessary assumption that age-specific rates and mortality distribution can vary independently of each other. Table 6 shows, first, the percentage of deaths due

TABLE 6 Distribution of Deaths by Major Cause in 1985 and Incremental Changes Expected by 2015 from Three Factors, World and Developed and Developing Countries

Region and Cause	1985 Percentage Distribution	Percentage Point Change by 2015 Due to		
		Age-Sex Structure	Mortality Change	Distribution Change
World				
Infections	29.6	–1.4	–3.3	–8.4
Neoplasms	9.8	1.1	1.1	2.6
Circulatory	26.5	3.3	4.4	5.3
Pregnancy	0.5	0.1	–0.2	0.0
Perinatal	6.7	–1.8	–1.6	0.6
Injury	7.4	–1.1	–0.7	1.1
Other	19.6	–0.1	0.2	–1.2
Developed Countries				
Infections	8.8	–1.1	–0.2	–0.6
Neoplasms	18.2	0.8	–0.2	–0.7
Circulatory	50.4	2.8	1.5	–1.8
Pregnancy	0.1	0.0	0.0	0.0
Perinatal	1.2	–0.4	–0.2	0.3
Injury	6.1	–0.9	–0.8	1.0
Other	15.3	–1.2	–0.1	1.9
Developing Countries				
Infections	36.2	–3.0	–3.0	–10.8
Neoplasms	7.2	1.8	1.0	3.6
Circulatory	18.8	5.2	3.9	7.4
Pregnancy	0.6	0.1	–0.2	0.0
Perinatal	8.4	–2.6	–1.8	0.7
Injury	7.8	–1.2	–0.6	1.1
Other	21.0	–0.2	0.6	–2.1

to each cause in 1985; second, the projected increase or decrease in this percentage by 2015 due to contemplated changes in the age-sex structure, with fixed mortality assumed; third, the further projected increase or decrease in this percentage if mortality is allowed to decline but the distribution of deaths by cause is fixed within age-sex groups; and fourth, the further projected increase or decrease due to changes in the distribution of deaths by cause within age-sex groups. Totaling the components for 2015 for any given cause and adding the 1985 figure give the projected percentage of deaths due to that cause by 2015.

Table 6 indicates that the three components can operate in the same or in opposite directions. For instance, population aging, lower mortality (especially at younger ages), and changes in the distribution of deaths all contribute to the decline in infectious diseases. On the other hand, population aging and lower mortality reduce the importance of injury and poisoning, but distribution change raises their importance in relation to other causes of death.

Which of the three components exerts the greatest effect varies considerably from cause to cause. The largest effect overall is that of distributional change on infectious and parasitic diseases, but in this case the other two components operate mostly in the same direction, namely, to reduce the proportion of deaths from this cause. The three components are also consistent in their effect on raising the importance of circulatory system diseases in developing countries, but in developed countries the components work in opposite directions. Therefore, both demographic and epidemiological change will have roles in modifying mortality by cause in the future.

Age-Sex Specific Patterns

Patterns by age and sex are roughly similar across regions but differ in many details. Between men and women, differences are small, except with regard to complications of pregnancy. Across ages, mortality is lowest at ages 5–14 and ages 15–44; about five times as high at 1–4 and 45–64 years; and about fifty times as high at 0 and 64 years and above. The cause-of-death patterns for each age group are roughly as follows: infectious and parasitic diseases decline in importance with age (though they are more prominent at age 1–4 than at 0, given the predominance of certain perinatal causes among infant deaths); circulatory system diseases and neoplasms increase in importance with age. Injury and poisoning are most prominent at age 15–44, perinatal conditions are of course significant at age 0, and complications of pregnancy are notable at age 15–44. Other causes are essentially stable across age groups.

Over time, cause-specific mortality rate projections show variable changes. For infectious and parasitic diseases and for the category of other causes, reductions are fairly constant across age groups, except for being somewhat smaller at age 65 and above. In contrast, for circulatory system diseases and for injury and poisoning, reductions over time are strongly linked to age, being much greater at younger ages. For neoplasms, increases over time are actually more frequent than reductions and are expected to occur in all regions, but most notably in sub-Saharan Africa.

To obtain the previously reported estimates for all ages, deaths were simply added up across age groups. Should deaths at different ages be given equal weight when using mortality figures in decision making? Several arguments to the contrary are possible. For instance, fewer deaths at the oldest ages are likely to be "premature" than at younger ages, and from the perspective of prevention, deaths at the oldest ages might therefore deserve less attention. Also, deaths at younger rather than older ages might be seen as depriving individuals of a larger number of potential years of life. To illustrate the effects of alternative weightings, Figures 4–6 compare the percentage distribution of deaths by cause with the percentage distribution of deaths under age 65 and with the percentage distribution across causes of death of potential years of life lost. Years lost are calculated under the simplifying assumptions that life expectancy is 75 and that deaths

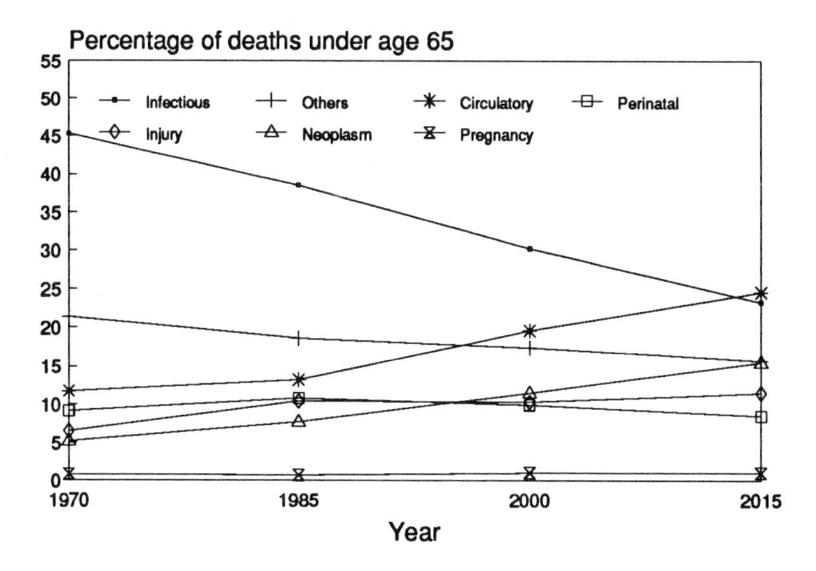

FIGURE 5 Percentage of deaths under 65 due to each major cause, world, 1970-2015.

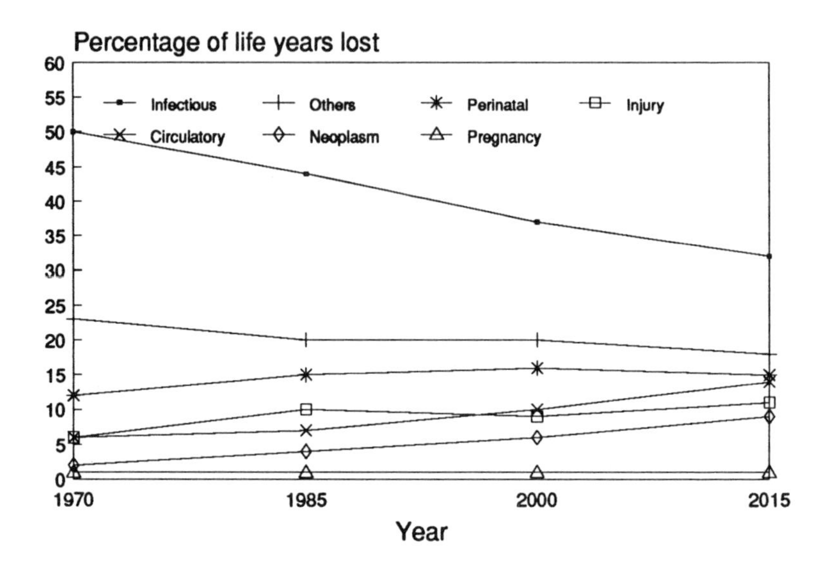

FIGURE 6 Percentage of life years lost due to each major cause, world, 1970-2015.

in each age group from each cause occur at the mean for that age group from all causes in the world as a whole in 1985.

Weighting deaths at younger ages more heavily increases the prominence of infectious and parasitic diseases, perinatal conditions, and injury and poisoning, and reduces the prominence of circulatory system diseases and neoplasms. The effects on the remaining categories are weak or inconsistent. Thus, infectious and parasitic diseases account for a little more than one-third of deaths in developing countries in 1985 but for one-half of all potential years of life lost. In comparison to infectious and parasitic diseases, circulatory system diseases will account for more deaths by 2000, but not for as many deaths under 65 until 2015, and even by 2015 for less than half as many potential years of life lost. Nevertheless, whether weighted or unweighted, the percentages mostly show similar trends over time, especially in decreases for infectious and parasitic diseases and increases for circulatory system diseases.

Reliability of Estimates

Since the expert assessments imply that at least some of the initial estimates are too low, the quality of these estimates and the biases that may

TABLE 7 Regional Population (percent) Covered by Reports to WHO or Sample Surveys, by Year

Region	1970	1985
World	28	59
Developed countries	74	76
Developing countries	10	53
Industrial market economies	98	100
Industrial nonmarket economies	29	32
Latin America and Caribbean	62	53
Sub-Saharan Africa	0	0
Middle East and North Africa	14	2
Asia	2	71

NOTE: For 1985, the former USSR is not counted as covered. China and rural India in 1985 are the only cases covered by sample surveys rather than registration. Urban India is not counted as covered.

exist in them are now considered. The source of particular estimates should be borne in mind. For several regions, the current and past estimates are based substantially on data reported to WHO. Table 7 shows the proportions of regional populations covered by reported data. (The former USSR is not counted as covered, but China and rural India are.) The 1970 and 1985 estimates for industrial market economies are drawn almost entirely from WHO reports, which is true to a lesser extent for the estimates for Latin America and the Caribbean and industrial nonmarket economies. The situation for Asian data is more ambiguous because of reliance on special survey data for China and India. For sub-Saharan Africa and for North Africa and the Middle East, on the other hand, practically all the 1970 and 1985 figures are produced from the regression models.

As noted earlier, estimates based entirely on reports to WHO are not free from potential bias. The general issues of reliability and comparability have already been noted, but in addition, some aspects of the coding appear not to conform with expert expectations. For example, substantial deaths from diarrhea at older ages were judged improbable. Nevertheless, on the average, across reporting countries in 1985, 40 percent of all deaths from this cause occurred at age 65 and older, and the proportion exceeded 80 percent in countries such as Norway and Japan, with presumably reliable reports. Misclassification cannot be excluded as an explanation but cannot be confirmed with available data.

Further potential problems exist with the regression-based estimates, where they are used for 1970 and 1985 for countries with no reported data, as well as for 2000 and 2015 for all countries. Both statistical and substantive criteria could be applied in assessing these results. Statistically, the equations for major causes of death produced patterns for 1970 and 1985 consistent with those produced by Hakulinen et al. (1986a,b) for 1980, using the same equations but different life tables and regional groupings. Hakulinen and colleagues argued that their results had many similarities to previous results by Preston (1976), who estimated equations that were not age specific. They also argued that the procedure was insensitive to choice of life tables, which appears to be borne out by the similarities between their results and these.

To assess the regression procedure, the equations were applied to the reporting countries for 1985 to see whether predictions would match reports. This comparison is permissible because the equations for major causes had been estimated separately (by Hakulinen et al.) with other data; the procedure is less informative regarding the equations for specific causes, which were estimated by using the reported data in the comparison. Table 8 shows, however, that the reported distribution by major causes is more closely approximated by predictions than is the distribution by specific causes. For the major causes, indices of dissimilarity between percentage distributions range from 5 to 13 among the four regions in Table 8. For specific causes under infectious diseases, these indices range from 12 to 34; for specific causes under circulatory system diseases, they range from 8 to 24; and for specific causes among the other causes, they range from 1 to 3. Generally, the distributions for nonmarket economies are more poorly predicted than those for other regions.

For specific causes, predicted percentages are higher than reported percentages in some regions, lower in others. For circulatory system diseases, for instance, predictions are too high in Asia and too low in nonmarket economies. One might draw implications from such comparisons about the possible directions of bias in the estimates for nonreporting countries, but only if one assumes similar mortality patterns in nonreporting as in reporting countries.

For the specific causes, the statistical adequacy of the equations varies by cause, as indicated earlier by using coefficients of determination. Those causes of death that have distinctive patterns in Africa and the Middle East, and possibly in Asia, may be poorly estimated for these regions, but this does not mean that diseases especially prevalent in these regions are underestimated: their prevalence might still be properly represented by extension of patterns across developed and Latin American countries. Rather, it means that causes of death that show important discontinuities between reporting and nonreporting countries may be poorly estimated for the nonreporting countries. Unfortunately, without reports for all regions, one cannot tell definitively which causes of death these are.

Even if the equations were entirely accurate for the present, projecting

TABLE 8 Predicted and Reported Percentage Distributions of Deaths by Cause for Reporting Countries Grouped by Region, 1985

	Industrial (24)[a]		Nonmarket (8)		LAC (26)		Asia (7)	
Cause	Predicted	Reported	Predicted	Reported	Predicted	Reported	Predicted	Reported
Percent of all causes								
Infections	8	8	20	11	23	20	31	32
Neoplasms	17	22	12	12	11	11	9	9
Circulatory	51	51	38	50	31	32	25	20
Pregnancy	0	0	0	0	0	0	1	1
Perinatal	1	1	2	2	7	7	6	8
Injury	6	6	6	6	7	10	6	11
Other	17	13	22	19	21	*b*	22	19
Percent of infections								
Diarrhea	7	1	16	3	22	28	25	9
Tuberculosis	4	2	8	5	6	6	5	8
Acute respiratory	42	49	43	30	41	31	43	33
Measles	1	0	2	0	2	1	3	1
COPD	33	45	19	17	16	*b*	12	16
Polio	0	0	0	0	0	*b*	0	0
Yellow fever	0	0	0	0	0	0	0	0
Malaria	0	0	1	0	1	0	1	2
Schistosomiasis	0	0	0	0	0	0	0	0
Intestinal parasites	0	0	1	0	1	1	1	1
Other infections	12	4	10	44	12	17	9	31

continued

TABLE 8 *Continued*

Cause	Industrial (24)[a]		Nonmarket (8)		LAC (26)		Asia (7)	
	Predicted	Reported	Predicted	Reported	Predicted	Reported	Predicted	Reported
Percent of circulatory								
Ischemic heart	30	38	29	43	29	28	27	17
Cerebrovascular	24	24	24	28	23	19	23	42
Other cardiovascular	34	29	34	22	34	37	34	23
Diabetes	6	3	6	1	6	8	6	3
Certain degenerative	7	6	7	5	9	13	9	15
Percent of other causes								
Mental disorders	2	4	1	1	1	[c]	1	1
Oral health diseases	0	0	0	0	0	[c]	0	0
Micronutrient	3	2	3	3	3	[c]	3	2
Malnutrition	1	1	2	2	2	[c]	3	5
Unspecified	94	93	94	94	94	[c]	93	91

[a]Number of countries included in the comparison.
[b]With no reported data for this category, it was assumed to be equal to the predicted value to permit comparisons for other categories.
[c]No data.

them into the future would still raise several issues. Future estimates also depend on assumptions about age structure, about current vital rates, and about trends in these variables. Furthermore, other unexpected changes could alter the outlook. Estimates for new causes of death cannot be generated by this procedure. For human immunodeficiency virus (HIV) infection, in particular, this limitation may have significance for the broader picture. Besides changes in diseases, changes in medical technology, in lifestyles, in health and safety measures, and in the delivery of health services, as well as in the nature and quality of cause-of-death reports, could change the picture. All that the projections provide is a hypothetical picture based on somewhat contradictory assumptions: that mortality decline will be extended into the future, extending past trends, but that historical patterns associating particular disease categories with particular mortality levels will remain as they are.

DISCUSSION

These projections suggest quite substantial changes in the causes of mortality from 1970 to 1985, and continuing changes for the following 30 years. The contrast between infectious and parasitic diseases, on the one hand, and circulatory system diseases, on the other, is the sharpest: the first group is in decline as a cause of death, whereas the second will increasingly be ascendant. These two major causes were responsible for about equal numbers of deaths in Latin America and the Caribbean by 1985. They caused equal numbers of deaths in Asia around 1990, and will do so in the Middle East and North Africa by around 2005, and in sub-Saharan Africa sometime after 2015. Other causes of death will increase or decrease in importance, depending not only on the technology available for control and cure, but also on demographic factors. For instance, as populations move through the demographic transition, the importance of infant and childhood diseases will decrease and the importance of neoplasms as a cause of death will increase.

Obtained from regression models that predict the distribution of causes of death from the overall mortality level, these estimates and projections have clear limitations. However, despite the caveats noted above, the broad patterns are consistent with actual reports and appear generally plausible.

What they imply for health systems is not immediately obvious. Over the medium term, shifts in services to focus on causes of increasing importance would seem to be appropriate. Yet many other factors besides numbers of deaths need to be taken into account, and new diseases of major significance may also command attention. That the distribution of causes of death is itself subject to interpretation was demonstrated by contrasting alternative percentage distributions of deaths, deaths under 65, and life years lost: from different perspectives, priorities can look somewhat different. Careful policy analysis is needed before practical implications can be drawn. One additional implication from any perspective is that better data on cause of death are essential.

REFERENCES

Bulatao, R.A., and E. Bos

1989 Projecting mortality for all countries. *Policy, Planning, and Research Working Papers.* No. 337. Washington, D.C.: World Bank.

Bulatao, R.A., and P.W. Stephens

1992 Estimates and projections of mortality by cause: A global overview, 1970–2015. *Policy Research Working Papers.* Washington, D.C.: World Bank.

Bulatao, R.A., E. Bos, P.W. Stephens, and M.T. Vu

1990 *World Population Projections, 1989–90 Edition: Short- and Long-Term Estimates.* Baltimore, Md.: Johns Hopkins University Press.

Coale, A.J., and P. Demeny, with B. Vaughn

1983 *Regional Model Life Tables and Stable Populations*, 2nd ed. New York: Academic Press.

Frenk, J., J.L. Bobadilla, J. Sepúlveda, and M. López Cervantes

1989 Health transition in middle-income countries: New challenges for health care. *Health Policy and Planning* 4(1):29–39.

Hakulinen, T., H. Hansluwka, A.D. Lopez, and T. Nakada

1986a Global and regional mortality patterns by cause of death in 1980. *International Journal of Epidemiology* 15(2):226–233.

1986b Estimation of global mortality patterns by cause of death. Pp. 179–205 in H. Hansluwka, A.D. Lopez, Y. Porapakham, and P. Prasartkul, eds., *New Developments in the Analysis of Mortality and Causes of Death.* Bangkok: World Health Organization and Mahidol University.

Omran, A.R.

1971 The epidemiological transition: A theory of the epidemiology of population change. *Milbank Memorial Fund Quarterly* 49:509–538.

Parkin, D.M., E. Laara, and C. S. Muir.

1988 Estimates of the worldwide frequency of sixteen major cancers in 1980. *International Journal of Cancer* 41:184–197.

Preston, S.H.

1976 *Mortality Patterns in National Populations, with Special Reference to Recorded Causes of Death.* New York: Academic Press.

Walsh, J.A.

1988 *Establishing Health Priorities in the Developing World.* Boston: Adams Publishing Group.

World Health Organization

1977 *Manual of the International Statistical Classification of Diseases, Injuries, and Causes of Death*, Vols. 1 and 2. Geneva: World Health Organization.

Childhood Precursors of Adult Morbidity and Mortality in Developing Countries: Implications for Health Programs

W. Henry Mosley and Ronald Gray

INTRODUCTION

The developing countries of the world are in the midst of a demographic and epidemiologic transition that is profoundly transforming their health profile (Mosley and Cowley, 1991). Prior to World War II, most developing countries experienced high rates of mortality, with infectious diseases of childhood dominating the epidemiologic picture. In the postwar period, largely as a result of advancements in medical technology directed against infectious and parasitic diseases, there have been rapid declines in infant and child mortality that, coupled with the high levels of fertility, have produced rapidly growing populations with a very young age structure. Beginning in the 1960s and accelerating through the 1970s and 1980s, birth rates declined in much of the developing world, initiating a process of slower population growth. This reduction in the growth rates, however, initially occurs among infants and children; the population of adults will continue to grow for decades into the future because of the large numbers of children already born who will survive to reach the older age groups (Chenais, 1990).

There were dramatic changes in the age structure of the world's population between 1960 and 1990 that will continue into the first quarter of the next century, according to estimates and projections by the United Nations

---

W. Henry Mosley and Ronald Gray are at the Department of Population Dynamics, the Johns Hopkins University, School of Hygiene and Public Health, Baltimore, Maryland. The authors acknowledge the assistance of Dr. Aida Abashawl and Dr. Laura F. Robin in the preparation of this paper. Partial support for the work was provided by the U.S. Agency for International Development under Child Survival Cooperative Agreement DPE-5951-A-00-5051.

(1991). For example, in developing countries in particular, the population under age 15 will have only slightly more than doubled over this 60-year time span, but the population age 15 to 64 will have increased by almost four times to 4,441 million in 2020, and the population over age 65 will have increased almost six times to 472 million in 2020. This rapid aging of the population will have a profound effect on the health system, which will have to shift its priorities toward the prevention and management of chronic diseases among adults (Mosley et al., 1993).

This paper examines only one aspect of the health transition in developing countries. It looks at the emerging health problems among the adults and the aged, and assesses to what degree these chronic diseases and disabilities might be a consequence of infectious diseases and other adverse conditions that were experienced decades earlier in infancy and childhood. A recognition of these relationships can enhance our understanding of the cost-effectiveness and cost-benefits of programs to promote child health. Child health interventions are not only cost-effective in saving lives and preventing disabilities in the short run but, more importantly, in the long run can result in major cost savings to health systems and can accelerate national development by improving the health and productivity of these children when they become adults.

BACKGROUND

Recently, Elo and Preston (1992) completed a review of the literature examining the effects of early life conditions on adult mortality. Their review begins with a discussion of the epidemiologic evidence for some of the major mechanisms whereby exposures and morbidity in childhood may have health consequences for adults. Initially, they examine a number of specific infectious diseases of childhood with well-documented, long-term health effects among adults (tuberculosis, hepatitis B, rheumatic heart disease) and then look at the growing literature suggesting that a number of chronic cardiovascular and pulmonary diseases may be related to a range of risk factors beginning in the intrauterine environment (e.g., intrauterine growth retardation) and extending through disease exposures and behavior patterns acquired in childhood (e.g., acute respiratory infections, dietary consumption of fat and salt). They examine other associations including a number of studies postulating that viral infections acquired in childhood may be linked to a wide variety of chronic diseases ranging from cancer to multiple sclerosis, juvenile diabetes, rheumatoid arthritis, and presenile dementia, as well as the extensive literature linking short stature and adult mortality. Elo and Preston's review then turns to population-based studies among cohorts of adults that seek to link conditions around birth and early childhood to differentials and subsequent mortality. They find that a wide variety of studies based on data from nineteenth and twentieth century Europe with findings that are generally consistent with the hypothesis that the childhood environment plays a substantial role in adult mortality.

The analysis in this paper extends the work of Elo and Preston (1992) in several ways. First, it takes a more epidemiological approach, looking at a broader range of disease conditions in infancy and childhood where the evidence supports a direct relationship to adult morbidity and mortality. Second, our analysis is oriented to the current situation in developing countries with the objective of trying to assess the probable magnitude of the health effects of selected childhood diseases on adult morbidity and mortality. Our assessment admittedly is more speculative, given the data limitations in most developing countries. Our purpose will be achieved, however, if this analysis highlights the need for more research on these issues as well as the importance of maintaining and expanding programs to promote child health in the developing world.

CLASSIFICATION OF DISEASES OR CONDITIONS OF INFANCY AND CHILDHOOD WITH CONSEQUENCES FOR ADULTS

There are a wide range of health conditions affecting infants and children in developing countries that have long-term consequences for adult health. Table 1 classifies these conditions into four groups: (1) conditions acquired in the perinatal period; (2) infectious diseases of childhood; (3) nutritional deficiencies of infancy and childhood; and (4) environmental hazards. This classification system is by no means comprehensive, but it does include many of the major diseases and conditions that have substantial effects on adult health and survival.

The first part of this paper briefly discusses each of these conditions, focusing particularly on the available information relating childhood diseases to adult health consequences. Where data are available, the magnitude of the problem in terms of effect on adult health is provided. In the concluding section of this paper we take a more integrated approach by examining some of the interactions among childhood risk factors in producing adult diseases. Also, recent trends in adult cause-of-death data from selected developing countries are examined to assess how mortality profiles may be related to conditions acquired in childhood several decades earlier.

Perinatal Conditions

Low Birthweight

Twenty million newborns per year, or 16 percent of all children born worldwide, are considered to be low birthweight as defined by a weight of

TABLE 1 Consequences of Selected Infant and Childhood Health Problems for Morbidity and Mortality in Adults

Conditions in Children	Consequences in Adults
Perinatal conditions	
Low birthweight	Growth stunting, chronic obstructive pulmonary disease
Birth trauma, asphyxia, metabolic disorders	Brain damage, cerebral palsy, mental retardation
Congenital and perinatal infections	
Hepatitis B	Liver cancer, chronic liver diseases
Syphilis	Blindness, deafness, paralysis, bone disease
Gonorrhea	Blindness
Infectious diseases of childhood	
Tuberculosis	Tuberculosis
Rheumatic fever	Chronic rheumatic heart disease
Poliomyelitis	Residual paralysis
Trachoma	Blindness
Chagas' disease	Heart failure
Schistosomiasis	Liver cirrhosis, general debility
Helicobacter pylori	Stomach cancer
Epstein-Barr virus	Nasopharyngeal cancer, Burkitt's lymphoma
Nutritional deficiencies in infancy and childhood	
Protein-energy malnutrition	Growth stunting, obstetrical complications, cardiovascular disease, chronic pulmonary diseases, intellectual impairment
Micronutrient deficiency	
Iodine	Cretinism, intellectual impairment
Iron	Learning disabilities, intellectual impairment
Vitamin A	Blindness
Environmental hazards	
Indoor air pollution	Chronic obstructive pulmonary disease, lung cancer
Lead exposure	Intellectual impairment

less than 2,500 grams (World Health Organization, 1990). Ninety percent of low-birthweight infants are born to mothers in developing countries. More than two-thirds of these occur in the countries of South Asia where approximately one birth in four is low birthweight. The overall risk of delivering a low-birthweight infant in a developing country is three times that in an industrialized country. In South Asia the risk is four times greater.

In developing countries, approximately 80 percent of low-birthweight infants are a result of intrauterine growth retardation (IUGR) rather than prematurity (Villar and Belizan, 1982). IUGR is primarily a consequence of inadequate energy and protein intake during pregnancy, often coupled with excessive energy expenditure during the later stages of pregnancy because of the heavy work load of most poor women in the developing world (Kramer, 1987). Adolescent pregnancy and maternal stunting are associated with low birthweight (Herrera, 1985). Additional factors are traditional practices of dietary restrictions during pregnancy, maternal infections such as malaria, and possibly close spacing of births (Kramer, 1987). Cigarette smoking and smoke from biomass cooking fuels may also be implicated (Ferraz et al., 1990; Mavalankar et al., 1993).

Studies in Guatemala, Colombia, India, Mexico, the United States, and Canada have confirmed that supplemental nutrition can increase birthweight (Pinstrup-Anderson et al., 1993). Improvement in birthweight appears to be greatest if supplementation is provided in the third trimester of pregnancy. It is noteworthy that most low-birthweight newborns in societies experiencing high levels of chronic malnutrition are found to remain stunted at below the tenth percentile for height and weight at 3 years of age (Mata, 1978).

Elo and Preston (1992) review the evidence indicating that stunted growth is associated with higher risks of mortality among adults, particularly from cardiovascular disease and chronic obstructive pulmonary disease (COPD). The former relationship is examined below in the discussion of protein energy malnutrition. Here we look at the evidence specifically relating low birthweight to respiratory infection in childhood and COPD in adults.

Low-birthweight infants have a higher incidence of lower respiratory tract infections than infants with normal birthweight (McCall and Acheson, 1968). As a consequence, low birthweight has been shown to be associated with a higher prevalence of cough and poor lung function in later childhood (Chan et al., 1989). Recently, Barker and colleagues (1991) completed a study relating birthweight and childhood respiratory infections to risk of death from chronic obstructive pulmonary disease and to pulmonary function among men ages 59-67 years in England. They confirmed that low birthweight and severe respiratory infections in infancy were associated with higher risks of death from COPD as well as with compromised lung function among the survivors. They note that an association between low birthweight and obstructive lung disease is biologically plausible, because fetal lung growth, particularly growth of the airways, is largely completed in utero (Bucher and Reid, 1961). Barker et al. (1991:674) conclude from their study that "prevention of chronic obstructive airway disease may partly depend on promotion of fetal and infant lung growth and reduction in the incidence of lower respiratory tract infection in infancy."

COPD is a leading cause of death among adults in developing countries, and the high incidence of low birthweight in these settings is undoubtedly a contributing factor. Because there are other important contributing factors in developing countries (see below), COPD is discussed in more detail in the second section of this paper.

Birth Trauma, Asphyxia, Metabolic Disorders

In developing countries only about 50 percent of the births are attended by trained personnel (World Health Organization, 1990). One consequence is a perinatal mortality rate four to six times higher than that seen in developed countries, where more than 99 percent of births take place in the presence of a trained attendant, and typically in a hospital setting. Unfortunately, data are lacking on the incidence of birth injury, asphyxia, and preventable metabolic disorders (such as hyperbilirubinemia secondary to physiologic jaundice) that can produce permanent disabilities among surviving infants in developing country settings. Brain damage leading to mental retardation, cerebral palsy, and other neurological disabilities would be among the most serious consequences with a lifelong influence on health status.

Although incidence data are not available, there are some clinical studies suggesting that birth injury is a significant contributor to chronic neurological disease. Nottidge and Okogbo (1991) found that among 413 children presenting with cerebral palsy in Ibadan, Nigeria, 41 percent appeared to be related to bilirubin encephalopathy and 20 percent to birth asphyxia. The patients seen in this urban referral center are by no means representative of the population; however, the data do suggest that a high proportion of brain damage seen in infants may be attributable to conditions preventable in the perinatal period. It is not clear how these observations may relate to neurological disability seen among adults, but the data are at least consistent with the thesis that inadequate antenatal and childbirth care can contribute significantly to the level of chronic disability in a population. This thesis requires far more research.

Congenital and Perinatal Infections

There are a number of maternal infections that may be transmitted to the fetus in utero or to the newborn around the time of childbirth that have significant consequences for adult health.

Hepatitis B By far the most prevalent and serious disease in this category is related to the maternal-infant transmission of hepatitis B virus (HBV) (Francis, 1986; Kane et al., 1993). The World Health Organization (1990) estimates that more than two billion individuals have been infected with HBV, of whom 280 million are chronically infected carriers of the virus. Prospective population-based studies indicate that ultimately, approximately one-quarter of these chronically infected individuals will die from chronic active hepatitis, cirrhosis, or primary liver cancer. HBV infection is directly related to one to two million deaths per year (World Health Organization, 1990). The prevalence of chronic HBV infection ranges from 6 to 10 percent throughout much of East and Southeast Asia and sub-Saharan Africa. For the rest of Asia, HBV prevalence is 3 to 5 percent, and it is 1 to 2 percent in Latin America (Francis, 1986).

Mother-infant transmission in the perinatal period is the primary reason for the high carrier rates in areas where hepatitis B is prevalent. Figure 1 from Beasley (1982) provides a schematic representation of the cycle of HBV infections and liver cancer from generation to generation. If the mother is an HBV carrier, approximately 50 percent of newborns will be infected, 95 percent of whom will become carriers. The daughters will grow up to transmit the virus to the next generation. Ultimately, about half the sons and 14 percent of the daughters will die of chronic liver disease and liver cancer later in life.

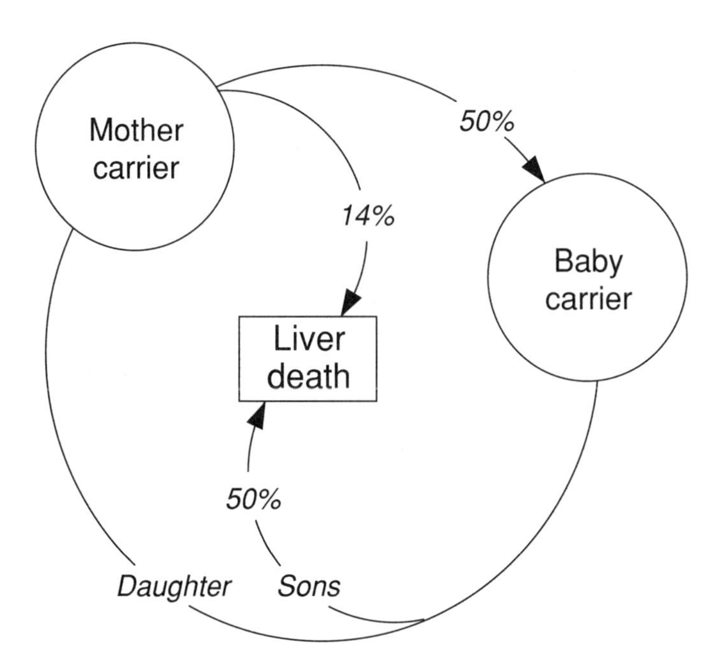

FIGURE 1 Schematic representation of the intergenerational cycle of hepatitis B infection, chronic liver disease, and liver cancer. SOURCE: Beasley (1982:22S). Permission to reprint granted. From "Hepatitis B virus as the etiologic agent in hepatocellular carcinoma: epidemiologic considerations". *Hepatology* 2(2):21S-26S.

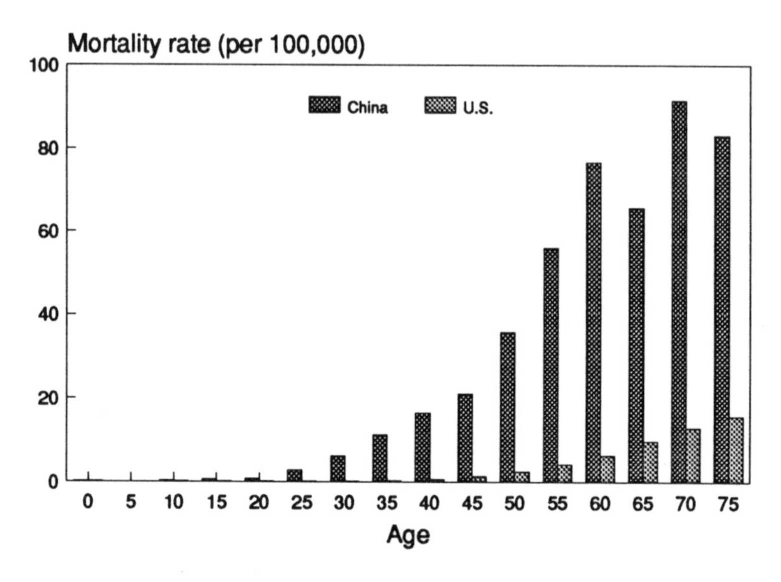

FIGURE 2 Liver cancer: Age-specific mortality rates per 100,000 population. SOURCE: Barnum and Greenberg (1993).

Demographically, HBV is an important cause of mortality among adults in developing countries. Primary liver cancer is a leading cause of cancer death in males in most of sub-Saharan Africa and much of East and Southeast Asia and the Pacific Basin. Figure 2 (from Barnum and Greenberg, 1993) compares the age-specific liver cancer mortality rates from China, where HBV is prevalent, to those from the United States, where maternal-infant HBV transmission is rare, to illustrate the relative importance of this condition in developing country settings. A two-year prospective study of 22,707 Chinese men in Taiwan documented that primary hepatocellular carcinoma and liver cirrhosis associated with HBV accounted for approximately 20 percent of all deaths (Beasley et al., 1981). Consistent with this, Elo and Preston (1992) review a number of demographic studies in East Asia and suggest that the Far Eastern pattern of mortality, characterized by very high death rates at older ages (30+) relative to younger ages, and present primarily among males, may relate to excess mortality as a consequence of a high prevalence of chronic carriers of HBV.

Hepatitis B vaccine is now available, and studies have documented that it is highly effective in preventing maternal-newborn transmission of HBV when administered to newborns (Francis, 1986). With recombinant genetic techniques, the cost of production of this vaccine has dropped to approximately $1 per dose, making this a highly cost-effective health intervention in most developing country settings.

Syphilis Syphilis and gonorrhea are two other infections transmitted from mothers to infants that can have consequences for adult health. Both of these problems are most serious in sub-Saharan Africa (Over and Piot, 1993). The prevalence of syphilis seroreactivity among pregnant women attending antenatal clinics has been found to range from 4 to 15 percent in a number of regions in eastern and central Africa (Schulz et al., 1987). Based on prospective studies in a variety of settings, from 50 to 80 percent of the pregnancies in these infected women will have an adverse outcome caused by syphilis. In the large majority of cases, congenital syphilis will result in spontaneous abortion or perinatal deaths; however, in 10 to 20 percent of cases, there will be a surviving infant with latent congenital syphilis who may develop active manifestations later in life (Hira et al., 1990). These may include blindness, deafness, paralysis, and a variety of bone lesions. Therefore, in some African populations where about 10 percent of childbearing women are infected, approximately 1 percent of newborns may have congenital syphilis that, if untreated, will result in disabling disease and premature death in adulthood (Schulz et al., 1987).

Gonorrhea Maternal newborn transmission of gonorrhea can lead to gonococcal ophthalmia neonatorum (GON) which, if untreated, often leads to blindness. Although prophylaxis or treatment of the eyes with antibiotics is simple and highly effective, it is not available in most poor areas of the world where the vast majority of births occur at home.

The World Health Organization (1990) gives a minimal estimate of the annual incidence of gonorrhea at 25 million cases. Again, as with syphilis, a high proportion of these will be in sub-Saharan Africa where diagnosis and treatment are not generally available. The prevalence of *Neisseria gonorrhoeae* in pregnant women has been reported as ranging between 3 and 22 percent in a dozen countries in sub-Saharan Africa (Schulz et al., 1987). These reported studies were undertaken in urban settings, and some researchers believe that gonorrhea is more prevalent in towns than in rural settings. Because about one-third of the infants exposed to *N. gonorrhoeae* during birth will develop GON if prophylaxis is not given, one can estimate that the incidence of GON in neonates in Africa may range from 0.5 percent to 6 percent (Schulz et al., 1987). Given that sub-Saharan Africa has more than 20 million births annually, this percentage represents a very large number of children who are exposed to the risk of blindness. Unfortunately, there are no data on the incidence of blindness related to GON in developing countries.

Infectious Diseases of Childhood

Tuberculosis

Tuberculosis represents the classical example of an infection acquired in childhood that manifests itself predominantly with disease among adults. The epidemiological features of tuberculosis were elucidated by Frost in the 1930s (Frost, 1939). Tuberculin skin test surveys in developing countries generally reveal a rather consistent increase in the proportion testing positive for infection with each year of age up to about age 20. The general picture, as represented by a cohort studied in the Netherlands, is that in populations where tuberculosis is endemic, approximately 40 percent of the infections will occur before the age of 5, 67 percent before age 10, and 90 percent by age 19 (Sutherland, 1976). The clinical symptoms of tuberculosis however, are not common with the onset of the infection; rather, after a latent period of some years, approximately 6 to 10 percent of infected individuals will go on to develop active tuberculosis. Eighty-five percent of these cases will be among adults in the most productive age group 15-59 years, as is shown in Figure 3 for several African populations. About 45 percent of the cases will be sputum positive, continuing the cycle of disease transmission to the next generation of children. The economic consequences

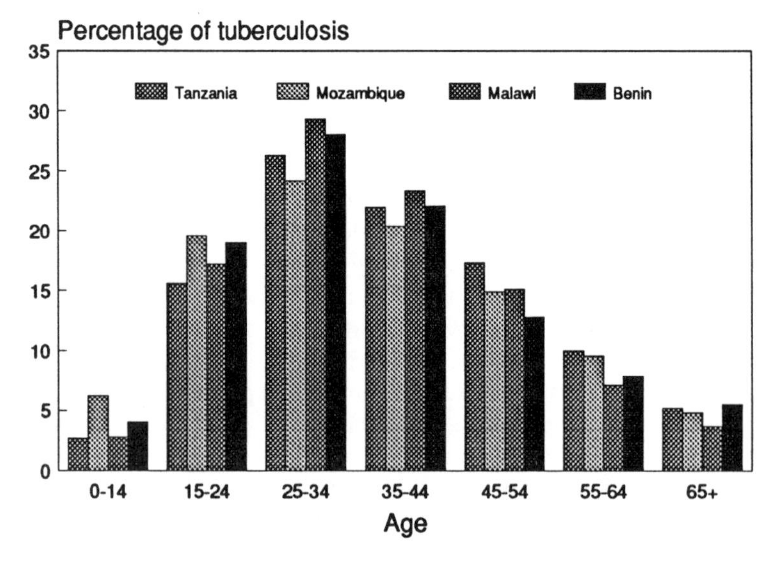

FIGURE 3 Age distribution of smear-positive tuberculosis in four sub-Saharan tuberculosis programs. SOURCE: Murray et al. (1993:Fig.2).

of this disease are enormous when one considers the estimates that tuberculosis accounts for 18.5 percent of all deaths in the 15-59 age group or 26 percent of all avoidable adult deaths (Murray and Feachem, 1990).

Tuberculosis is the single most serious infectious disease in the developing world (Murray et al., 1993). Annual infection rates are highest in sub-Saharan Africa and Asia, ranging from 1 to 2.5 percent; in South and Central America, North Africa, and Western Asia the range is 0.5 to 1.5 percent. Murray et al. have estimated for the developing world in 1990 an annual incidence of 7.3 million cases and 2.7 million deaths.

With the diagnostic technology and chemotherapeutic agents currently available, demonstration projects in a number of developing countries have shown that short-course chemotherapy can be applied on a national scale with cure rates approaching 90 percent (Styblo, 1989). Treatment of smear-positive tuberculosis will rapidly accelerate the decline in disease incidence. Analysis of health intervention programs has shown that tuberculosis case therapy is one of the most cost-effective health interventions available (Jamison, 1993).

Rheumatic Fever

Rheumatic fever is a systemic complication of pharyngitis due to group A streptococcal infection, which can result in inflammatory manifestations principally in the joints and the heart. Infection in children is associated with low socioeconomic status and crowding, and continues to be prevalent in developing countries. Although significant mortality accompanies the acute disease, the chronic consequences of rheumatic heart disease—resulting in disability and ultimately death among young adults in the economically productive ages—represent a significant cost to society. A recent World Health Organization (1988) report notes that ". . .among the majority of the world's population, rheumatic heart disease remains the most common cardiovascular cause of death in the first four decades of life."

Rheumatic heart disease remains a significant problem in the developing world (Michaud et al., 1993). Prevalence rates per 1,000 among school-age children included in surveys in different regions and countries of the world were North Africa, 9.9 to 15.0; Nigeria, 0.3 to 3.0; Latin America, 1.0 to 17.0; Asia, 0.4 to 21.0; Pacific, 4.7 to 18.6. Hospital studies in nine sub-Saharan African countries revealed that rheumatic heart disease accounted for 10 to 35 percent of all cardiac admissions (Hutt, 1991).

The complications of group A streptococcal pharyngitis (GASP) can be prevented by early diagnosis and treatment with antibiotics. Community-based approaches to promote early detection of pharyngitis, coupled with selection of cases for antibiotic therapy based on the use of a clinical algorithm, have been proposed; at present, however, these are not cost-effective because of the rarity (0.4 percent) with which GASP is followed by rheumatic fever (Michaud et al., 1993.) With the growing evidence of a genetic risk factor for rheumatic heart disease, there is an urgent need for more research to simplify the identification of susceptible persons so that more specific preventive interventions can be developed.

Polio

Polio is a viral illness transmissible through fecal-oral and pharyngeal-oral routes. Although highly effective oral and injectable vaccines are available and the international community is moving toward universal childhood immunization, approximately 50 percent of the world's children have not yet been reached, particularly in sub-Saharan Africa and South Asia (Jamison et al., 1993). The majority of the unimmunized children in developing countries will be infected in the first few years of life, although the majority of infections remain asymtomatic. In the 1980s, the annual incidence of poliomyelitis was estimated at 200,000 to 250,000 cases, approximately 25,000 of whom died (World Health Organization, 1990). Residual paralysis with lameness is the health condition of consequence for adults.

During the late 1970s and early 1980s, lameness surveys were carried out in many regions of the world. The median prevalence of lameness in Asia and Africa due to polio ranged from 3 to 6 per 1,000, with considerable variation in each of these settings (Jamison et al., 1993). Based on these surveys, it is estimated that between 10 and 20 million people are currently living with disability due to polio.

The international community, with national governments, has embarked upon a program of global polio eradication (Grant, 1990). Eradication efforts are already proving highly effective in Latin America. China has also reached very high levels of vaccine coverage. It is likely that by the turn of the century, polio will become a rare disease.

Trachoma

Trachoma is a chronic infectious conjunctivitis caused by *Chlamydia trachomatis*. The disease is characterized by progressive exacerbations and remissions that, over a period of many months, result in gradual scarring of the cornea with progressive corneal opacity resulting in varying degrees of permanent vision loss or blindness. The infectious agent is transmitted among children by direct contact or by sharing contaminated articles such as towels and handkerchiefs. The disease can be treated effectively with antibiotic eye ointments, although application two to four times a day for four to six weeks is required. Advanced disease with scarring requires surgical treatment.

Trachoma is one of the major causes of blindness in the world today. It accounts for 6 to 9 million blind persons, representing about 25 percent of all the blind in the world (World Health Organization, 1990). The disease is endemic throughout large parts of East and West Asia. It is estimated that 500 million people live in areas with endemic blinding trachoma (World Health Organization, 1990). Given the conditions of transmission, prevention will require education of the population to reduce disease transmission through improved hygienic conditions, early recognition of infection manifestations, and ready availability of treatment through a primary health care system.

Chagas' Disease

Chagas' disease is a chronic disease caused by the protozoan *Trypanosoma cruzi*. This disease, which is limited to South and Central America, is also called South American trypanosomiasis (Marsden, 1986). (Another form of trypanosomiasis causes sleeping sickness in Africa.) The agent of Chagas' disease is transmitted by contamination of the bite of the "assassin" or "kissing" reduviid bugs (triatoma and related Reduviidae) with the infected feces of the insect. The bug vector typically lives in cracks in the walls, floor, or ceiling of primitive brick or wood houses, most often in rural areas. The bug can be killed by insecticides; however, a control program requires a comprehensive approach involving application of insecticide, monitoring of bug infestation, and housing improvement to eliminate cracks that harbor the bug (Marsden, 1986).

Small children are typically infected while sleeping at night, when the bug will leave its habitat to obtain a blood meal. The acute phase of infection in humans typically passes unnoticed, although the child may have some fever and an enlarged spleen or liver. The disease then progresses to the so-called indeterminate phase manifest only by positive serology. After two decades or more, signs of damage to target organs begin to appear, principally the heart. Destruction of the muscle fibers produces heart failure and cardiac arrhythmias leading to death. Heart failure appears mainly between ages 20 and 50.

Based on epidemiological studies, the World Health Organization (1990) estimates the number of infected people in Latin America to be on the order of 15 to 18 million. Of infected individuals, approximately 10 percent go on to develop chronic Chagas' cardiopathy. Recent evidence suggests that chronic Chagas' disease may be responsible in some endemic areas for up to 10 percent of deaths among the adult population.

Chagas' disease is strongly associated with poverty. Control measures will require a concerted and sustained effort to upgrade housing conditions, particularly among the rural poor.

Schistosomiasis

Schistosomiasis is a visceral parasitic disease caused by blood flukes of the genus Schistosoma (Warren, 1986; Warren et al., 1993). Freshwater snails in streams polluted by feces or urine are the intermediate hosts. Human infection follows contact by bathing or wading with the free-swimming cercariae of the parasite that penetrate the skin and are carried by the bloodstream to the liver where they mature. Adult worms then migrate to the venules of the bladder or intestines. Three species cause clinical disease: S. haematobium affects the bladder, whereas S. mansoni and S. japonicum involve the intestine. In these sites, the worms lay their eggs, which penetrate the mucosal surface to be excreted in the urine or stool, continuing the cycle of transmission if the eggs enter fresh water with an intermediate snail host.

Because these worms do not multiply in the human host, the severity of symptoms relates to the intensity of infection, which is governed by the rate of acquisition of new worms and the life span of the worms in the body (less than five years). Infections are acquired through the course of childhood so that the heaviest worm burdens are typically seen in adolescence and young adults. Clinical symptoms relate to low-grade disability among adults and to immune responses in the host, producing some tissue destruction and fibrosis in the liver with intestinal infection, and in the bladder and ureter with genital- urinary infection. On a population basis, the primary health effect of schistosomiasis is a decreased capacity for heavy work (Warren et al., 1993). In a number of areas, heavy infection has been clearly implicated in reduced labor productivity. Death is rare.

Schistosomiasis is endemic in 76 countries in Asia, Africa, and Latin America. The World Health Organization (1990) estimates that about 200 million people are infected with schistosome parasites. Elimination of schistosomiasis from the population will require major changes in human behavior and environmental improvement in many populations to reduce the contact with infected water sources. A more practical and cost-effective intermediate-term measure that is currently being considered is mass chemotherapy with the drug praziquantel (Warren et al., 1993). Mass administration of this chemotherapeutic agent to school-age children at intervals of about two years, would not interrupt transmission, but could dramatically reduce the intensity of infection and, thus, the load of morbidity in the population.

Helicobacter Pylori

Helicobacter pylori (H. pylori) are bacteria that are associated with chronic atrophic gastritis, an inflammatory precursor of stomach cancer.

Stomach cancer is estimated to be the world's second most common cancer (after lung cancer; Parkin et al., 1988). In the 1930s it was the most common cancer in the United States. Over the past 50 years there has been a dramatic decline in the incidence of stomach cancer in the United States and Western Europe, leading some to proclaim an "unplanned triumph" (Howson et al., 1986). Stomach cancer rates, however, remain very high in much of Asia and Latin America (Barnum and Greenberg, 1993) as shown in Figure 4, which compares age-specific mortality rates for stomach cancer in China and the United States.

The relationship between infection with H. pylori and stomach cancer has only recently begun to be elucidated. More than two decades ago, pioneering studies by Haenszel et al. (1972) of Japanese who had migrated to Hawaii and California showed that the risk of gastric carcinoma was determined largely by environmental factors early in life. It is now known that one difference between populations at high risk and those at low risk of gastric carcinoma is that in high-risk populations there is a high prevalence of H. pylori infection among children, apparently associated with poor environmental sanitation (Correa, 1991). Once an individual acquires H. pylori, infection persists for life if not treated, producing the chronic atrophic gastritis associated with gastric carcinoma.

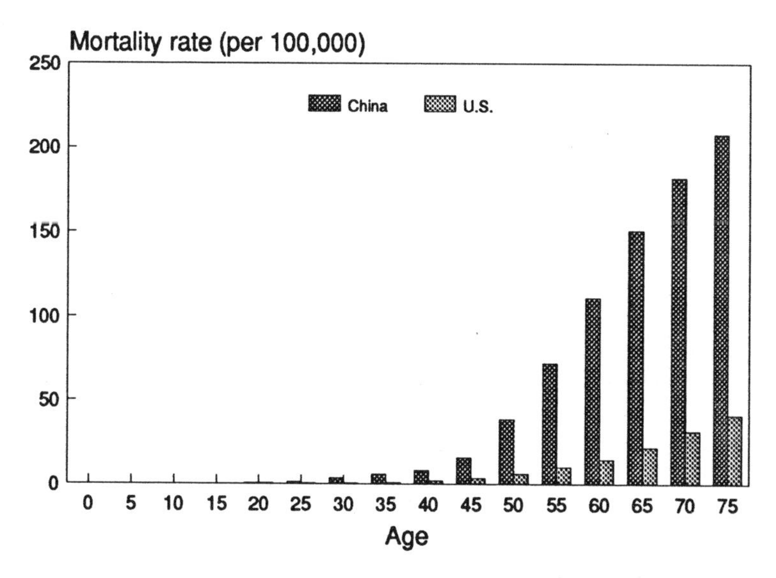

FIGURE 4 Stomach cancer: Age-specific mortality rates per 100,000 population. SOURCE: Barnum and Greenberg (1993).

Because H. pylori infection is prevalent among adults in the populations that have been studied, a number of epidemiologic studies were required to establish a causal relationship with gastric carcinoma. Initially, these were case-control studies documenting that the risk of having stomach cancer was higher among persons who were currently infected than among uninfected persons (Correa, 1991). More definitive evidence for a causal relationship came from recent investigations by Parsonnet et al. (1991) and Nomura et al. (1991), which demonstrated a higher risk of gastric carcinoma in individuals in whom infection with H. pylori could be documented by serological tests on blood samples collected 20 years earlier as compared to individuals who were uninfected then. Based on migrant studies cited above and the fact that H. pylori is a lifelong infection, it appears that the risk of gastric cancer is primarily due to H. pylori acquired early in childhood. It should be noted that although H. pylori is very prevalent in the adult populations, over a 20-year period the risk of gastric carcinoma among infected individuals is relatively low, amounting to 2.5 percent. It is likely that, in addition to H. pylori infection as an initiator, cofactors, possibly excessive salt intake and a diet low in fresh fruits and vegetables, are important as promoters in inducing gastric carcinoma.

The data so far suggest that up to 60 percent of stomach cancers are attributable to H. pylori infection. Although this implies that approximately 60 percent of the gastric carcinomas in these populations could be prevented if H. pylori infection were eliminated (by antibiotic treatment), such treatment is not a practical measure. The dramatic decline in stomach cancer in the developed world is an encouraging sign; it suggests that by improving environmental sanitation to reduce the risk of acquiring H. pylori infection early in life and by promoting better diets, we may expect to see corresponding declines in gastric cancer in the developing regions of the world. These interventions will, of course, have immediate health benefits for the children as well.

Epstein-Barr Virus

Epstein-Barr (EB) virus is the agent commonly associated with infectious mononucleosis in children and young adults. Once EB virus infection occurs, a persistent (lifelong) infection follows. EB virus is spread through close contact, mainly by the oral-respiratory route. In areas of poor sanitation and hygiene in developing countries, primary EB virus infections usually occur in infancy and are silent or too mild to be diagnosed. In higher socioeconomic groups, primary exposure to EB virus is often delayed until adolescence or later, when infections usually lead to infectious mononucleosis.

Persistent EB virus infection acquired in childhood is relevant to the health of adults because of the epidemiological evidence that this infection is involved in the etiology of Burkitt's lymphoma and nasopharyngeal cancer (Barnum and Greenberg, 1993). Burkitt's lymphoma is essentially confined to sub-Saharan Africa. Nasopharyngeal carcinoma, although rare in most of the world, is the most common cause of cancer death in some southern Chinese populations. Nasopharyngeal cancer occurs with peak frequency among adults in the 35- to 65-year age category.

As with other cancers, it seems clear that factors in addition to EB virus are necessary for the induction of malignant disease. A suggested cofactor for nasopharyngeal cancer is traditionally prepared Chinese salted fish. Immunization with an EB virus vaccine has been proposed as a preventive measure in the southern Chinese population, where nasopharyngeal cancer occurs at high frequency; however, an effective vaccine for EB virus has not yet been developed. Dietary change may be helpful, although this is problematical because the precise cofactors are not known. Regarding Burkitt's lymphoma, epidemiological evidence suggests that malaria might be a cofactor. So far, no preventive measures have been proposed.

Nutritional Deficiencies in Infancy and Childhood

Protein-Energy Malnutrition

Chronic protein-energy malnutrition (PEM) is a serious condition that continues to affect both children and adults in developing countries. The sequelae of PEM among children include excess morbidity and mortality, with growth stunting among survivors. The World Health Organization (1990) estimates that globally, 25 percent, or 1.3 billion, of the world's population are stunted (low height for age). Regionally in the developing world, the prevalence of stunting ranges from 48 percent in Asia and 38 percent in Africa to 26 percent in Latin America (Table 2).

PEM and the accompanying stunting have a variety of health consequences for adults (Pinstrup-Anderson et al., 1993; Gopalan, 1989). In terms of mental development, PEM has been associated with poor school performance and possibly delayed cognitive development. In working-age adults, stunting has been associated with lower productivity. Among pregnant women, short stature is a risk factor for life-threatening pregnancy complications, particularly obstructed labor due to pelvic insufficiency. Further, as noted earlier, maternal stunting is an important determinant of low birthweight; thus, there is an intergenerational consequence of undernutrition.

As summarized in the review by Elo and Preston (1992), in recent years there has been growing evidence that height is related to risk of death among adults in developed countries. Waaler (1984), in an analysis of the relation between height and mortality among Norwegians, observed that the risk of death at ages 40-59 for men who were less than 165 centimeters in

TABLE 2 Global Estimates of the Prevalence of Stunting by Region, 1985

Region[a]	Approximate Total Population (millions)	Percentage Stunted	Total Stunted (millions)
Africa	448	37.9	125
Americas	722	18.5	134
Southeast Asia	1309	47.8	626
Europe	842	3.8	32
Eastern Mediterranean	369	26.4	97
Western Pacific	1562	18.7	293

[a]World Health Organization Regions.

SOURCE: World Health Organization (1990).

height was 71 percent higher than for men who were greater than 182.5 centimeters. This relationship was especially marked for cardiovascular diseases, tuberculosis, and chronic obstructive lung disease. A similar investigation by Marmot et al. (1984) of British civil servants revealed a strong relationship between short stature and mortality, particularly a higher risk for coronary artery disease. Elo and Preston (1992) summarize other work in Finland and the United States supporting a relationship between short stature and coronary artery disease mortality among both men and women. The difference in relative risks of death between the shortest and tallest groups in these studies was generally a factor of three. Elo and Preston (1992) also report on a recent study of 22,000 male physicians in the United States by the American Heart Association showing that the risk of heart attack declined by 3 percent for every inch of height, a relationship that could not be accounted for by known risk factors such as obesity, high cholesterol, and elevated blood pressure.

Based on their review, Elo and Preston (1992:9) conclude that because "height is probably the best single indicator of nutritional conditions and disease environment in childhood . . . . [these relationships] represent at present the firmest statistical support for the belief that childhood conditions can make a good deal of difference for adult death rates." With the available data, it is not possible to measure the potential magnitude of the effect growth stunting may have on adult mortality in developing countries. Given the very high prevalence of stunting that is reported above, however, it is probable that the effect is substantial and that significant reductions in adult mortality may be expected with improvements in childhood nutritional status among populations of developing countries.

Micronutrient Deficiencies

Deficiencies in iodine, iron, and vitamin A during infancy and childhood can affect adult morbidity, particularly as it relates to intellectual development (Levin et al., 1993).

Iodine Approximately 1 billion persons are at risk of iodine deficiency in the developing world with the highest risks in South and East Asia (Levin et al., 1993). The World Health Organization (1990) estimates that approximately 20 million people suffer from measurable mental and/or motor retardation due to iodine deficiency, and 5.7 million suffer from full cretinism. Iodine deficiency disorders (IDDs) are prevalent in highland areas in many countries. IDD is due either to inadequate intake of iodine because the soil and water are deficient or to local diets that contain foods high in naturally existing "goitrogens," which interfere with the utilization of iodine.

The primary manifestations of severe iodine deficiency during pregnancy for the offspring are dwarfism and severe mental retardation known as cretinism. Of more concern than these extreme forms of deficiency are the possibility that noncretinist children may be mentally and neurologically handicapped in endemic areas. This milder impairment may go unnoticed in many poor communities, although it can limit social and economic growth (Stanbury, 1987).

Cretinism is obviously irreversible. It is likely that mild mental retardation resulting from impaired structural development of the brain during fetal life is also irreversible. Thus, correcting iodine deficiency in reproductive-age women is of highest priority. In the short run it can be accomplished by injection of iodized oil (Lipiodol); over the long term, fortification of commonly used foods (salt) is the most cost-effective strategy.

Iron Iron deficiency anemia affects approximately 800 million people worldwide (World Health Organization, 1990). The regions with the highest prevalence are Africa and South Asia, where upwards of 40 percent of the population is anemic. Lower rates in the range of 10 to 30 percent are seen in Latin America and East Asia. Major associated causes of iron deficiency anemia besides dietary deficiency of iron are heavy parasitic infections (hookworm and schistosomiasis) and repeated pregnancies and lactation (Levin et al., 1993).

A significant consequence of iron deficiency anemia in infancy and childhood for adults is its potential effect on mental development. A number of investigations have clearly documented that children with anemia score lower on tests of mental development than children without anemia (Soewondo et al., 1989). Of interest and concern in the long term is the fact that after a period of iron supplementation therapy, which results in a good hematologic response, previously anemic infants have not consistently shown improvement on their mental test scores (Levin et al., 1993).

Recently, Lozoff et al. (1991) reported on a four-year follow-up of children who had iron deficiency anemia in infancy that had been corrected with iron treatment. These carefully controlled studies suggested that the previously anemic children had long-lasting developmental disadvantages as assessed by a variety of tests of mental and motor development when compared to a control group without anemia in infancy. These developmental disadvantages persisted when the studies were statistically controlled for a variety of other background risk factors. The authors concluded that although they could not rule out the possibility that earlier detection and more vigorous treatment of iron deficiency anemia during infancy and childhood could be effective in preventing a developmental disadvantage later in life, the safest approach, given current knowledge, would be vigorous efforts directed to the primary prevention of iron deficiency in the population.

Vitamin A Vitamin A deficiency afflicts around 40 million preschool children in 37 countries, producing an estimated 250,000 to 500,000 cases of blindness annually (West and Sommer, 1987). Approximately two-thirds of these, however, die within weeks to months after becoming blind (Sommer, 1982). Cumulatively the survivors account for an estimated 2.8 million, or 10 percent, of blind persons in the world today (World Health Organization, 1990). In the short term, vitamin A deficiency can be prevented by the administration of one vitamin A capsule every six months, the strategy used in many developing countries. In the long run, dietary change and food fortification programs will have to be established.

Environmental Hazards

Indoor Air Pollution

Contrary to the general belief that air pollution is more severe in the cities of developed countries, recent studies by the United Nations Environment Program/World Health Organization Global Environment Monitoring Systems are demonstrating that the worst ambient conditions are in the cities of developing countries (Chen et al., 1990). More importantly, studies of indoor air quality reveal that the largest pollutant concentrations and exposures are found in the houses in developing countries in both rural and urban areas.

The major source of indoor air pollution in developing countries is the cooking stove. On a global scale, Chen et al. (1990) estimate that more than half of the world's households cook daily with unprocessed solid fuels such as dried animal dung, crop residues, wood, charcoal, and coal. In a high proportion of these households, cooking takes place under situations where much of the smoke is released into the living area. A second, somewhat less prevalent source of indoor pollution is space heating with biomass fuels, which is common, at least part of the year, in high-altitude areas of Africa, Asia, and Latin America.

Chen et al. (1990) review a wide range of epidemiological studies relating household air pollution to acute respiratory infection in children and chronic obstructive pulmonary disease among adults. Their review describes studies in China, India, Nepal, The Gambia, and other countries documenting a strong relationship between the frequency of respiratory symptoms among children and their exposure to household smoke from cooking with wood and other biomass fuels. Correspondingly, adults in these settings had higher rates of chronic bronchitis and chronic obstructive lung disease, but it is not possible to determine whether adult COPD is due to childhood exposures or to the cumulative effects of smoke at later ages.

COPD is a very serious health problem in most developing countries where there is heavy exposure to household smoke from open fires using biomass fuels. Figure 5 compares age-specific mortality rates for COPD in China and the United States for males and for females (Bumgarner and Speizer, 1993). In the United States, COPD is due almost entirely to cigarettes so that resultant death rates are approximately three times higher for males than for females. As the figure illustrates, in China, COPD mortality rates are four to six times higher than in the United States, with death rates essentially the same among males and females. Furthermore, in China, death rates in rural areas are more than three times higher than in urban areas, again reflecting the very high rates of exposure to indoor household smoke.

In the context of this review on the childhood precursors of adult disease, it must be noted that chronic obstructive lung disease typically occurs after two or three decades of smoke exposure. Thus, childhood exposure alone cannot be blamed for these adverse consequences. On the other hand, it is likely that when exposure begins in infancy and childhood, resulting in recurrent acute respiratory infections, and continues for a lifetime, the onset of disabling symptoms will begin earlier among adults and lead to chronic disability and death at much younger ages.

Lead Exposure

The addition of lead to gasoline has been called "the mistake of the 20th century" (Shy, 1990). Combustion of leaded gasoline since 1925 accounts for about 90 percent of total atmospheric lead. In the United States in the peak year 1972, 250,000 metric tons of lead were utilized for leaded fuel, amounting to an average of 2.4 pounds of lead per person per year (U.S. Environmental Protection Agency, 1986). National household surveys between 1976 and 1980, when lead-free fuels were being introduced, docu-

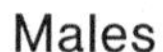

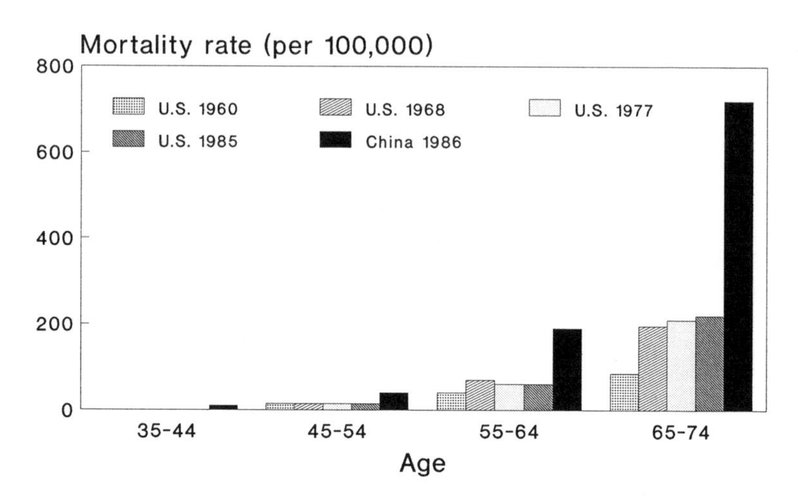

Females

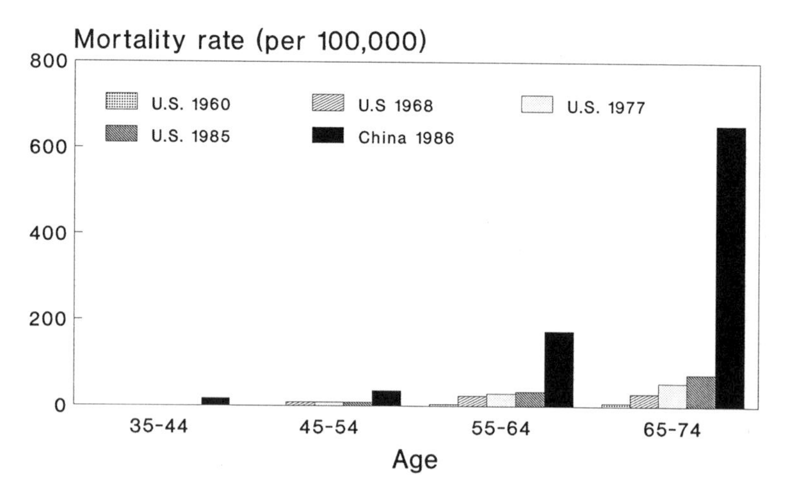

FIGURE 5 Chronic obstructive pulmonary disease: Age-specific mortality rates, China and the United States.

mented a direct correlation between declining ambient lead concentrations and blood lead levels in the U.S. population (Shy, 1990).

It is important to recognize how exposure to lead occurs in the population. Although combustion of leaded gasoline initially disperses lead into the atmosphere, actually inhalation of lead from the air contributes only 1 to 2 percent of the total lead intake of humans. More important is indirect exposure to atmospheric lead via ingestion and inhalation of lead in dust, soil, food, and water affected by the fallout of atmospheric lead. One study in Italy confirmed that an estimated 60 percent of blood lead levels in the city of Turin was attributable to inhalation or ingestion of leaded fuel emission in dust, food, and water (Facchetti and Geiss, 1982). Not surprisingly, lead exposure is highest among children in urban areas where there is a high density of air, soil, and dust lead levels.

A number of epidemiological studies have documented that the developmental effects of chronic low-level lead exposure in early life include low birthweight, impaired mental development in the first two years of life, I.Q. deficits in school-age children, and disturbances in sensory pathways within the central nervous system persisting for five or more years (Shy, 1990). These effects, particularly the neurological and cognitive ones, occur at very low blood lead levels. For example, studies in the United States and Australia in the early 1980s documented evidence of measurable declines in cognitive functions among infants at blood lead levels that were lower on the average than those detected in U.S. school children based on measurements taken in the National Health and Nutrition Examination Survey II (Bellinger et al., 1987; McMichael et al., 1988). The data from these and other studies lead Shy (1990:174) to conclude that "with respect to lead, there should be as little human exposure as possible, and all evidence points to a greater risk of a variety of adverse effects, particularly on cognition and hematological function at what were formerly considered normal blood lead levels."

The adverse effects of lead on human health is well documented in developed countries. Unquestionably the cognitive and neurological deficiencies detectable in children will have consequences for their intellectual development in school and their mental abilities as adults. There are essentially no data on the risks to lead exposure in developing countries; however, the rapid urbanization and increase in the use of motor vehicles indicate that it will be a growing problem in the future. In this context it is noteworthy that in the United States, lead-free gasoline was introduced in the 1970s to protect catalytic converters rather than to prevent disease in human beings. Catalytic converters have not been mandated in most developing countries because of cost considerations; therefore, the use of leaded fuel is the norm. Consequently, one can predict that there will be a growing problem with lead exposure in these settings.

SYNERGISM OF CHILDHOOD RISK FACTORS PRODUCING ADULT DISEASE

The preceding discussion examines a series of infections and other conditions in childhood in isolation from each other, focusing on their established or possible biological links to morbidity and mortality among adults. This approach, however, oversimplifies the situation because typically there are common underlying risk factors for many of these conditions that are associated with the impoverished living conditions in developing country settings. Chronic obstructive pulmonary disease is used as an example to illustrate how multiple risk factors in childhood can be operating simultaneously and even synergistically to produce disability and death among adults (Samet et al., 1983).

Figure 6 illustrates schematically some of the possible underlying childhood determinants of COPD in developing country settings. The use of low-grade, biomass fuels for cooking results in heavy indoor air pollution, which has been well established as a direct contributor to a high rate of acute respiratory infections among infants and children. Indirectly, indoor air pollution may contribute to low birthweight if there is poor ventilation so that women in pregnancy are exposed to significant concentrations of carbon monoxide (Mavalankar et al., 1993). More importantly, under impoverished circumstances the mothers may already be stunted, and this condition, along with poor diets and heavy exertion during pregnancy, can result in low-birthweight infants. Low birthweight, as noted earlier, is associated with impaired lung development, which also increases the risk of acute respiratory infection. In the long run, all of these conditions in combination become precursors of chronic airway obstruction leading to COPD.

A similar scenario may be sketched for infant malnutrition, which can result in growth faltering in childhood to produce the long-term health consequences of stunting among adults noted earlier. As with COPD, there are social and environmental determinants of growth faltering and stunting, including poor hygiene and sanitation leading to a high incidence of diarrheal disease.

A key point about these theoretical examples is that curative interventions limited to the treatment of acute respiratory infections and episodes of diarrhea can be lifesaving in the short run but may not produce major reductions in adult morbidity and mortality in the long run unless the underlying risk factors are addressed. In the cases cited above, improvements in stove construction, household ventilation, and water and sanitation programs might be expected to produce both short-term and long-term health gains in the population. Relevant in this context is an analysis by Preston and van de Walle (1978) of the gains in survival in a number of French cities in the last century following improvements in the water supply. Data were avail-

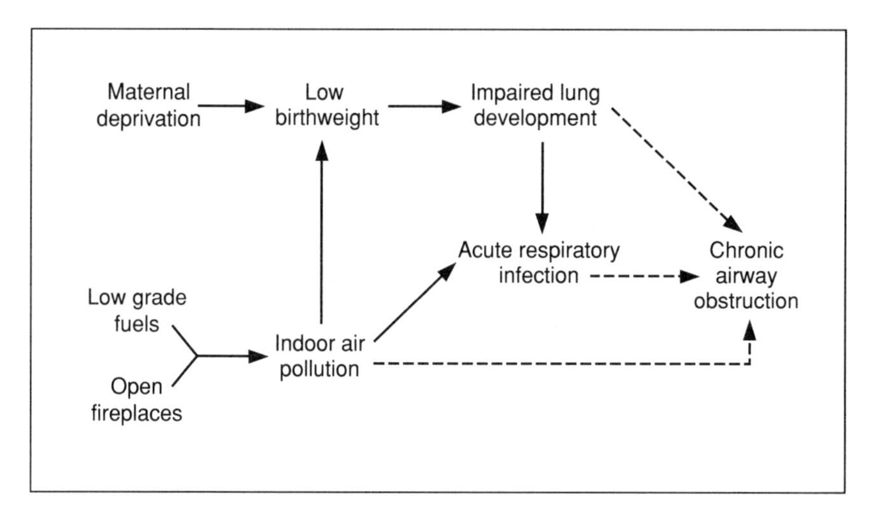

FIGURE 6 Underlying childhood determinants of chronic obstructive pulmonary disease.

able to document that over several decades after sanitary improvements were instituted, gains in survival were initially observed in infants and children and then successively in older groups as the young cohorts aged over time.

INFLUENCE OF CHILDHOOD-ACQUIRED DISEASES ON ADULT MORTALITY—COUNTRY STUDIES

The data presented above on individual diseases and conditions provide a general assessment of the morbidity and mortality consequences of these conditions for adult health. Although the numbers of persons affected on a global scale are in the tens of millions, it is difficult to assess from such data the relative importance of these childhood conditions compared to other diseases acquired later in life that contribute to adult morbidity and mortality. One problem with making such assessments is the fact that very few developing countries have adequate data at the national level on cause of death. India does have a national sample registration system for vital events that in recent years has included cause of death. These data have limitations because cause of death is based on lay reporting. Indian data do reveal that among adults ages 15-54, tuberculosis alone accounted for 18 percent of deaths among males and 11 percent of deaths among females, indicating that this disease is not inconsequential in contributing to premature mortality (Feachem et al., 1992).

Much better data are available from China, which has a national sample registration system providing cause-of-death information, most of it is medically certified, for more than 100 million people. Table 3 from Feachem et al. (1992) summarizes the leading causes of death for Chinese men and women between the ages of 15 and 60 in the year 1988. Noteworthy, cancers of the liver and stomach, due primarily to infections acquired in infancy, account for 13 percent of deaths in men and 9 percent in women. COPD accounts for 11 percent in both men and women. Tuberculosis and rheumatic heart

TABLE 3 Distribution of Deaths by Cause for Chinese Women and Men Ages 15-59, 1988

Causes of Death	Women (%)	Men (%)
Communicable	7.1	7.8
Tuberculosis	3.5[a]	3.8[a]
Maternal	1.8	
Cancer	23.6	27.3
Liver	4.3[a]	8.3[a]
Stomach	4.8[a]	5.0
Lung	3.8	3.9
Esophagus	2.5	2.9
Colon-rectum	1.4	1.4
Nasopharynx	0.3[a]	0.9
Breast	1.7	
Cervix	0.8	
Cardiovascular	23.8	20.4
Cerebrovascular	11.2	10.8
Ischemic	4.3	3.6
Rheumatic	4.3[a]	2.2[a]
Hypertensive	2.0	2.3
Respiratory	9.9	10.4
Chronic obstructive pulmonary disease[b]	9.5[a]	9.3[a]
Digestive	5.6	7.5
Chronic liver disease	2.6[a]	4.2[a]
Endocrine	0.8	0.8
Diabetes	0.6	0.8
Other noncommunicable diseases	6.5	5.7
Injuries	20.9	20.1
All causes	100.0	100.0
Probability of dying (percent) between ages 15 and 59	11.87	14.29

[a]These causes are largely related to childhood condition.

[b]Pulmonary heart disease is included with chronic obstructive pulmonary disease.

SOURCE: Derived from Feachem et al. (1992: Table 2.14).

disease together account for 6 to 7 percent of deaths, whereas chronic liver disease, much of which is related to hepatitis B virus, accounts for another 3 to 4 percent. Overall, conditions that are largely related to childhood precursors accounted for more than 30 to 34 percent of all of the premature and generally preventable deaths in this age group.

CONCLUSION

Typically, when one considers health conditions in developing countries, the focus of attention is on the high levels of infant and child mortality. This focus is reasonable because children under 5 years of age generally account for 15 to 20 percent of the population and the vast majority of deaths in this age group are preventable. What is less appreciated is that the surviving adults in these populations also experience very high rates of preventable morbidity and premature mortality. For example, although we may expect to see 6 to 10 percent of adults dying between the ages of 15 and 60 in developed countries, in developing countries upwards of 25 to 35 percent of adults may die in this period of life. As this review suggests, as many as one-third of these premature deaths may be the consequence of infections and other conditions acquired in infancy and childhood. Although not discussed here, it should be clear that because most of these fatal conditions produce death only after a prolonged chronic illness, the burden of morbidity in the population is far greater. Added to this burden must be that lifetime disability from nonfatal conditions of childhood that produce blindness, paralysis, and mental retardation.

The recent child survival revolution in the developing world promoted by UNICEF, WHO, and the international donor community, has brought to the forefront of the world's attention the cost-effectiveness of a number of selected technical interventions such as immunization and oral rehydration therapy in saving the lives of infants and children. More recently, additional interventions such as antibiotic therapy for acute respiratory diseases have been added to the child survival strategy. For the most part, the goal of child survival programs has been to produce an immediate mortality reduction, and the accomplishments have been noteworthy in many countries (Grant, 1990). A recent exception to this short-term strategy has been the introduction of hepatitis B vaccine into childhood immunization programs in a number of countries in Africa and Asia, including China.

The premise of this review is that far more attention should be given to the long-term as well as short-term benefits of programs to promote child health. Attention should be given not only for direct child health interventions such as vaccines but particularly for interventions that will have cross-cutting effects on reducing the risks of multiple conditions simultaneously. Interventions such as reducing indoor air pollution, upgrading housing and sanitation, and improving pregnancy care and nutrient intake would fit in this category. Too often, when only narrowly defined, short-term benefits are taken into account, such broad-based intervention programs are considered too costly. However, as shown by Briscoe (1978) in terms of improving the water supply, when the multifaceted and long-term health benefits are considered, intervention programs in these areas become quite cost-effective.

A major limitation of this analysis is the paucity of empirical data from population-based studies, particularly from developing countries, which could provide a firm basis for establishing the links between childhood exposures and adult morbidity and mortality. More precise knowledge of these linkages would be important for policy and programmatic purposes as well as having scientific significance. Although we can generally expect health conditions to improve in developing countries with rising incomes and better diets and living conditions, in a resource-constrained environment it would be invaluable for health policymakers to have better information about specific linkages between childhood conditions and adult morbidity and mortality so that development strategies could be formulated that would maximize the health gains to the population. In this context, as noted in this paper as well as in the review by Elo and Preston (1992), such health policies and programs may be directed toward not only reducing the current burden of disease seen in developing countries, for example, by the introduction of hepatitis B vaccine, but also limiting the emergence of the "diseases of development" such as cardiovascular disease by promoting the maintenance or adoption of healthy dietary practices in infancy and childhood as economies grow. Given the potential magnitude of the health gains in populations that could be achieved by directing more attention to risks and exposures in childhood, the importance and need for far more research in this area should be self-evident.

REFERENCES

Barker, J.P., K.M. Godfrey, C. Fall, C. Osmond, P.D. Winter, and S.O. Shaheen
1991 Relation of birth weight and childhood respiratory infection to adult lung function and death from chronic obstructive airways disease. *British Medical Journal* 303:671-675.

Barnum, H., and R. Greenberg
1993 Cancers. In D.T. Jamison and W.H. Mosley, eds., *Disease Control Priorities in Developing Countries*. New York: Oxford University Press for the World Bank.

Beasley, R.P.
1982 Hepatitis B virus as the etiologic agent in hepatocellular carcinoma: Epidemiologic considerations. *Hepatology* 2(2):21S-26S.

Beasley, R.P., L-Y. Hwang, C-C. Lin, and C-S. Chien
1981 Hepatocellular carcinoma and hepatitis B virus. *Lancet* 1129-1133.

Bellinger, D., A. Leviton, C. Waternaux, H. Needleman, M. Rabinowitz
1987 Longitudinal analyses of prenatal and postnatal lead exposure and early cognitive development. *New England Journal of Medicine* 316:1037-1043.

Briscoe, J.
1978 The role of water supply in improving health in poor countries (with special reference to Bangladesh). *American Journal Clinical Nutrition* 31:2100-2113.

Bucher, U., and L. Reid
1961 Development of the intrasegmental bronchial tree: The pattern of branching and development of cartilage at various stages of intrauterine life. *Thorax* 16:207-218.

Bumgarner, J.R., and F.E. Speizer
1993 Chronic obstructive pulmonary disease. In D.T. Jamison and W.H. Mosley, eds., *Disease Control Priorities in Developing Countries*. New York: Oxford University Press for the World Bank.

Chan, K.N., C.M. Noble-Jamieson, A. Elliman, E.M. Bryan, and M. Silverman
1989 Lung function in children of low birth weight. *Archives of Disease in Childhood* 64:1284-1293.

Chen, B.H., C.J. Hong, M.R. Pandey, and K.R. Smith
1990 Indoor air pollution in developing countries. *World Health Statistics Quarterly* 43(3):127-137.

Chenais, J-C.
1990 Demographic transition patterns and their impact on the age structure. *Population and Development Review* 16(2):327-336.

Correa, P.
1991 Is gastric carcinoma an infectious disease? *New England Journal of Medicine* 325(16):1170-1171.

Elo, I.T., and S.H. Preston
1992 Effects of early-life conditions on adult mortality: A review. *Population Index* 58(2):186-212.

Facchetti, S., and F. Geiss
1982 Isotopic lead experiment—Status report. *Publication No. EUR 8352 EN*. Luxembourg: Commission of the European Communities.

Feachem, R.G.A., T. Kjellstrom, C.J.L. Murray, M. Over, and M.A. Phillips, eds.
1992 *The Health of Adults in the Developing World*. Oxford: Oxford University Press for the World Bank.

Ferraz, E.M., R.H. Gray, and T.M. Cunha
1990 Determinants of preterm delivery and intra-uterine growth retardation in NE Brazil. *International Journal of Epidemiology* 19:101-108.

Francis, D.P.
1986 Hepatitis B virus and its related diseases. Pp. 289-297 in J.A. Walsh and K.S. Warren, eds., *Strategies for Primary Health Care*. Chicago: University of Chicago Press.

Frost, W.H.
1939 The age selection of mortality from tuberculosis in successive decades. *American Journal of Hygiene* 30:91-96.

Gopalan, C.
1989 Stunting: Significance and implications for public health policy. In *Nutrition, Health, and National Development*. New Delhi: Nutrition Foundation of India.

Grant, J.
1990 *State of the World's Children 1991*. New York: UNICEF.

Haenszel, W., M. Kurihara, M. Segi, and R.K. Lee.
1972 Stomach cancer among Japanese in Hawaii. *Journal of the National Cancer Institute* 49:969-988.

Herrera, M.G.
1985 Maternal nutrition and child survival. Paper presented to UNICEF Conference on Child Health and Survival, Harvard School of Public Health, Boston, May 30-31.

Hira, S.K., G.J. Bhat, D.M. Chikamata, B. Nkowane, G. Tembo, P.L. Perine, and A. Meheus
1990 Syphilis intervention in pregnancy: Zambian demonstration project. *Genitourinary Medicine* 66:159-164.

Howson, C.P., T. Hiyama, and E.L. Wynder
1986 The decline in gastric cancer: Epidemiology of an unplanned triumph. *Epidemiology Review* 8:1-27.

Hutt, M.S.R.
1991 Cancer and cardiovascular diseases. Pp. 221-240 in R.G. Feachem and D.T. Jamison, eds., *Disease and Mortality in Sub-Saharan Africa*. New York: Oxford University Press for the World Bank.

Jamison, D.T.
1993 Disease control priorities in developing countries: An overview. In D.T. Jamison and W.H. Mosley, eds., *Disease Control Priorities in Developing Countries*. New York: Oxford University Press for the World Bank.

Jamison, D.T., A. Torres, L. Chen, and J. Melnick
1993 Poliomyelitis. In D.T. Jamison and W.H. Mosley, eds., *Disease Control Priorities in Developing Countries*. New York: Oxford University Press for the World Bank.

Kane, M., J. Clements, and D. Hu
1993 Hepatitis B. In D.T. Jamison and W.H. Mosley, eds., *Disease Control Priorities in Developing Countries*. New York: Oxford University Press for the World Bank.

Kramer, M.S.
1987 Determinants of low birthweight: Methodological assessment and meta-analysis. *Bulletin of the World Health Organization* 65:663-737.

Levin, H.M., E. Pollitt, R. Galloway, and J. McGuire
1993 Micronutrient deficiency disorders. In D.T. Jamison and W.H. Mosley, eds., *Disease Control Priorities in Developing Countries*. New York: Oxford University Press for the World Bank.

Lozoff, B., E. Jimenez, and A.W. Wolf
1991 Long-term developmental outcome of infants with iron deficiency. *New England Journal of Medicine* 325(10):687-694.

Marmot, M.G., M.J. Shipley, and G. Rose
1984 Inequalities in death-specific explanations of a general pattern. *Lancet* May 5:1003-1006.

Marsden, P.D.
1986 Chagas' disease. Pp. 128-139 in J.A. Walsh and K.S. Warren, eds., *Strategies for Primary Health Care*. Chicago: University of Chicago Press.

Mata, L.J.
1978 *The Children of Santa María Cauqué: A Prospective Field Study of Health and Growth*. Cambridge, Mass. and London: MIT Press.

Mavalankar, D.V., R.H. Gray, and C.R. Trivedi
1993 Risk factors for pre-term and term low birth weight in Ahmedabad, India. *International Journal of Epidemiology*. Forthcoming.

McCall, M.G., and E.D. Acheson
1968 Respiratory disease in infancy. *Journal of Chronic Diseases* 21:349-359.

McMichael, A.J., P.A. Baghurst, N.R. Wigg, G.V. Vimpani, E.F. Robertson, and R.J. Roberts
1988 Port Pirie cohort study—Environmental exposure to lead and children's abilities at the age of four years. *New England Journal of Medicine* 319:468-475.

Michaud, C., J. Trejo-Gutierrez, C. Cruz, and T.A. Pearson
1993 Rheumatic heart disease. In D.T. Jamison and W.H. Mosley, eds., *Disease Control Priorities in Developing Countries.* New York: Oxford University Press for the World Bank.

Mosley, W.H., and P. Cowley
1991 The challenge of world health. *Population Bulletin* 46(4)(December).

Mosley, W.H., J-L. Bobadilla, and D.T. Jamison
1993 The health transition: Implication for health policy in developing countries. In D.T. Jamison and W.H. Mosley, eds., *Disease Control Priorities in Developing Countries.* New York: Oxford University Press for the World Bank.

Murray, C.J.L., and R.G. Feachem
1990 Avoidable adult mortality in the developing world. *Transactions of the Royal Society of Tropical Medicine* 84(1):1-2.

Murray, C.J.L., K. Styblo, and A. Rouillon
1993 Tuberculosis. In D.T. Jamison and W.H. Mosley, eds., *Disease Control Priorities in Developing Countries.* New York: Oxford University Press for the World Bank.

Nomura, A., G.N. Stemmermann, P-H. Chyou, I. Kato, G.I. Perez-Perez, and M.J. Blaser
1991 Helicobacter pylori infection and gastric carcinoma among Japanese Americans in Hawaii. *New England Journal of Medicine* 325(16):1132-1136.

Nottidge, V.A., and M.E. Okogbo
1991 Cerebral palsey in Ibadan, Nigeria. *Developmental Medicine and Child Neurology* 33(3):241-245.

Over, M., and P. Piot
1993 HIV infection and sexually transmitted diseases. In D.T. Jamison and W.H. Mosley, eds., *Disease Control Priorities in Developing Countries.* New York: Oxford University Press for the World Bank.

Parkin, D.M., E. Laara, and C.S. Muir
1988 Estimates of the worldwide frequency of sixteen major cancers in 1980. *International Journal of Cancer* 41:184-197.

Parsonnet, J., G.D. Friedman, D.P. Vandersteen, Y. Chang, J.H. Vogelman, N. Orentreigh, and R.K. Sibley
1991 Helicobacter pylori infection and the risk of gastric carcinoma. *New England Journal of Medicine* 325(16):1127-1131.

Pinstrup-Anderson, P., S. Burger, J-P. Habicht, and K. Peterson
1993 Protein-energy malnutrition. In D.T. Jamison and W.H. Mosley, eds., *Disease Control Priorities in Developing Countries.* New York: Oxford University Press for the World Bank.

Preston, S.H., and E. van de Walle
1978 Urban French mortality in the nineteenth century. *Population Studies* 32:275-298.

Samet, J.M., I.B. Tager, and F.E. Speizer
1983 The relationship between respiratory illness in childhood and chronic air-flow obstruction in adulthood. *American Review of Respiratory Disease* 127:508-523.

Schulz, K.F., W. Cates, Jr., and P.R. O'Mara
1987 Pregnancy loss, infant death, and suffering: Legacy of syphilis and gonorrhoea in Africa. *Genitourinary Medicine* 63:320-325.

Shy, C.M.
1990 Lead in petrol—The mistake of the XXth century. *World Health Statistics Quarterly* 43(3):168-175.

Soewondo, M., M. Husaini, and E. Pollitt
1989 Effects of iron deficiency on attention and learning processes in preschool children: Bandung, Indonesia. *American Journal of Clinical Nutrition* 50(supplement):667-674 .

Sommer, A
1982 *Nutritional Blindness, Xerophthalmia and Keratomalacia.* New York: Oxford University Press.

Stanbury, J.B.
1987 The iodine deficiency disorder: Introduction and general aspects. In B.S. Hetzel, J.T. Dunn, and J.B. Stanbury, eds., *The Prevention and Control of Iodine Deficiency Disorders.* New York: Elsevier.

Styblo, K.
1989 Overview and epidemiological assessment of the current global tuberculosis situation with an emphasis on control in developing countries. *Reviews of Infectious Diseases 2* (supplement 2; March-April):S339-S346.

Sutherland, I.
1976 Recent studies in the epidemiology of tuberculosis, based on the risk of being infected with tubercle bacilli. *Advances in Tuberculosis Research* 19:1-63.

United Nations
1991 *World Population Prospects 1990.* New York: United Nations.

U.S. Environmental Protection Agency
1986 *Air Quality Criteria for Lead.* EPA Report No. EPA-600/8-83028aF-dF. Research Triangle Park, N.C.: Office of Health and Environmental Assessment.

Villar, J., and J.M. Belizan
1982 The relative contribution of prematurity and fetal growth retardation to low birth weight in developing and developed societies. *American Journal of Obstetrics and Gynecology* 143:793.

Waaler, H.T.
1984 Height, weight and mortality. *Acta Medica Scandinavica* No. 679(supplement):3-56 .

Warren, K.S.
1986 Schistosomiasis. Pp. 72-83 in J.A. Walsh and K.S. Warren, eds., *Strategies for Primary Health Care.* Chicago: University of Chicago Press.

Warren, K.S., D. Bundy, R. Anderson, A.R. Davis, D.A. Henderson, D.T. Jamison, N. Prescott, and A. Senft
1993 Helminth infection. In D.T. Jamison and W.H. Mosley, eds., *Disease Control Priorities in Developing Countries.* New York: Oxford University Press for the World Bank.

West, K.P., Jr., and A. Sommer
1987 Delivery of oral doses of vitamin A to prevent vitamin A deficiency and nutritional blindness. *ACC/SCN State-of-the-Art Series.* Nutrition Policy Discussion Paper 2. Geneva: World Health Organization.

World Health Organization
1988 Rheumatic fever and rheumatic heart disease. Study Group Report. P. 28 in *WHO Technical Report Series.* No. 764. Geneva: World Health Organization.
1990 *Global Estimates for Health Situation Assessment and Projections 1990.* Publication WHO/HST/90.2 (April). Geneva: World Health Organization.

Projecting Morbidity and Mortality in Developing Countries During Adulthood

Kenneth G. Manton and Eric Stallard

INTRODUCTION

Forecasting chronic disease and health problems in adulthood requires different models and data than those for infant mortality and infectious disease because chronic diseases are often associated with long-term exposure to risk factors and age changes in host physiology. Many infectious diseases have both acute and chronic health consequences, and often are cofactors for chronic disease incidence and progression. Lifestyle and dietary habits are also important risk factors for chronic and degenerative diseases. Thus, in projecting the prevalence of these diseases, as well as resulting disabilities and deaths, it is necessary to consider the level of exposure to the risk factors and the consequences of other diseases and conditions of poor health.

Two examples of infectious diseases that contribute to chronic illnesses are malaria and helicobacter pylori. Chronic malarial infection alters the immune system so that the Epstein-Barr virus (EBV) causes Burkitt's lymphoma in East Africa, rather than infectious mononucleosis as in developed countries (Lam et al., 1991; Prevot et al., 1992). Helicobacter pylori (H. pylori), a waterborne bacteria, causes an infection that may be asymptomatic for decades (Barthel et al., 1988). It is a major causative agent for duodenal ulcers (Blaser, 1988) and gastric cancer (Forman, 1991; Talley et al., 1991), one of the most prevalent cancers in developing countries (Forman et al., 1990; Parsonnet et al., 1991). Prevention or treatment of H. pylori could

---

Kenneth G. Manton and Eric Stallard are with the Center for Demographic Studies, Duke University. This research was supported by National Institute on Aging Grant No. 5R01AG01159.

reduce gastric cancer (and possibly other chronic gastric disorder) rates by up to 60 percent in developing countries (Forman, 1991).

Communicable viral infections also contribute to chronic diseases. Although atherosclerosis and coronary heart disease (CHD) are etiologically linked to blood lipids, other factors explain more of the geographic, temporal, and cultural distribution of CHD. An etiology of cardiovascular disease (CVD) based on food-borne viral infection appears to be associated with the global distribution of risk factors and their change over time. There is evidence of viral activity in atherosclerosis' association with immunological factors (Muscari et al., 1990; Tertov et al., 1990), which might explain why Chinese men with heart attacks have average cholesterol levels (i.e., 194 milligrams per deciliter (mg/dl)) lower than the "desired" level of 200 mg/dl (Schwartzkopff et al., 1990). Thus, viral and bacterial diseases have chronic effects on cancer (e.g., EBV and retroviruses), neurological disease (e.g., poliomyelitis and late effects of encephalitis), CVD, and autoimmune disorders (e.g., rheumatoid arthritis and rheumatic heart fever).

Predisposition to a number of chronic diseases may be the result of nutritional insults during gestation and infancy. Maternal "deprivation," for example, increases the risk of type I diabetes in children (Crow et al., 1991). Other studies show that the ratios of birth to placental weight, and to body weight at 1 year, have strong associations with several chronic diseases (including diabetes) at later ages (Barker and Martyn, 1992). A low ratio (and low weight at 1 year) implies fetal growth dysfunction, favoring the development of the brain and heart at the expense of other organs (e.g., lungs or liver). Thus, malnutrition may cause fetal growth dysfunction, which contributes to the risk of CVD, pulmonary, and hepatic diseases through adulthood (Barker et al., 1991a,b, 1992a,b).

Many chronic diseases (cancer, CVD, stroke, diabetes mellitus) are associated with nutritional or lifestyle factors: fat and protein consumption, micronutrient deficiencies (Choi et al., 1990; Tonglet et al., 1992), alcohol use, smoking, and levels of physical activity (Dodu, 1988; Trowell and Burkitt, 1991). In developing countries, especially rural areas, fat intake and serum cholesterol tend to be low, thus reducing CHD risk. Among males in rural Nigeria, the mean cholesterol level was almost 40 mg/dl lower than in men living in urban areas, and similar differences were noted in Ghana and Côte d'Ivoire (Kesteloot et al., 1985; Knuiman et al., 1982). Mean cholesterol is low in China (e.g., Chen et al., 1991) where CHD is 7 percent of total mortality. Among the Tarahumara Indians of Mexico, cholesterol rose from 121 to 159 mg/dl over five weeks after changing from a "traditional" (2,700 kilocalories (kcal), low cholesterol and fat, high complex carbohydrate and fiber) to an "affluent" (4,100 kcal, high fat, cholesterol, sugar, and energy) diet (McMurray et al., 1991). Though cholesterol increased in the Tarahumara, the ratio of high- to low-density cholesterol did not change because of high levels of physical activity.

On the other hand, low levels of exposure to risk factors can also have adverse effects on health. Low serum cholesterol levels (especially low-density lipoprotein) is associated with gallbladder disease (Mohr et al., 1991), and with liver (Chen et al., 1991), colon (Cowan et al., 1990; Lee et al., 1991; Nomura et al., 1991), and lung (Isles et al., 1989) cancer. These associations may be mediated by low vitamin C intake (Choi et al., 1990; Jacques et al., 1987), low serum albumin (Kimura et al., 1979), viral infection (Mozar et al., 1990), rapid weight fluctuation (Hamm et al., 1989), or free-iron overload (Sullivan, 1989). The association of low cholesterol with hemorrhagic stroke and cancer is found in select population studies. Thus, diets consumed in developing countries need to be carefully examined for favorable and unfavorable elements, especially during pregnancy, infancy, and childhood, and old age (McGill, 1988; Tonglet et al., 1992).

Physical activity is a problem for the elderly in developing countries because after "retirement," activity declines rapidly (e.g., Dowd and Manton, 1992; Wilson et al., 1991). In Zimbabwe, mortality rises after retirement because of the rapid onset of impairments of activities of daily living (ADLs) due to activity reduction and malnutrition, especially vitamin B deficiency (Wilson et al., 1991; Evans, 1990). Zimmet et al. (1991) found that reduced physical activity increased risk factors for CHD and diabetes in Mauritius. Maintenance of physical activity with limited impairment is difficult in developing countries because of a lack of the physical and housing aids available in developed countries. Thus, promotion of physical activity (with nutritional supplementation) is important at postreproductive ages, both for risk factor reduction and for health maintenance.

Nutrition, physical activity, and metabolic factors are important in chronic disease forecasts. Exposures such as viral and bacterial infection, alcohol, and smoking, also need to be modeled either directly or through effects on measurable parameters (e.g., effect of smoking on pulmonary function). Once disease (and mortality) is predictable from measured risk factors, it can be related to interventions and used in policy development. Disease burden can be translated into effects on human capital (Manton et al., 1991d) by forecasting the physical and cognitive impairments generated by chronic disease. This paper discusses a three-part model to forecast chronic disease, disability, and mortality: the first part describes changes in risk factors; the second predicts disability, morbidity, or mortality as functions of risk factors; and the third assigns costs for health events that reduce productivity or incur medical costs.

COMBINING MULTIPLE DATA SOURCES

To conduct health forecasts and simulations, data are needed. Below we review types of data available in developed and developing countries.

Developed Countries

Developed countries have national health surveys and longitudinal studies of select populations. Some U.S. health surveys are longitudinal (e.g., the Longitudinal Studies of Aging in 1986, 1988, and 1990, based on the 1984 Supplement on Aging to the National Health Interview Survey (NHIS); National Center for Health Statistics (NCHS), 1987). Some surveys measure risk factors (e.g., National Health Examination Survey (NHES), National Health and Nutrition Examination Survey (NHANES) and the NHANES-I ten year follow-up). Some community studies longitudinally follow risk factors and health outcomes (e.g., studies in Framingham, Mass; Evans County, Ga.; Albany, N.Y.; and Charleston, S.C.). Epidemiological and health survey data are common in Britain and Scandinavian countries (e.g., the Swedish Götebörg Study; the Finnish North Karelia project and East-West studies). Scandinavian countries have population-based disease registries (e.g., the Swedish Tumor Registry; Manton et al., 1986). The National Cancer Institute's SEER program covers a large portion of the United States.

A number of surveys now describe the functional status of the elderly either by supplementing the sample with older persons (e.g., the Supplement on Aging - Longitudinal Survey on Aging (SOA-LSOA) or use of specialized survey designs (e.g., the 1982 to 1994 National Long Term Care Surveys (NLTCS)). Epidemiological studies of elderly populations were started (e.g., National Institute on Aging's Establishment of a Population for Epidemiologic Studies of the Elderly (EPESE) program) and instrumentation was added to existing studies (e.g., functional assessment in Framingham and the 30-year follow-ups of the Finnish, Dutch, and Italian components of the Seven Countries Study). In addition, vital statistics data on mortality and administrative data on health service use are generally of good quality. Because of the availability of data, health can be compared across culturally and socioeconomically diverse populations in developed countries (e.g., persons of Japanese ancestry in Hawaii: Reed et al., 1988; blacks and whites in Charleston, S.C.; Lackland et al., 1992).

Developing Countries

Developing countries often have health survey data due to World Health Organization (WHO) and United Nations programs. Most surveys rely on self-reported conditions and symptoms, and lack risk factor measurement. The 1976-1977 Indonesian disability survey used local physicians as interviewers but did not have formal clinical exams or measure risk factors (Dowd and Manton, 1992). There are now health surveys of the elderly in 17 countries in three WHO regions (e.g., Andrews et al., 1986; Manton et al., 1987). WHO's noncommunicable disease program sponsored Monitoring of Trends and Determinants in Cardiovascular Disease (MONICA) risk factor studies in 45 sites and cross-sectional surveys of CHD risk factors in Cuba, Ghana, Mauritius, Sri Lanka, Tanzania, and Thailand (Dowd and Manton, 1990). WHO and the National Institutes of Health sponsored stroke surveys in Taiwan, China, India, the United States, Nigeria, Colombia, Ecuador, Mexico, Venezuela, and Peru (Bharucha et al., 1988). However, with few longitudinal studies in developing countries, cross-sectional data on risk factor distributions may have to be combined with parameter estimates made from longitudinal studies in developed countries. Such a combination assumes that relations estimated from risk factor time-series data in developed countries represent biologically invariant characteristics of chronic disease processes. If this assumption "holds" (relative to the precision of other data employed) the model can legitimately integrate data and parameters from multiple sources.

A major methodological problem is to "mix" parameters estimated from ancillary longitudinal data sets to describe risk conditions in the reference population. Such a procedure is logically similar to "indirect standardization" (i.e., distributional differences are controlled by reweighting cell-specific rates) except that, within each cell population, we have a model describing the evolution of risk factors. Using models within each cell population exploits far more information than modeling a cell population by a single probability assuming the population is homogeneous. If the process is well described, inferences about health changes may be unconfounded from differences in the distribution of risk factors; that is, aggregate-individual interactions (conditional on individual parameters; Hoem, 1985, 1989) produce biases that are "negligible" relative to the precision of other estimates.

FORECASTING MODEL BASED ON INDIVIDUAL HEALTH CHANGES

To forecast health changes for n years, we use a cohort component projection model,

$$\mathbf{P}_{t+n} = \mathbf{G}_{t+n} \cdots \mathbf{G}_{t+1} \mathbf{P}_t \tag{1}$$

where $\mathbf{P}_t$ is a vector of age-specific population counts. The $\mathbf{G}$ matrix contains probabilities of surviving from one age category to the next for A age categories. One can produce projections for males and females or for ethnic groups by having **G**s and **P**s for each group. Survival probabilities are predicted from information on specific diseases and risk factors. The five-year probability of death is the sum of the probabilities of death for each of K causes. If we can eliminate a cause of death by intervention (e.g., influenza deaths may be eliminated among young and old persons by vaccination, nutritional supplements (e.g., vitamin A), and antiviral drugs) then we can eliminate (or reduce by a fixed amount) the probability of dying from influenza. How information is used in predicting each element of **G** differentiates forecasting models. We used a flexible model (Manton et al., 1992a) with components for risk factor change, i.e., the relation of risk factors to mortality. Below, the components are integrated in a comprehensive model to forecast health status.

Risk Factor Regressions

Risk factor regressions describe changes over time. Changes are due to lifestyle modification (cessation of smoking, less physical labor at work, reduction of stress); nutrition (change in protein-energy balance, fat consumption, micronutrient intake); environment (both general and job-related exposure); and health care access. The regressions describe changes over a fixed time period for each of J risk factors (and variables that either can be modified or are naturally undergoing changes we want to anticipate) as a function of age (many risk factors such as disability or cholesterol change with age), the prior value of risk factors (i.e., the person's health at the beginning of the period), factors affecting a person's ability to change (e.g., education, income), and exogenous factors (e.g., health programs).

The regression predicts risk factor values as a linear function of current age, risk state, and factors that can be changed to improve health:

$$x_{it+1} = u_0+(u_1 \cdot age_{it})+R_1x_{it}+(R_2x_{it} \cdot age_{it})+R_3z_{it}+e_{it}(age_{it})^d \qquad (2)$$

In the equation, u_0 is a constant (it may reflect genetic determinants of risk factor level), u_1 represents age effects, x_{it} are risk factor values at time t; d is the parameter that allows diffusion effects, e_{it}, to change with age. Many risk factors (R) interact and are correlated over time so all risk factors must be included in each equation. For example, smoking may raise blood pressure and reduce lung capacity, but reduce weight. Weight gain may increase blood glucose (a measure of diabetes and a CVD risk factor; Modan et al., 1991, 1992), serum cholesterol, and blood pressure. Thus, it is unrealistic to model changes in one risk factor at a time. For example, the Multiple Risk Factor Intervention Trial (MRFIT) Research Group (1990) found no improvement in mortality in 6.8 years of intervention; by 10.5 years, the medications had been changed and total mortality had dropped significantly. The original antihypertensive drug worsened cardiac arrythmias and adversely altered glucose metabolism, raising certain mortality risks.

We include interactions with age (i.e., $x_{it} \cdot age_{it}$) because risk factor effects may change with age. For example, reducing blood pressure may have adverse effects in an elderly person with preexisting heart disease. The z_{it} represents other factors such as education, income, employment, and public health efforts at disease prevention. Thus, Equation (2) both describes risk factor change with time and variables through which one might intervene. Only if intervention variables are modeled can their effects be assessed. This methodology differs from strict "cause elimination" in which all (or a fixed proportion of) deaths from a cause are assumed to be averted by an intervention. Cause elimination indicates the *potential* effect of intervention. Risk factor regressions *forecast* the size of the health effect and, possibly, help us understand why some effects fail to materialize.

The last term in Equation (2) represents the interaction of error with age (e.g., there may be less stability of blood pressure in elderly persons (McLean et al., 1992)) and adjusts regressions for age-related heteroscedasticity (systematically unequal variances).

To estimate each regression requires longitudinal data. Though such data are rare in developing countries, often age- and sex-specific distributions of risk factors are available from surveys (e.g., the six countries in Dowd and Manton, 1990; the 45 MONICA sites; or the 13 countries in Knuiman et al., 1982). Initial conditions (i.e., age-specific and sex-specific risk factor means and variances) can be combined with regression coefficients describing risk factor changes estimated from longitudinal studies in developed countries (e.g., Framingham, Kaunas, and Finnish East-West studies; Dowd and Manton, (1992)). In addition, socioeconomic factors may improve a regression's applicability to the population of interest.

Studies of risk factors in special populations can be used to assess assumptions of physiological invariance of the cross-temporal regressions (e.g., Lackland et al., 1992). Thus, coefficients describing the relation of two physiological variables, if socioeconomic status and demographic factors are controlled, may be less variable across countries than age- and sex-specific risk factor means and variances. Thus, if no longitudinal data exist, regressions estimated from studies in developed countries may be combined with data on age, sex, and socioeconomic population distributions, and age-specific and sex-specific risk factor distributions in the country. Later, we show how life tables are adjusted for country-specific mortality differences. Model assumptions can be verified in cross-national studies (Reed et al., 1991; Choi et al., 1990).

Multivariate Hazard Functions

Multivariate hazard functions describe mortality as functions of age and risk factors. The model below is based on the Gompertz function used to describe adult mortality:

$$\mu(age_{it}) = \alpha \cdot \exp(\theta \cdot age_{it}) \tag{3}$$

where α determines the mortality level (the scale parameter) and θ determines the shape of its age dependence (i.e., $\theta \times 100$ is the percentage that mortality increases per year). A θ of 0.0805 means mortality increases 8.05 percent per year. Equation (3) does not include risk factors. We generalized Equation (3) by substituting a scalar function of risk factor values (predicted from the regressions) for α. Thus, instead of a fixed-scale parameter, we use a scalar function of J time-varying risk factors, or

$$\mu(x_{it}, age_{it}) = (\mu_0 + \mathbf{b}^T x_{it} + \frac{1}{2} x_{it}^T \mathbf{B} x_{it}) \exp(\theta \cdot age_{it}) \tag{4}$$

where a quadratic function of risk factors is substituted for α. In Equation (4) there are terms describing mortality rates independent of age and risk factors (i.e., μ_0, expressed as a rate of deaths per 100,000 persons in a year); linear risk factor effects (i.e., **b**, a vector containing a linear coefficient for each risk factor scaled as a change in the annual mortality rate); and nonlinear effects (i.e., the matrix **B**, whose diagonals represent the effect on the mortality rate of risk factor values squared and whose off-diagonals represent the effect on mortality of the pairwise product of risk factors). The T superscript indicates that the vector or matrix should be transposed. In a Gompertz function, α is time invariant. In Equation (4) at each time, a new set of risk factor values (with or without interventions) estimated from the regressions is substituted. Each term is multiplied by the exponential function, representing the percentage increase in mortality per year of age. Thus, the constant can be evaluated for persons aged 45, 60, or 75 by substituting a value for age_{it} in the exponential and multiplying it by μ_0. This procedure is done for every coefficient in the hazard so that all risk factor effects are age dependent. Thus, we can examine the effect on the annual mortality rate of a risk factor change predicted by the regressions (e.g., a 5 percent reduction in cholesterol over two years due to dietary changes) at specific ages.

The addition of the J time-varying risk factors affects the values of other coefficients (i.e., if risk factors explain some of the age dependence of mortality, θ is correspondingly reduced). With a lot of risk factor information, mortality might be modeled with $\theta = 0$ (i.e., no age effect). It is more likely that some age-dependent risk factors are unmeasured, and country-specific unmeasured factors affect the age dependence of mortality. When we do not have measures of the risk factors causing the age dependence of mortality, their effect must be represented by μ_0 (the constant) and θ (i.e., μ_0 and θ represent the average constant and age-dependent effects, respectively, of unobserved risk factors on mortality).

The quadratic form of the hazard allows risk factor functions to be estimated for each cause of death and corresponding coefficients added to obtain a total mortality function:

$$\mu(x_{it}, age_{it}) = \sum_{k=1}^{K} \mu_k(x_{it}, age_{it}) = \sum_{k=1}^{K} (\mu_{0k} + \mathbf{b}_k^T x_{it} + \frac{1}{2} x_{it}^T \mathbf{B}_k x_{it}) \cdot \exp(\theta \cdot age_{it}). \tag{5}$$

Thus, if $K = 3$ (e.g., cancer, heart disease, and other), we estimate three equations like Equation (5) where μ_{0k}, $\mathbf{b}_k$, $\mathbf{B}_k$ differ by cause. They are summed to obtain total mortality. The same risk factor values are used in each equation.

In developing countries, age-specific and sex-specific means and variances of risk factors (e.g., smoking, body weight, blood pressure, cholesterol, blood glucose), estimates of the age dependence of total mortality, and the proportion of all deaths due to (exhaustive and exclusive) causes of death can be combined with regressions and hazard coefficients estimated with data from longitudinal studies in developed countries. The output is a cohort life table that shows, for example, how changing a risk factor affects life expectancy, the risk of death from each cause, and ages at which mortality is affected by direct and indirect risk factor effects. The life table also describes age changes in risk factor means and variances due to the deaths of persons with adverse risk factor values, as well as risk factor means and variances for *survivors*. Interventions are simulated by changing the initial risk factor distribution (a short-lived effect) or coefficients in the regression or mortality functions.

Cost Estimation

Forecasts are useful for public health planning in developing countries because adverse lifestyle habits (smoking) and dietary practices (fat consumption) may not have been adopted and may be prevented by central action (e.g., import taxes on cigarettes or alcohol). Clinical and epidemiological studies suggest that early (and low-cost) action on nutrition and physical activity can reduce disease and mortality at later ages (Blair et al., 1989; Lindsted et al., 1991; Paffenbarger et al., 1986; Zimmet et al., 1991).

Many developing countries lack adequate resources to deal with *current* health problems (e.g., infant and maternal health)—let alone future problems. To prioritize the allocation of scarce resources we must compare diverse, long-range outcomes. Two metrics for comparison are life expectancy (active life expectancy, if adjusted for disability), and changes in risk factors. Both represent health-adjusted "human capital." Active life expectancy is the productive *potential* of the population over its remaining lifetime. Risk factors represent the earliest factors in the causal chain leading to disease and disability.

To make decisions about interventions, the costs of different scenarios must be evaluated—possibly assigning different values to each year of life gained or lost. For example, one way to assign value is to see what an average person earns at all ages past t. If a person dies at t then lost wages, representing the value of the worker's production to the economy (i.e., what society was willing to pay for the labor), represent the indirect cost of death. Direct costs are the cost of trying to avert death and of the disposition of the individual and his property at death.

There are problems in translating human capital into monetary terms in economies with surplus labor. Human capital may be measured directly by a person's functional capacity. Such calculations are important in evaluating interventions in groups not active in the labor force (i.e., the young and the elderly). Thus, independent of labor force conditions, human capital is assumed to have intrinsic productive value. The problem is to estimate this intrinsic, but latent, value. The measure considered here is "active" life expectancy—life expectancy decomposed into disability categories.

EXAMPLES

Risk Factor Intervention

The regression and hazard coefficients are estimated from longitudinal data in developed countries and combined with country-specific mortality and risk factor data from developing countries to make forecasts. Illustrative life tables and age-specific risk factor values projected from parameters estimated from longitudinal data are given in Table 1.

The survival probability (l_t), life expectancy (e_t), and means (v_t) for eight risk factors are presented for survivors to age t. Estimates of age-specific risk factor means are presented for both independent and dependent elimination of CVD. In independent elimination, the resulting change in overall mortality does not change risk factor means and variances. Dependent elimination means that we calculate cause-specific life tables where risk-factor change and mortality functions interact, i.e., risk factor values for persons who would have died from the eliminated cause of death no longer died and are not subtracted from the risk factor means and variances so that mortality for the non-eliminated causes is increased.

Risk factor means differ over age between the two computations because eliminating CVD reduces mortality selection at later ages. For males at age 90, dependent elimination increases life expectancy 3.1 years (6.0 – 2.9). Under independence it increases 4.3 years (7.2 – 2.9). The decrease is 1.2 years less under dependence because persons with adverse risk factor values for CVD (e.g., smokers) now no longer die of CVD but die at later ages from the remaining diseases—if we assume that the eliminated cause had risk factors in common with one or more of the retained causes. Ignoring the effect of CVD mortality on risk factor means and variances overestimates CVD's effect on life expectancy by 26 percent.

In Tables 2A and 2B (Dowd and Manton, 1990), descriptive and risk factor statistics are presented for six developing countries, along with composite statistics for developed countries. Male life expectancy varies from

TABLE 1 Observed (baseline) and Cause Elimination Life Table Values for Males of Selected Ages if No Change in Risk Factors is Assumed

				v_{1t}	v_{2t}	v_{3t}	v_{4t}	v_{5t}	v_{6t}	v_{7t}	v_{8t}
	l_t	e_t	Age (years)	Pulse Pressure	Diastolic Blood Pressure	Body Mass Index	Serum Cholesterol	Blood Sugar	Hemoglobin	Vital Capacity Index	Cigarettes per Day
Baseline	100,000	43.9	30	45.0	80.0	260.0	215.0	80.0	145.0	140.0	14.0
Independence	100,000	54.8		45.0	80.0						
Dependence	100,000	53.9		45.0	80.0						
Baseline	68,108	10.8	70	63.0	82.8	266.1	223.0	98.5	150.7	100.8	4.9
Independence	86,701	18.8		63.0	82.8	266.1	223.0	98.5	150.7	100.8	4.9
Dependence	86,595	17.7		63.3	83.0	265.7	223.4	99.0	150.7	100.2	5.2
Baseline	5,754	2.9	90	77.3	80.8	250.3	204.7	111.9	151.9	78.0	0.0[a]
Independence	39,520	7.2		77.3	80.8	250.3	204.7	111.9	151.9	78.0	0.0[a]
Dependence	36,146	6.0		79.4	81.7	242.3	205.6	115.0	151.3	78.3	0.0[a]

NOTES: Independence and altering the risk factor distribution (dependence): CVD elimination, males, Framingham Heart Study (20-year follow-up).

Pulse pressure = difference between systolic and diastolic blood pressures, in millimeters of mercury.
Diastolic blood pressure = in millimeters of mercury.
Body mass index = hectograms (weight) per height squared (squared meters).
Serum cholesterol = milligrams of cholesterol per deciliter of blood.
Blood sugar = milligrams of glucose per deciliter of blood.
Hemoglobin = grams of hemoglobin per liter of blood.
Vital capacity index = centiliters of air volume per height squared (squared meters).

[a]Cigarette smoking was fixed at zero to prevent negative values.

49 years in Ghana to 72 years in Cuba. Proportionate mortality for CVD is lowest (21 percent) in Sri Lanka and highest (50 percent) in the developed country composite. Cancer risks are high in Cuba (22 percent; with the most smoking) and Tanzania (18 percent; with the lowest cholesterol). Cholesterol varies from 135 mg/dl in Tanzania to 215 mg/dl in Mauritius. The U.S. National Cholesterol Education Program identified cholesterol levels below 200 mg/dl as desirable, with values between 200 and 239 mg/dl as borderline but not requiring treatment unless other risk factors (e.g., hypertension, obesity, smoking) are present. This borderline area occurs because much of the risk of CVD comes from the effect of jointly elevated risk factors. Per capita smoking varics from 1.4 cigarettes per day in Sri Lanka to 11 per day in Cuba. Body mass index (BMI) varies little (206 – 220 hectograms per

TABLE 2A Mean Levels of Risk Factors in Six Developing Countries for Males Age 30-35

	Risk Factors Means				
	Systolic BP (mm/Hg)	Diastolic BP (mm/Hg)	BMI (hg/m^2)	Total Cholesterol (mg/dl)	Cigarettes per Day
Cuba[a]	125	80	220	200	11.0
Ghana[b]	134	82	206	180	2.3
Mauritius[a]	121	76	215	215	3.7
Sri Lanka[a]	120	75	206	211	1.4
Tanzania[b]	124	75	210	135	4.0
Thailand[a]	125	75	211	189	8.2
Developed[c]	125	80	260	215	10.0
Framingham	125	80	260	215	14.0
Framingham optimum[d]	110	74	255	212	0.0
Ideal[e]	120	75	250	200	0.0

NOTES: BP = blood pressure; BMI = body mass index; dl = deciliter; hg = hectogram; m^2 = square meter; mg = milligrams; mm = millimeters.

[a]World Health Organization (1987).

[b]Estimates for Ghana and Tanzania from United Nations Population Division (e_0, e_{15}, e_{30}) and from World Health Organization working documents (proportional mortality for those over 30 years).

[c]Developed country average: average of risk factor levels for males (age 30-35) from Framingham, Finnish East, Finnish West, and Kaunas, Lithuania studies.

[d]Manton et al. (1993)

[e]Ideal: target values generally accepted when a reduction in mortality from all causes is desired.

SOURCE: Dowd and Manton (1990:Table 1). By permission of Oxford University Press.

TABLE 2B Demographic and Epidemiologic Characteristics in Six Developing Countries for Males

Country	Population Size 1986 (millions)	Percentage 15-64 Years	Life Expectancy (years) at Age		Proportional Mortality for Those Over 30 Years (%)		
			0	30	Cancer	CVD	Other Causes
Cuba[a]	10.1	65.7	72	44	22	44	34
Ghana[b]	14.0	50.5	49	35	13	22	65
Mauritius[a]	1.1	65.0	65	43	10	45	45
Sri Lanka[a]	16.5	61.0	67	43.5	5	21	74
Tanzania[b]	23.3	49.0	50	37	18	22	60
Thailand[a]	52.3	60.0	63	40	15	30	55
Developed[c]	—	67.0	71	44	25	50	25

NOTE: CVD = cardiovascular disease

[a]World Health Organization (1987).

[b]Estimates for Ghana and Tanzania from United Nations Population Division (e_0,e_{15},e_{30}) and from WHO internal working documents (proportional mortality for those over 30 years).

[c]Developed country: average of risk factor levels for males age (30-35) from Framingham, Finnish East, Finnish West, and Kaunas, Lithuania studies.

SOURCE: Dowd and Manton (1990:Table 2). By permission of Oxford University Press.

square meter), but these levels are low (e.g., the average for developed countries is 260). Blood pressure is highest in Ghana (134/82). CVD in developing countries is often due to untreated hypertension.

In Table 3 the economic benefits of interventions are illustrated along with changes in total and cause-specific mortality achieved by restricting risk factors to an "ideal" profile. These calculations were carried out for males age 30 years and older in six countries with cross-sectional (age-specific and sex-specific) risk factor and proportional mortality data. The population was projected to extinction by using Equation (1), both with ("ideal") and without (baseline) interventions in each of the cohort equa-

TABLE 3 Projected Changes in Median Age at Death and Total Mortality When Risk Factors Take on "Ideal" Values[a]

Median Age at Death	Cuba	Ghana	Mauritius	Sri Lanka	Tanzania	Thailand
			Total Mortality			
Baseline (years)	73.10	65.99	73.90	71.51	68.97	70.61
"Ideal" (change in years)	(3.51)	(4.51)	(2.09)	(4.99)	(6.40)	(4.33)
			Cancer Mortality			
Baseline (years)	72.73	63.80	72.36	72.13	67.89	69.56
"Ideal" (change in years)	(3.87)	(4.47)	(2.06)	(3.92)	(5.67)	(4.73)
Percent of total mortality						
Baseline	26.0	12.5	10.0	8.0	18.0	15.0
"Ideal"	23.5	11.5	9.5	8.0	14.0	14.0
			Cardiovascular Mortality			
Baseline (years)	72.80	63.73	73.84	71.91	68.29	69.99
"Ideal" (change in years)	(3.40)	(4.88)	(1.88)	(4.40)	(5.54)	(4.53)
Percent of total mortality						
Baseline	40.0	22.0	45.0	20.0	22.0	28.0
"Ideal"	42.5	24.5	45.0	24.0	34.0	32.0
			Residual Mortality			
Baseline (years)	73.74	67.01	74.27	71.34	69.52	71.15
"Ideal" (change in years)	(3.37)	(4.48)	(2.25)	(5.28)	(5.40)	(4.19)
Percent of total mortality						
Baseline	34.0	65.5	45.0	72.0	60.0	57.0
"Ideal"	34.0	64.0	45.5	68.0	52.0	54.0
Gain in "ideal" scenarios						
U.S. $	678.38	153.35	163.32	133.12	83.64	247.67
Percent GNP	36.4	41.5	14.9	35.0	29.9	31.0

[a]For males age 30 and older.

SOURCE: Dowd and Manton (1990:Table 4). By permission of Oxford University Press.

tions for risk factor changes and mortality used to generate elements of **G**. The six developing countries have life expectancies from near those of the United States (i.e., Cuba) to those of extremely poor countries. Risk factor effects vary in different country conditions. The greatest gain in median age at death for the ideal risk factor profile is in Tanzania (6.4 years). In Ghana the gain in median age at death is less (4.5 years) but the proportionate gain in GNP is highest, 41.5 percent. This results occurs because the distribution of cause-specific mortality was close to that predicted by the ideal profile (a cancer excess did not exist); the population was younger than in Tanzania so that young persons were affected. Thus, the most important risk factors are associated with differences in the age-specific and sex-specific means and variance of risk factors across countries (e.g., in the least developed countries, cholesterol and BMI are low and blood pressure is elevated; in developed countries the level of detection and treatment of hypertension is high). Economic impact depends on the age profile of mortality (cancer generally affects younger persons than CVD) and the population age distribution (i.e., demographic parameters relevant to labor force activity interact with health parameters in determining economic effects). The ideal risk factor profile improved total and cause-specific mortality for all countries. GNP (converted to U.S. dollars) also increased in all countries.

Active Life Expectancy (ALE)

In evaluating interventions, the gain in life expectancy may not be the most relevant measure. A measure directly representing a person's physical and mental capacity may be more appropriate. One measure weights health by subjective factors (e.g., quality adjusted life years, QALYs; Wright, 1990). QALYs are criticized because weights are determined subjectively (LaPuma and Lawlor, 1990) and calibrating instruments are not validated (Carr-Hill and Morris, 1991).

A second approach decomposes life expectancy into the time expected to be lived in states defined by level and type of functional ability. To define these states we calculate scores on multiple dimensions of physical and cognitive functioning identified from self-reported items. The scores are then used in the forecasts. Table 4 presents male and female active life expectancy (ALE) estimates based on functional dimensions identified from (a) 27 measures of physical and mental performance for 25,541 respondents to the 1982 and 1984 NLTCS, and (b) 31 health and functioning measures on 16,600 Medicare-eligible, noninstitutionalized U.S. respondents in four sites. By presenting results from two studies, we can compare functional dimensions derived from different survey instruments and different populations (the Medicare sample excluded institutional residents and was not a national sample).

TABLE 4 Active Life Expectancy Estimates from 1982-1984 NLTCS and 1985-1989 Experience in Four U.S. Counties

				Active[b]		Frail[c]	
Age	Source	Population	e_t (years)[a]	Mean Residual Lifetime (years)	Initial Proportion Alive	Mean Residual Lifetime (years)	Initial Proportion Alive
Males							
65	Medicare	100,000	15.2	12.94	.86	.46	.03
	NLTCS	100,000	15.4	13.42	.93	.73	.05
75	Medicare	63,192	11.4	8.42	.86	.60	.05
	NLTCS	66,272	10.7	8.75	.92	.59	.06
85	Medicare	33,593	7.1	4.73	.72	.81	.12
	NLTCS	32,587	6.6	4.69	.78	.88	.13
95	Medicare	9,093	3.6	2.69	.52	.81	.23
	NLTCS	7,061	4.4	2.89	.65	1.08	.24
Females							
65	Medicare	100,000	21.4	16.06	.94	.58	.03
	NLTCS	100,000	20.5	16.20	.91	.79	.03
75	Medicare	81,487	15.2	9.74	.90	.60	.04
	NLTCS	80,560	14.2	10.01	.88	.98	.08
85	Medicare	57,951	9.2	4.54	.73	.90	.09
	NLTCS	53,931	8.5	4.72	.69	1.77	.20
95	Medicare	24,695	4.7	2.58	.46	1.36	.29
	NLTCS	18,192	5.5	2.61	.47	2.08	.38

[a]Life expectancy at age *t*.
[b]Functional class 1 in NLTCS and functional classes 1 and 5 in Medicare-eligible respondents.
[c]Functional classes 5, 6, and institutional in NLTCS and functional classes 3 and 6 in Medicare-eligible respondents.

The dimensions of ability/disability are identified by a multivariate procedure (i.e., grade of membership analysis; Woodbury and Clive, 1974; Woodbury et al., 1978) from measures reported with error. If the 27 and 31 measures define a small number of "similar" dimensions, scores may be compared between populations. "Comparison" of dimensions in two populations can be done either by matching the association of each self-reported item with each dimension in the two analyses or by conducting an analysis on data pooled from the two data sets. In the first case, validation depends on the correlation of the dimensions with independent measures (e.g., mortality, acute and long-term care (LTC) service use, age and sex; Manton et al., 1991c). In the second, the analysis is performed by using the missing-information principle (Orchard and Woodbury, 1971) to infer scores for the developing country. The procedure used is robust to differences in sampling; other multivariate procedures such as principle components are not. If dimensions that represent functioning in the combined populations are defined, the disability scores can be compared (Manton et al., 1991a) and used to project change in function.

The dimensions derived from the two analyses were similar. They are less subject to measurement error than the original items; because they are statistically weighted averages, averaging over multiple items by using optimized weights improves reliability. These dimensions have excellent predictive validity for health service use, mortality, and sociodemographic measures in the United States (e.g., Manton and Stallard, 1990, 1991; Manton et al., 1992b). Life tables calculated from the two populations (labeled Medicare and NLTCS) appear in Table 4 (Manton et al., 1991a).

Both the total life expectancy (e.g., male e_t in the NLTCS is 15.4 years at age 65) and the decomposition of e_t into the proportion expected to be lived with given levels and types of impairment are presented. Of the 15.4 years in NLTCS, about 93 percent, or 14.3 years, is expected to be lived free of disability. These people could continue to work or perform social functions (e.g., provide child care within the family or care for other disabled persons). As in the case of risk factors, we can "intervene" in the progression of disability with aging to forecast what life expectancy and costs would be if intervention goals are met.

For the purposes of illustration, we present ALE as estimated for U.S. cohorts representing all ages 65 and above for a given date, for 1990 and 2020.

We conducted two simulations: persons remaining "active" to death, and persons remaining frail to death (both from age 65). In the first case, male life expectancy was 23.6 years and female life expectancy was 33.4 years. For frail males, life expectancy was 5.1 years and for frail females, life expectancy was 7.4 years.

The strategy used for risk factors can be used to estimate ALE for developing countries when longitudinal data on disability are missing. From cross-sectional surveys of functioning in developing countries (which exist in many cases), we calculate scores specific to age and sex that may be similar in substantive content to scores calculated from longitudinal surveys of disability in developed countries. The age and sex distribution of scores in the developing country can be combined with parameters describing age-specific rates of change in disability, and the dependence of mortality on the scores, estimated from a longitudinal study in a developed country.

A concern is that functional measures may be more culturally dependent than risk factors such as blood pressure (although there are measurement effects for risk factors such as "white coat" hypertension; anxiety over a medical visit also acutely raises hematocrit and cholesterol). The 27 measures in the NLTCS involve well-defined physical tasks (e.g., hold a 10-pound package, climb one flight of stairs, rise from a seated position) and ADLs (Katz and Akpom, 1976; Katz et al., 1983). ADLs are based on a sociobiological model of the acquisition during childhood (and loss with age in reverse order) of biologically fundamental self-maintenance skills (e.g., toileting, bathing, eating, dressing, and walking). Thus, these functions have to be performed in developing countries (they are basic to human existence), but the social and physical environment may make some harder or easier to do. Instrumental activities of daily living (IADLs) also represent tasks necessary for self-maintenance (e.g., laundry, cooking). With appropriate adjustments, ADLs and IADLs could be meaningfully assessed in rural and developing country settings.

SUMMARY

We have discussed strategies for combining multiple data sets to forecast morbidity, disability, and mortality, and presented a three-part model based on mortality and cross-sectional risk factor or disability data from a developing country, and longitudinal risk factor and survival parameter estimates from a developed country. This model assumes invariance of health and functional *process* parameters (but not distributions) across socioeconomic and cultural conditions. Such assumptions are reasonable for physiological risk factors. For functional measures, the validity of the assumption is improved if socioeconomic covariates are available.

A health forecasting model is useful in planning health interventions for developing countries. A model is necessary because successful strategies should consider all elements of a health care system simultaneously—public health efforts at primary prevention; access to primary health care facilities; and modern health care facilities to treat serious diseases. Often strategies in developing countries have emphasized one sector of health care over another at different times. This single-sector, sequential strategy has seldom proved successful (Cox, 1992). To identify the optimal balance and timing of interventions in different health service sectors requires evaluating multiple demographic, health, and economic parameters. This complexity requires a model to reflect interrelations of factors to determine the most efficient service mix for specific conditions.

Without a dynamic model it is difficult to guage accurately the quantitative effects of intervention. Clearly, reducing smoking has broad and large health benefits. However, there are small (relative to benefits) but real adverse consequences of smoking reduction that must be considered (e.g., persons who quit smoking may gain weight, leading to increases in blood pressure, cholesterol level, and blood sugar). Furthermore, without a model, one will have difficulty in assessing the "true" level of risk for an individual from a single risk factor measurement (Keli et al., 1992). People may be misclassified in risk categories and estimates may be distorted so that choosing between such qualitatively different health strategies as "high-risk" (i.e., screening and then treatment) versus "population-based" (i.e., reducing risk factor levels in the population) approaches is difficult. The evaluation of these two strategies is affected by the form of the risk function and the population distribution of risk factors (Strachan and Rose, 1991). Thus, biologically accurate models are necessary to make good qualitative policy choices.

Finally, models provide tools to monitor population health change and intervention effects in a systematic way. One may initially have to select a strategy using "uncertain" long-range projections. The use of models in surveillance can aid in the management of programs and in the "fine tuning" of interventions by tracking real-time effects. For example, the elderly in the United States and other countries are very health conscious (e.g., the greatest changes in risk factors have been for persons aged 65 to 74). However, U.S. public health interventions have been directed toward *avoiding* risk factors rather than optimizing nutrition in target groups. Thus, although cholesterol levels declined in the United States between 1977 and 1987, there was little recognition of the special nutritional needs of the elderly—who are often malnourished (Popkin et al., 1992). Thus, health interventions have to be crafted for specific country conditions and for the special health problems of target groups.

REFERENCES

Andrews, G.R., A.J. Esterman, A.J. Braunack-Mayer, and C. Runge
1986 *Aging in the Western Pacific: A Four-Country Study*. Manila: Western Region World Health Organization.

Barker, D.J.P., and C.N. Martyn
1992 The maternal and fetal origins of cardiovascular disease. *Journal of Epidemiology and Community Health* 46:8-11.

Barker, D.J.P., A.R.Bull, C. Osmond, and S.J. Simmonds
1991a Fetal and placental size and risk of hypertension in adult life. *British Medical Journal* 301:259-262.

Barker, D.J.P, K.M. Godfrey, C. Fall, C. Osmond, P.D. Winter, and S.O. Shaheen
1991b Relation of birth weight and childhood respiratory infection to adult lung function and death from chronic obstructive airways disease. *British Medical Journal* 303:672-675.

Barker, D.J.P., K.M. Godfrey, C. Osmond, and A. Bull
1992a The relation of fetal length, ponderal index and head circumference to bloodpressure and the risk of hypertension in adult life. *Pediatric and Perinatal Epidemiology* 6:35-44.

Barker, D.J.P., T.W. Meade, C.H.D. Fall, A. Lee, C. Osmond, K. Phipps, and Y. Stirling
1992b Relation of fetal and infant growth to plasma fibrinogen and factor VII concentrations in adult life. *British Medical Journal* 304:148-152.

Barthel, J.S., T.U. Westblom, A.D. Havey, F. Gonzalez, and E.D. Everett
1988 Gastritis and *Campylobacter pylori* in healthy, asymptomatic volunteers. *Archives of Internal Medicine* 148:1149-1151.

Bharucha, N.E., E.P. Bharucha, A.E. Bharucha, A.V. Bhise, and B.S. Schoenberg
1988 Prevalence of stroke in the Parsi community of Bombay. *Stroke* 19(1):60-62.

Blair, S.N., H.W. Kohl, R.S. Paffenbarger, D.G. Clark, K.H. Cooper, and L.W. Gibbons
1989 Physical fitness and all-cause mortality: A prospective study of healthy men and women. *Journal of the American Medical Association* 262:2395-2401.

Blaser, M.J.
1988 Type B gastritis, aging, and *Campylobacter pylori*. *Archives of Internal Medicine* 148:1021-1022.

Carr-Hill, R.A., and J. Morris
1991 Current practice in obtaining the "Q" in QALYs: A cautionary note. *British Medical Journal* 303:699-701.

Chen, Z., R. Peto, R. Collins, S. MacMahon, J. Lu, and W. Li
1991 Serum cholesterol concentration and coronary heart disease in population with low cholesterol concentrations. *British Medical Journal* 303:276-282.

Chiang, C.L.
1968 *Introduction to Stochastic Processes in Biostatistics*. New York: John Wiley & Sons.

Choi, E.S., R.B. McGandy, G.E. Dallal, R.M. Russell, R.A. Jacob, E.J. Schaefer, and J.A. Sadowski
1990 The prevalence of cardiovascular risk factors among elderly Chinese Americans. *Archives of Internal Medicine* 150:413-420.

Cowan, L.C., D. O'Connell, M.H. Criqui, et al.
1990 Cancer mortality and lipid and lipoprotein levels. *American Journal of Epidemiology* 131(3):468.

Cox, P.S.V.
1992 Prevention vs cure in developing countries: The pendulum syndrome. *Lancet* 339:664-665.

Crow, Y.J., K.G.M. Alberti, and J.M. Parkin
1991 Insulin dependent diabetes in childhood and maternal deprivation in northern England, 1977-86. *British Medical Journal* 303:158-160.

Dodu, S.R.A.
1988 Emergence of CVD in developing countries. *Cardiology* 75:56-64.

Dowd, J.E., and K.G. Manton
1990 Forecasting chronic disease risks in developing countries. *International Journal of Epidemiology* 19(4):1018-1036.
1992 Projections of disability consequences in Indonesia. *Journal of Cross-Cultural Gerontology* 7(3):237-258.

Evans, J.
1990 The economic status of older men and women in the Javanese household and the influence of this upon their nutritional level. *Journal of Cross-Cultural Gerontology* 5:217-242.

Forman, D.
1991 Helicobacter pylori infection: A novel risk factor in the etiology of gastric cancer. *Journal of the National Cancer Institute* 83(23):1702-1703.

Forman, D., F. Sitas, N.G. Newell, A.R. Stacey, J. Boreham, R. Peto, T.C. Campbell, J. Li, and J.Chen
1990 Geographic association of Helicobacter pylori antibody prevalence and gastric cancer mortality in rural China. *International Journal of Cancer* 46:608-611.

Hamm, P., R.B. Shekelle, and J. Stamler
1989 Large fluctuations in body weight during young adulthood and twenty-five-year risk of coronary death in men. *American Journal of Epidemiology* 129:312-318.

Hoem, J.M.
1985 Weighting, misclassification and other issues in the analysis of survey samples of life histories. Pp. 249-293 in J.J. Heckman and B. Singer, eds., *Longitudinal Analysis of Labor Market Data*. Cambridge, Mass.: Cambridge University Press.
1989 The issue of weights in panel surveys of individual behavior. Pp. 539-559 in D. Kasprzyk, G. Duncan, G. Kalton, and M.P. Singh, eds., *Panel Surveys*. New York: John Wiley & Sons.

Isles, C.G., D.J. Hole, C.R. Gillis, V.M. Hawthorne, and A.F. Lever
1989 Plasma cholesterol, coronary heart disease, and cancer in the Renfrew and Paisley survey. *British Medical Journal* 298:920-928.

Jacques, P.F., S.C. Hartz, R.B. McGandy, R.A. Jacob, and R.M. Russell
1987 Ascorbic acid, HDL, and total plasma cholesterol in the elderly. *Journal of the American College of Nutrition* 6:169-174.

Katz, S., and C.A. Akpom
1976 A measure of primary sociobiological functions. *International Journal of Health Services* 6:493-508.

Katz, S., L.G. Branch, M.H. Branson, J.A. Papsidero, J.C. Beck, and D. S. Greer
1983 Active life expectancy. *New England Journal of Medicine* 309:1218-1223.

Keli, S., B. Bloemberg, and D. Kromhout
1992 Predictive value of repeated systolic blood pressure measurements for stroke risk. *Stroke* 23(3):347-351.

Kesteloot, H., D.X. Huang, X.S. Yang, J. Claes, M. Rosseneu, J. Goboers, and J. V. Joossens
1985 Serum lipids in the People's Republic of China: Comparison of western and eastern populations. *Arteriosclerosis* 5:427-433.

Kimura, N., H. Toshima, Y. Nakayama, K. Takayama, H. Tashiro, and M. Takagi
1979 Fifteen-year follow-up population survey on stroke: A multivariate analysis of the risk of stroke in farmers of Tanushimaru and fisherman of Ushibuka. Pp. 505-510 in Y. Yamori, W. Lovenberg, and E.D. Freis, eds., *Prophylatic Approach to Hypertensive Diseases*. New York: Raven Press.

Knuiman, J.T., C.E. West, and J. Burema
1982 Serum total and high density lipoprotein cholesterol concentrations and body mass

index in adult men from 15 countries. *American Journal of Epidemiology* 116(4):631-642.

Lackland, D.T., J.J. Orchard, J.E. Keil, D.E. Saunders, F.C. Wheeler, L.L. Adams-Campbell, R.H. McDonald, and R.G. Knapp
1992 Are race differences in the prevalence of hypertension explained by body mass and fat distribution? A survey in a biracial population. *International Journal of Epidemiology* 21:236-245.

Lam, K.M.C., N. Syed, H. Whittle, and D.H. Crawford
1991 Circulating Epstein-Barr virus-carrying B cells in acute malaria. *Lancet* 337:876-878.

LaPuma, J., and E.F. Lawlor
1990 Quality-adjusted life-years. *Journal of the American Medical Association* 263:2917-2921.

Lee, I-M., R.S. Paffenbarger, and C-C Hsieh
1991 Physical activity and risk of developing colorectal cancer among college alumni. *Journal of the National Cancer Institute* 83:1324-1329.

Lindsted, K.D., S. Tonstad, and J.W. Kuzma
1991 Self-report of physical activity and patterns of mortality in Seventh-Day Adventist men. *Journal of Clinical Epidemiology* 44:355-364.

Manton, K.G., H. Malker, and B. Malker
1986 Comparison of temporal changes in U.S. and Swedish lung cancer, 1950-51 to 1981-82. *Journal of the National Cancer Institute* 77(3):665-675.

Manton, K.G., G.C. Myers, and G. Andrews
1987 Morbidity and disability patterns in four developing nations: Their implications for social and economic integration of the elderly. *Journal of Cross-Cultural Gerontology* 2:115-129.

Manton, K.G., and E. Stallard
1990 Changes in health functioning and mortality. Pp. 140-162 in S. Stahl, ed., *The Legacy of Longevity: Health and Health Care in Later Life*. Newbury Park, Calif.: Sage Publications.
1991 Cross-sectional estimates of active life expectancy for the U.S. elderly and oldest-old populations. *Journal of Gerontology* 48:S170-182.

Manton, K.G., J.E. Dowd, and M.A. Woodbury
1991a Methods to identify geographic and social clustering of disability and disease burden. Pp. 61-84 in A.G. Hill, and J. Caldwell, eds., *Measurement of Health Transition Concepts*. Canberra: Australian National University Press.

Manton, K.G., E. Stallard, and S. Wing
1991b Analyses of black and white differentials in the age trajectory of mortality in two closed cohort studies. *Statistics in Medicine* 10:1043-1059.

Manton, K.G., E. Stallard, and M.A. Woodbury
1991c A multivariate event history model based upon fuzzy states: Estimation from longitudinal surveys with informative nonresponse. *Journal of Official Statistics* 7:261-293.

Manton, K.G., M.A. Woodbury, and E. Stallard
1991d Statistical and measurement issues in assessing the welfare status of aged individuals and populations. *Journal of Econometrics* 50:151-181.

Manton, K.G., E. Stallard, and B. Singer
1992a Sources of uncertainty in projecting the size and health status of the U.S. elderly population. *International Journal of Forecasting* 8(3):433-458.

Manton, K.G., M.A. Woodbury, E. Stallard, and L.S. Corder
1992b The use of Grade of Membership techniques to estimate regression relationships. In P. Marsden, ed., *Sociological Methodology*. London: Blackwell.

Manton, K.G., J.E. Dowd, and E. Stallard

1993 The effects of risk factors on male and female cardiovascular risks in middle and late age. In K.G. Manton, B. Singer, and R. Suzman, eds., *Forecasting the Health of Elderly Populations*. New York: Springer-Verlag.

McGill, H.C.

1988 Cerebral artery atherosclerosis and diet. *Stroke* 19(7):801.

McLean, K.A., P.A. O'Neill, I. Davies, and J. Morris

1992 Influence of age on plasma osmolality: A community study. *Age and Ageing* 21:56-60.

McMurray, M.P., M.T. Cerqueira, S.L. Connor, and W.E. Connor

1991 Changes in lipid and lipoprotein levels and body weight in Tarahumara Indians after consumption of an affluent diet. *New England Journal of Medicine* 325(24):1704-1708.

Modan, M., S. Almog, Z. Fuchs, A. Chetrit, A. Lusky, and H. Halkin

1991 Obesity, glucose intolerance, hyperinsulinemia, and response to antihypertensive drugs. *Hypertension* 17(4):565-573.

Modan, M., J. Or, A. Krasik, Y. Drory, Z. Fucha, A. Lusky, A. Chetrit, and H. Halkin

1992 Cardiovascular disease in men. *Circulation* 85(3):1220.

Mohr, G.C., D. Kritz-Silverstein, and E. Barrett-Connor

1991 Plasma lipids and gallbladder disease. *American Journal of Epidemiology* 134(1):78-85.

Mozar, H.N., D.G. Bal, and S.A. Farag

1990 The natural history of atherosclerosis: An ecologic perspective. *Atherosclerosis* 82:157-164.

Multiple Risk Factor Intervention Trial (MRFIT) Research Group

1990 Mortality rates after 10.5 years for participants in the multiple risk factor intervention trial. *Journal of the American Medical Association* 263:1795-1801.

Muscari, A., C. Bozzoli, G.M. Puddu, C. Rovinetti, G.P. Fiorentini, R.A. Roversi, and P. Puddu

1990 Correlations between serum lipids and complement components in adults without demonstrated atherosclerotic disease. *Atherosclerosis* 81:111-118.

National Center for Health Statistics

1987 The Supplement on Aging to the 1984 National Health Interview Survey. In J. Fitti and M.G. Kovar, eds., *Vital and Health Statistics*. Series 1, No. 21. DHHS Pub. No. (PHS) 87-1323, Public Health Service. Washington, D.C.: U.S. Government Printing Office.

Nomura, A.M.Y., G.N. Stemmermann, and P-H. Chyou

1991 Prospective study of serum cholesterol levels and large-bowel cancer. *Journal of the National Cancer Institute* 83:1403-1407.

Orchard, R., and M.A. Woodbury

1971 A missing information principle: Theory and application. Pp. 697-715 in L.M. LeCam, J. Neyman, and E.L. Scott, eds., *Proceedings Sixth Berkeley Symposium on Mathematical Statistics and Probability*. Berkeley: University of California Press.

Paffenbarger, R.S., R.T. Hyde, A.L. Wing, and C.C. Hsieh

1986 Physical activity, all-cause mortality, and longevity of college alumni. *New England Journal of Medicine* 314:605-613.

Parsonnet, J., G.D. Friedman, D.P. Vandersteen, Y. Chang, J.H. Vogelman, N. Orentreich, and R. K. Sibley

1991 Helicobacter pylori infection and the risk of gastric carcinoma. *New England Journal of Medicine* 325(16):1127-1131.

Popkin, B.M., P.S. Haines, and R.E. Patterson
1992 Dietary changes in older Americans, 1977-1987. *American Journal of Clinical Nutrition* 55:823-830.

Prevot, S., S. Hamilton-Dutoit, J. Audoouin, P. Walter, G. Pallesen, and J. Diebold
1992 Analysis of African Burkitt's and high-grade B cell non-Burkitt's lymphoma for Epstein-Barr virus genomes using in situ hybridization. *British Journal of Haematology* 80:27-32.

Reed, D.M., J.A. Resch, T. Hayashi, C. MacLean, and K. Yano
1988 A prospective study of cerebral artery atherosclerosis. *Stroke* 19:820-825.

Reed, T., J. Quiroga, J.V. Selby, D. Carmelli, J.C. Christian, R.R. Fabsitz, and C.E. Grim
1991 Concordance of ischemic heart disease in the NHLBI twin study after 14-18 years of follow-up. *Journal of Clinical Epidemiology* 44:797-805.

Schwartzkopff, W., J. Schleicher, I. Pottins, S-B. Yu, C-Z Han, and D-Y. Du
1990 Lipids, lipoproteins, apolipoproteins and other risk factors in Chinese men and women with and without myocardial infarction. *Atherosclerosis* 82:253-259.

Strachan, D., and G. Rose
1991 Strategies of prevention revisited: Effects of imprecise measurement of risk factors on the evaluation of "high-risk" and "population-based" approaches to prevention of cardiovascular disease. *Journal of Clinical Epidemiology* 44(11):1187-1196.

Sullivan, J.L.
1989 The iron paradigm of ischemic heart disease. *American Heart Journal* 117:1177-1188.

Talley, N.J., A.R. Zinsmeister, A. Weaver, E.P. DiMagno, H.A. Carpenter, G.I. Perez-Perez, and M.J. Blaser
1991 Gastric adenocarcinoma and helicobacter pylori infection. *Journal of the National Cancer Institute* 83:1734-1739.

Tertov, V.V., A.N. Orekhov, K.S. Sayadyan, S.G. Serebrennikov, A.G. Kacharava, A.A. Lyakishev, and V.N. Smirnov
1990 Correlation between cholesterol content in circulating immune complexes and atherogenic properties of CHD patients' serum manifested in cell culture. *Atherosclerosis* 81:183-189.

Tonglet, R., P. Bourdoux, T. Minga, and A-M. Ermans
1992 Efficacy of low oral doses of iodized oil in the control of iodine deficiency in Zaire. *New England Journal of Medicine* 326:236-241.

Trowell, H.C., and D.P. Burkitt
1991 *Western Diseases: Their Emergence and Prevention.* Cambridge, Mass.: Harvard University Press.

Wilson, A.O., D.J. Adamchak, and A.C. Nyanguru
1991 A study of well-being of elderly people in three communities in Zimbabwe. *Age and Ageing* 20:275-279.

Woodbury, M.A., and J. Clive
1974 Clinical pure types as a fuzzy partition. *Journal of Cybernetics* 4:111-121.

Woodbury, M.A., J. Clive, and A. Garson
1978 Mathematical typology: A grade of membership technique for obtaining disease definition. *Computers and Biomedical Research* 11:277-298.

World Health Organization
1987 *World Health Statistics Annual 1987.* Geneva: World Health Organization.

Wright, L.
1990 The role of aging in establishing social priorities: An economic perspective. Pp. 647-658 in R.L. Kane, J.G. Evans, and D. MacFadyen, eds., *Improving the Health of Older People: A World View*. Oxford: World Health Organization and Oxford University Press.

Zimmet, P.Z., V.R. Collins, G.K. Dowse, G.M.M. Alberti, Z. Tuomilehto, H. Gareeboo, and P. Chitson
1991 The relation of physical activity to cardiovascular disease risk factors in Mauritians. *American Journal of Epidemiology* 134:862-875.

Health Indices as a Guide to Health Sector Planning: A Demographic Critique

Samuel H. Preston

Cruel choices have got to be made, and it seems to me utterly irresponsible in a public official to make these choices without tracing their consequences to the fullest extent possible.

Milton Russell (1990)

INTRODUCTION

This paper examines, from a demographic perspective, the index of healthy years of life saved by health interventions. This index has been widely applied to summarize the expected gains from health programs in developing countries. The paper attempts to identify the demographic circumstances under which this index does and does not provide reliable information. It compares existing practices to the demographic accounting identities that describe how populations change over time. Problems that are revealed in using the index as a planning instrument include imprecision about the time sequence and age pattern of health program effects; inconsistency of assumptions; failure to incorporate interactions among disease processes; and failure to make explicit potentially valuable information. These problems are averted by the use of population projection to demonstrate the expected effects of health programs.

Samuel H. Preston is at the Population Studies Center, University of Pennsylvania.

BACKGROUND

In 1981, a useful and very detailed analysis of diseases in Ghana developed a measure of the years of healthy life lost to various diseases (Ghana Health Assessment Project Team, 1981). Although similar measures had been proposed earlier, the careful and imaginative application of this measure to a concrete situation drew attention to the procedure as a possible device for health planning. It was quickly recognized that what was needed for planning purposes was not an index of the total burden of a disease but that portion of the burden that could be eliminated by a health program. It was also recognized that the healthy years saved by a program would have to be related to the cost of the program. The measure of healthy years of life saved became the numerator of a cost-effectiveness calculation that permitted comparisons across various kinds of health programs (e.g., Prost and Prescott, 1984; Barnum, 1987).

These and other analyses have elaborated on this measure and considered whether to treat all healthy years lost to a disease (i.e., potentially saved through health interventions) equally (Murray, 1990; Mooney and Creese, 1990). The main issues here are:

(1) whether to discount years saved beyond the initial year by a social discount rate, which has become a conventional procedure in assessing many government programs;

(2) whether to count years saved in the "productive" age interval (typically, 15-60 or 15-65) in the same fashion as years saved outside this interval;

(3) whether disabled or unhealthy years of life should be treated in the same way as years lost to premature death (some have argued that disability actually exacts a higher social cost than death and should be given greater negative weight (Prost and Prescott, 1984), whereas most other analysts would take the point of view of the potential victim and apply a lower weight to disabled years than to years lost to death); and

(4) whether to recognize different degrees of disability, morbidity, and quality of life in arriving at a single index. A great deal of attention has been devoted to the development of health status indicators in developed countries (for recent reviews, see Patrick and Deyo, 1989; Loomes and McKenzie, 1989).

One way of dealing with these issues is to present different measures embodying the distinctions raised above and allow health planners to choose among them. Such an elaboration proved unwieldy in the World Bank's massive Health Sector Priority Review. This valuable assessment of 48 types of health interventions in developing countries settled on an index of the cost-effectiveness of discounted years of healthy life for making inter-program comparisons. That is, the questions identified above were resolved in favor of discounting future years (a discount rate of .03 was recommended); treating years inside and outside the productive range equally; treating years lost to disability and death equally; and ignoring distinctions among degrees of disability (Jamison and Mosley, 1991:Chapter 1). Individual chapters in the review often use a wider variety of indicators.

These choices inevitably affect the relative value of interventions targeted at children and those targeted at adults. The decision to discount increases the relative cost-effectiveness of adult interventions, because the years of healthy life gained by children lie further in the future, on average, than those gained by adults. The choice of a low discount rate, however, makes this tilt less consequential. The decision not to give higher weight to years saved in the productive age span clearly promotes the relative cost-effectiveness of interventions aimed at children. This decision seems more vulnerable to criticism than others. Neonatal deaths (nearly half of childhood deaths in developing countries) are often "replaced" by additional births that would not otherwise have occurred. Such replacement is clearly not possible among adults. Furthermore, an infant's net contribution to other members of a society is obviously less than that of older children and adults.

The consequences of some of these choices for the relative importance of programs aimed at children and those aimed at a wider spectrum of ages are illustrated nicely by Prost and Prescott (1984). Table 1 reproduces their comparison of a measles control program and a program of onchocerciasis control in the Côte d'Ivoire. If an index of *discounted* years of *productive* life is used, as advocated by the authors, onchocerciasis control is more cost-effective than measles immunization. For any of the three remaining versions of the index, measles immunization is more cost-effective.

The purpose of this paper is not to express views on the set of choices required in constructing an index of years saved by health programs. Nor does it assess the different means available to place a value on the years of life gained (e.g., Torrance, 1986; Mishan, 1988), an operation that is ultimately required if the benefits of health programs are to be compared to those of other government programs. Rather, it examines the demographic adequacy of existing health indices as guides to evaluating the potential effects of programs (i.e., in measuring what they purport to measure). By using the same information and data that are required to construct such an index, population projections can generally supply more accurate and detailed information with little added effort on the analyst's part. Under certain circumstances, the information provided by this approach can be collapsed into one of the health indices now in common use.

TABLE 1 Cost-Effectiveness of Onchocerciasis Control and Measles Immunization in the Côte d'Ivoire Under Various Procedures Regarding Discounting and Weighting of Productive Years

Index of Cost per	Cost of Onchocerciasis Control ($)	Cost of Measles Immunization ($)
Year of healthy life added	20	10
Productive year of healthy life added[a]	20	15
Discounted year of healthy life added[b]	150	49
Discounted year of productive life added[a,b]	150	190

SOURCE: Prost and Prescott (1984:Table 7).

[a]The age range 15-59 is considered productive. No distinctions are made among ages within this range.
[b]A discount rate of .10 is used.

EVALUATING THE EFFECTIVENESS OF HEALTH INTERVENTIONS

The information required to evaluate the effectiveness of a health program includes the following elements:

(1) How many more years of life will be lived as a result of this program?
(2) How many of those years of life will be lived in a healthy state?
(3) How many of those years will be lived in an unhealthy state?
(4) At what ages will those additional years of total, healthy, and unhealthy life be lived?
(5) How will those added years be distributed over time?

Item 4 is needed if different ages are to be weighted differently, and item 5 is needed if time discounting is to be used. Even if neither of these conditions prevails, the information in items 4 and 5 may still help planners understand the full implications of undertaking a program.

To answer these questions explicitly, population projection is necessary. The elements required for population projection are the following:

$N(a,0)$ = number of people aged a at time 0, when the health program is initiated,

${}_np_a$ = probability that a person aged a will survive n years in the absence of the health program,

$_{n}p'_{a}$ = probability that a person aged a will survive n years in the presence of the health program,

$h(a)$ = probability that someone aged a is healthy in the absence of the health program,

$h'(a)$ = probability that a person aged a is healthy in the presence of the health program.

These same data are required to construct one of the indices in common use, although various simplifications have been made to reduce the age detail required. For the time being, we set aside the important question of whether the effects on those unborn at the time the health program is initiated are to be included among its effects and assume that we are counting only the years of life added among the population alive at time 0.

Table 2 shows the formulas for projecting the population alive at time 0 forward in the presence and absence of the health program. They are presented in the form of summations across all age groups, but detail is required on each age group in order to produce the sum. Although the formulas can be expressed more compactly by using calculus, nothing more than simple algebra is required to apply them. Many applications of the procedures to alternative mortality scenarios have been made (e.g., United Nations, 1991; Preston, 1976).

Let us see how standard health indices relate to these procedures. In so doing, we rely mainly on the description by the Ghana Health Assessment Project Team (1981), which provides the most extensive exposition of this method and which appears to have been followed by subsequent analysts. First, we focus on mortality alone. In Ghana, 70 percent of the healthy years of life added by the array of interventions studied were a product of life extension rather than of morbidity reduction (Ghana Health Assessment Project Team, 1981).

Health Programs That Operate for One Year

We first show that the conventionally defined total years of life added by a health program can be derived from these procedures by making the assumption that the entire effect of the health program on mortality is realized in the program's first year. Under this condition, death rates change by $\Delta\mu(a)$ during the first year and then revert to their previous levels. The new probability of survival for one year is

$$ {}_{1}p'_{a} = e^{-\int_{a}^{a+1} \mu'(x)dx} = e^{-\int_{a}^{a+1} [\mu(x)+\Delta\mu(x)]dx} $$

$$ \cong [1-\Delta\mu(a)]e^{-\int_{a}^{a+1} \mu(x)dx} = [1-\Delta\mu(a)]\,{}_{1}p_{a}\,, $$

where $\mu(x)$ is the death rate (deaths divided by person-years of exposure) at age x. If all of the effect of a program is realized in the first year, then all survival probabilities beyond the first year are unaltered. Therefore,

$$_n p'_a = [1 - \Delta\mu(a)]\ _n p_a\ , \quad n \geq 1.$$

The total years of life added by the health program (the summation over time of the top right-hand column in Table 2) is therefore

$$\int_0^\infty \int_0^\infty N(a,0)\Delta\mu(a)\ _t p_a\, da\, dt$$

$$= \int_0^\infty D(a) e_a^0\, da\ ,$$

where $D(a)$ is the number of deaths averted in the first year of the program by the mortality reduction at age a and e_a^0 is life expectancy at age a in the absence of the program. This formula embodies the standard procedure for calculating the total years of life added by a health program: simply estimate the number of deaths that would be averted by the program and multiply them by life expectancy at each age. Clearly, this procedure assumes that the health program operates for only one year and that those "saved" by the program revert to the average level of mortality in the population (as embodied in the set of $_n p_a$'s) thereafter.

We have shown that the conventional procedure produces a reliable estimate of undiscounted years of life saved for programs that operate for only one year. When discounting is used, however, this approach introduces an unnecessary flaw. Many analysts have recognized that the time effect of a health program in terms of years of life saved is not uniform and that gains will diminish for the population alive at time 0. The conventional assumption is that those "saved" by the program at age a in year 0 will subsequently live e_a^0 years and that all will die at an age of $(a + e_a^0)$. Although this formulation is correct as an undiscounted average, it provides misleading information when the years of life saved are to be discounted. In reality, some of those saved will die before age $(a + e_a^0)$, whereas others will die at an older age. Because of discounting, however, the years lost before $(a + e_a^0)$ by people who die before that age have a higher present value than the years gained after that age by those who live beyond it. A procedure that assigns e_a^0 additional years to all those saved thus overstates the gains from the health program.

To illustrate what error the assumption can introduce, let us assume that those "saved" are subject thereafter to an annual age-specific death rate of .03. Thus, their life expectancy is 33.33 years and their probability of surviving n years beyond the start of the program is $e^{-.03n}$. We will assume

TABLE 2 Formulas Used in Population Projections in Absence and Presence of a Health Program (population alive at time 0)

Years Since Program Was Initiated	Population Size in Absence of Program (1)	Population Size in Presence of Program (2)	Years of Life Added (3) = (2) – (1)
0	$\int_0^\infty N(a,0)da$	$\int_0^\infty N(a,0)da$	0
1	$\int_0^\infty N(a,0)\,{}_1p_a\,da$	$\int_0^\infty N(a,0)\,{}_1p'_a\,da$	$\int_0^\infty N(a,0)[{}_1p'_a - {}_1p_a]da$
2	$\int_0^\infty N(a,0)\,{}_2p_a\,da$	$\int_0^\infty N(a,0)\,{}_2p'_a\,da$	$\int_0^\infty N(a,0)[{}_2p'_a - {}_2p_a]da$
n	$\int_0^\infty N(a,0)\,{}_np_a\,da$	$\int_0^\infty N(a,0)\,{}_np'_a\,da$	$\int_0^\infty N(a,0)[{}_np'_a - {}_np_a]da$

	Number of Healthy People Alive in Absence of Program	Number of Healthy People Alive in Presence of Program	Years of Healthy Life Added
0	$\int_0^\infty N(a,0)h(a)\,da$	$\int_0^\infty N(a,0)h(a)\,da$	0
1	$\int_0^\infty N(a,0)\,{}_1p_a\,h(a+1)\,da$	$\int_0^\infty N(a,0)\,{}_1p'_a h'(a+1)\,da$	$\int_0^\infty N(a,0)[{}_1p'_a h'(a+1) - {}_1p_a h(a+1)]\,da$
2	$\int_0^\infty N(a,0)\,{}_2p_a\,h(a+2)\,da$	$\int_0^\infty N(a,0)\,{}_2p'_a h'(a+2)\,da$	$\int_0^\infty N(a,0)[{}_2p'_a h'(a+2) - {}_2p_a h(a+2)]\,da$
n	$\int_0^\infty N(a,0)\,{}_np_a\,h(a+n)\,da$	$\int_0^\infty N(a,0)\,{}_np'_a h'(a+n)\,da$	$\int_0^\infty N(a,0)[{}_np'_a h'(a+n) - {}_np_a h(a+n)]\,da$

a discount rate of 10 percent. The present value of a life saved by the program is

$$\int_0^\infty \frac{e^{-.03n}}{e^{.10n}}\,dn = \int_0^\infty e^{-.13n}\,dn = -\frac{1}{-.13} = 7.69 \text{ years.}$$

If we assume erroneously that all of those saved die at their life expectancy, i.e., the probability of surviving n additional years is one, then the present value of a life saved is

$$\int_0^{33.3} \frac{1}{e^{.10n}}\,dn = 9.64 \text{ years.}$$

The conventional procedure overestimates the present value of years of life saved in this example by 25 percent. The bias will typically be smaller than this amount because mortality rates among those saved will not be constant but will rise with age. Nevertheless, an upward bias will result and it will vary across programs. The bias is obviously unnecessary because population projection provides an explicit indication of the time sequence of program effects.

Multiyear Health Programs

Although mass immunization campaigns or campaigns to screen for cervical cancer may operate in only one year, most health programs do not. Is it reasonable to assume that the gains from extending the program to later years will more or less replicate those of the first year? This assumption is required to use some measure of life years gained as a guide to implementing a multiyear or permanent program. Unfortunately, the index of years of life saved does not automatically provide reliable estimates for later years. The population alive at time 0 diminishes over time until all members are dead; any health program with constant features (in terms of $\Delta\mu(a)$) will eventually save many fewer lives among the population alive at time 0 and even fewer years of future life. The index of years of life gained will, in general, overstate the gains for future years unless those unborn at time 0 are admitted to the calculus.

Let us assume for the moment that they are not admitted and that health decisions are to be made on behalf of the population alive at the time a program is implemented. Then the conventional approach produces a major distortion in its assessment of the relative merits of interventions aimed at adults and those aimed at children. Age distributions in developing countries are typically very youthful. There are many more people aged 5, for example, than people aged 30. The assumption that the health program lasts for only one year means that there are many more potential beneficiaries at young ages than at older ages. However, if the program is permanent, then 30 birth cohorts of the existing population will benefit from a mortality improvement at age 30, and only 5 will benefit from an improvement at age 5 (by maintaining the assumption that we care only about the population alive at time 0). The fact that the benefits to younger cohorts of health improvements at older ages are not counted in the "years of life added" calculation can create a serious bias tilting calculations in favor of health interventions directed at children. It would not be a "bias" if programs lasted only one year, but few do.

To illustrate the bias against adult interventions under conventional procedures, let us perform two thought experiments:

(1) Assume that a health intervention succeeds in permanently reducing death rates at age 5 in developing countries by .001.

(2) Assume that a health intervention succeeds in permanently reducing death rates at age 30 in developing countries by .001.

In projecting the population forward to demonstrate the effects of these changes, we use the estimated age distribution of developing countries in 1990 (United Nations, 1989) and a life table with a life expectancy at birth of 63.1 years.[1] We assume that the benefits (i.e., added years of life) are to be registered only for the population alive at the initiation of the program. We then calculate the present value of years of life added without discounting and with discounting at a rate of .03. Results are shown in Table 3.

The relative gains in years of life are radically different according to the different methods. By the conventional measure, the number of years added by the mortality reduction at age 5 is 2.5 times greater than the number added by the reduction at age 30. This difference reflects the fact that there are more 5-year-olds than 30-year-olds, as well as the longer life expectancy at age 5 than at age 30. However, if the reduction in death rates is permanent (i.e., lasts 30 years), then the reduction at age 30 produces 2.7-3.0 times as many years of added life as the reduction at age 5, depending on whether discounting is used. The reason is that there are many more potential beneficiaries of the reduction at age 30.

If a population chooses its health programs on the basis of the interests of those alive at the time choices are made (including children whose interests may be represented by adults), then the conventional index will provide misleading information about relative gains from different programs. It is reasonable to suppose that social decisions are made by the living popula-

[1]The United Nations (1991) estimates life expectancy at birth in less developed countries during 1990-1995 as 63.3 years. To provide the requisite age detail on survivorship, we use a "West" model life-table level 19 (mean value of males and females), which has a life expectancy at birth of 63.1 years (Coale and Demeny, 1983:51).

TABLE 3 Comparisons of Total Years of Life Added by Permanent Health Programs That Reduce Death Rates by One per Thousand at Ages 5 and 30: Less Developed Countries, 1990

	Years Added (thousands)		
Total Years Added by	Reduction at Age 5 (1)	Reduction at Age 30 (2)	Ratio, (2)/(1)
Conventional method[a]	6,454	2,579	0.40
Projection of living population forward			
Undiscounted[b]	33,854	101,853	3.01
Discounted at 3%	13,637	36,086	2.70

[a]Years added as a result of mortality reduction at age $x = N(x)e_x^0(.001)$.

[b]Years added as a result of mortality reduction at age $x = .001\int_0^x N(a)_{x-a}p_a \cdot e_x^0\, da$.

tion primarily on behalf of the living population. Only if unborn generations have equal status—that is, they are given equal weight in social decisions—to those currently alive would the conventional approach embody a roughly appropriate representation of social decision making.

Useful information about how people actually value saving lives at different dates has emerged from three U.S. surveys (Cropper et al., 1992). Respondents were asked to choose between programs that would save, for example, 100 lives now or 1,000 lives 50 years from now. The length of time and the number of future lives saved were varied randomly among respondents. Basic results are presented in Table 4.

The table shows that attitudes toward the saving of lives are highly present oriented. For example, a life saved a decade hence is only one-third as valuable as a life saved in the present. The authors report that the implicit discount rates did not vary significantly with income or education, so the figures in the table may also be reasonable approximations to values in developing countries.

These results show that the saving of lives is discounted at a much higher rate than the 3 percent figure used by the World Bank in its Health Sector Priority Review. The discount rate is 17 percent during the first 5 years, 11 percent for the first 10 years, and diminishes thereafter. While the results do not bear directly on the issue of whether the unborn at time 0 are to be treated differently from those alive at time 0, it is reasonable to suppose that the high discount rate partially reflects the fact that they are not given a weight equal to those currently alive. If they are not, then the

TABLE 4 Average Value to Respondents of Lives Saved—Future Versus Present: United States

Years Since Program Initiation (t)	Value of Life Saved at Time t, Relative to Value of Life Saved in Present
0	1.00
5	.43
10	.33
25	.16
50	.09
100	.02

SOURCE: Adapted from Cropper et al. (1992:Table 1).

conventional approach is distorted away from adult and toward children's programs.

What if those unborn at the time of program initiation are in fact to be considered equal beneficiaries of health programs? That is to say, whatever discount rate is used, it is applied equally to all cohorts regardless of whether or not they were alive at the time program implementation decisions were made. Does the conventional index provide a fair representation of the relative benefits of different multiyear programs under this circumstance?

Under one circumstance, the index of years of life saved would be almost exactly correct: if the reduction in mortality induced by the program were constant with respect to age ($\Delta\mu(a) = K$), then it would induce no change in the population's age distribution (Keyfitz, 1968). If, in addition, the population to which the mortality change is applied is demographically "stable"—with constant fertility, mortality, and migration rates leading to a constant age distribution—then the age distribution of deaths averted by the program ($D(a)$) would not change over time. The only error in the index under this circumstance is that the preprogram $p(a)$ function is used to estimate e_a^0 instead of the postprogram $p'(a)$ function.

These conditions are, of course, highly restrictive. The most serious distortion that they introduce results from the assumption that age distributions are constant. Largely as a result of declining fertility, age distributions are growing older in nearly all developing countries, and the aging process will almost certainly continue (United Nations, 1989). Given a particular change in age-specific death rates, the deaths-averted function ($D(a)$) at baseline is thus younger than it would be in future years. The conventional index is thus biased toward health interventions at young ages in aging populations.

The amount of bias is directly proportional to impending changes in the age distribution. Table 5 displays the changes projected by the United

TABLE 5 Age Bias in Conventional Measures of Years of Lite Saved by Health Programs: Less Developed Countries

	Projected Ratio of Population in Age Interval to Population 0-4				Bias in 1990 Measure of Years of Lite Saved by Health Programs Targeted at Particular Ages, Relative to Age 0-4 (%)		
Age	1990	2000	2010	2020	2000	2010	2020
0-4	1.000	1.000	1.000	1.000	0	0	0
30-34	.533	.644	.680	.834	21	27	56
50-54	.265	.309	.434	.603	17	63	128
70-74	.096	.119	.154	.213	24	60	122

SOURCE: Compiled from United Nations (1989:8).

Nations. The assumption that the age distribution at baseline will not change, which is built into the conventional approach, produces large biases in favor of programs targeted at young ages, even during the first decade. Relative to health interventions targeted at ages 0-4, those directed at ages 50-54 or 70-74 would produce 17-24 percent more years of life saved in 2000 than would be indicated by the index computed for 1990. This bias grows rapidly to 60-63 percent in 2010 and to 122-128 percent in 2020.

It is widely recognized that age distributions in developing countries are growing older and that more attention should be paid to adult health issues. It is not so apparent that the index of years of life saved takes no account of these changes when applied to multiyear programs. The result of embedding the initial age distribution in concrete is to bias calculations in favor of youthful and against adult interventions. The only solution is to use population projection to provide a more reliable estimate of the age and time effects of various programs.

Adding Health to Years of Life

An additional problem with conventional procedures is their treatment of disability. Let us assume that we can agree on a definition of disability and that years of life added in the disabled state do not count toward the gain in "healthy" years of life. The correct formulas for calculating years of healthy life added are presented in the lower portion of Table 2.

Unfortunately, conventional practice deviates markedly from these formulas. The years of healthy life gained are calculated as the sum of two components, one resulting from the morbidity reduction and the other from the mortality reduction. In computing the latter component, the years of life saved by a health intervention (Equation (1) of Table 2) are all assigned to the healthy state (cf. Ghana Health Assessment Project Team, 1981:74,80). Even if the intervention had no effect on age-specific disability rates ($h'(a) = h(a)$), some of the years of life added by a program would be disabled years, simply because many disease processes that produce disability will not be affected by the intervention. The conventional procedure clearly overestimates years of healthy life gained. If disability rates are 20 percent at each age, then the gain in healthy years of life from the mortality reduction—the bulk of the total gain in years of healthy life—will be overestimated by this amount. In general, the conventional procedure will overestimate the value of interventions targeted at older ages more than those targeted at younger ages because rates of disability rise with age.

A second, less critical, problem with the treatment of ill-health in the Ghana team's procedures is that it concentrates the morbidity associated with a disease at one age, typically a youthful age (Barnum, 1987). This tactic means that the gains from morbidity reduction are too heavily concentrated in the first year of the program and are underrepresented in later years. The relative distortion in index values across diseases will, as a result, vary with the discount rate that is employed.

Program Interactions

The conventional procedure does not incorporate interactions among disease processes or programs (Barnum, 1987). Many such interactions are possible. The simplest situation arises when two potential programs would act "independently" to reduce mortality rates. Suppose that program 1 would reduce mortality rates by $\Delta\mu_1(a)$ and program 2 would reduce mortality rates by $\Delta\mu_2(a)$. Then the gain in years of life from introducing both programs will exceed the sum of gains from introducing each of them individually, unless they both operate at one and the same age. The reason is that those "saved" from death by one program will live more years as a result of implementation of the other program. Thus, the gains from the two programs are synergistic rather than additive. Synergy is particularly likely to involve programs spanning a variety of adult ages. Only if the two programs operate at exactly the same age—and early childhood is the most likely target of multiple programs—would this property be absent. To incorporate these interactions in population projection, it is only necessary to introduce both sets of effects into the ${}_np'_a$ function, which is a straightforward operation.[2]

More complex interactions are, of course, likely. These would typically involve not only mortality but morbidity. Mosley and Becker (1991) provide a lucid account of how changes in the intensity of one disease process

[2]Since ${}_np_a = e^{-\int_a^{a+n}\mu(x)dx}$, the new survivorship function would be ${}_np'_a = e^{-\int_a^{a+n}[\mu(x)-\Delta\mu_1(x)-\Delta\mu_2(x)]da}$.

can affect other processes. They note that, in general, interventions that alter the incidence of a disease would be expected to add more years of life than those that alter case-fatality rates, even though the initial effect on age-specific death rates may be equivalent. The reason is that alterations in case-fatality rates are more likely to raise levels of morbidity and hence leave the survivors more vulnerable to other disease processes. The problem is one not only of modeling the proper effects of interventions $h^j(a)$ but also of predicting their effects on ${}_np^j_a$. These are unquestionably important issues that bedevil not only a projection approach to planning but also the computation of conventional indices. The problems are, in fact, identical in the two cases. More complex models of disease and death processes involving disease interactions have been used to study health issues in developed countries (e.g., Manton and Stallard, 1984; Rogers et al., 1989), but Mosley and Becker's approach is better suited to yielding practical guidelines for developing country health programs.

How Should Births Added by Health Programs be Treated?

We have noted that the family of conventional measures of years of life gained assumes that a program lasts only one year. The measures work as crude approximations to the effects of a permanent program if those unborn at the time of program initiation are included among the beneficiaries. To make the approximation more exact, it would be necessary to use the new (i.e., postprogram) set of ${}_np_a$'s and $h(a)$'s and to project the number of births that will occur in the future. Meeting these requirements involves nothing more or less than performing a population projection.

In a projection framework, births will increase as a result of a successful health program that improves survivorship at any age less than 45 or 50. The question is not simply whether to allow the unborn to count as beneficiaries of the program but also how to count the births that would be added as a result of the program. Do their entire lives count toward years of life added by the program? If so, the most cost-effective health intervention would be a restriction of contraceptive availability, which would both save money and add years of life. Not surprisingly, advocates of contraceptive programs have used other indices and procedures.

The question is far from trivial because most of the years of life eventually added by most health programs will be lived by people who would not have been born in the program's absence. The huge expansion of the human population since 1940 is primarily a result of successful health programs; most of the years of life added represent births that would not otherwise have occurred, rather than longer lives for people who would have been born in any event. Put more concretely, saving the life of a 20-year-old woman in a typical developing country will lead to approximately four more births in the next two decades. The issue is not readily swept under the rug, as critics of expanded health programs are quick to point out (e.g., King, 1990).

This issue is contentious because of the presumed economic burden of additional births in poor countries. Although this burden may not be as great as once believed (National Research Council, 1986), it is unquestionably true that the "extra" births will not become productive citizens for 15 years or so, by which time their productive contribution will be heavily discounted under most accounting procedures. It is also true that most of these births will be "wanted" by their parents and will help to fulfill the aspirations of those whose lives may have been spared by health interventions. Most of the costs of raising children through their dependent years will be borne not by society at large but by the parents who voluntarily bore them.

When economic issues are introduced, it is appropriate—if not always politically expedient—to make them explicit. Once again, population projections are the most direct and straightforward means of making the underlying considerations operational. For example, by using the age distribution of projected populations at future dates together with age profiles of consumption and production, it is a simple matter to take a first cut at identifying the effects of a health program on the relative balance of the two and on per capita income. The effects are not likely to be large, although the short-term and long-term consequence of most mortality declines has been to increase the fraction of the population outside labor force age (Coale, 1972). The most complete consideration of the effects of health programs on a wide array of economic processes in a population projection framework remains Barlow's (1968) analysis of antimalarial programs in Sri Lanka.

The point, however, is not to make the comparative assessment of health programs so complex as to be impractical. The indices of years of life gained have achieved great currency because they provide relatively simple measures that allow cross-program comparisons. We have tried to show more precisely what assumptions are necessary in interpreting these indices. In so doing, we have identified certain problems, inconsistencies, and interpretive difficulties to which the measures are subject. These difficulties can be removed—without adding any data requirements—by the use of population projections. Such projections also serve as a solid and trustworthy vehicle for answering more complex questions if those are pertinent to the planning process.

DISCUSSION

The conventional measure of years of healthy life gained functions best as a guide to evaluating health interventions lasting one year. Can the measure simply be reapplied each year to evaluate whether a program should continue? There are two obvious difficulties with this approach. One is that most interventions involve both start-up costs and continuing costs. In order to properly evaluate whether start-up costs should be invested, an assessment is needed that stretches over the full life of a program. The second problem is that as a practical matter, government agencies do not engage in continuous self-reflection. Planning is sporadic, and careful evaluation of existing programs is impeded by the constituencies that develop around them. It is realistic to suppose that careful health planning by using quantitative measures of expected program effects will occur infrequently in developing countries. When it does occur, it is best that the methods used take full advantage of the information available.

SUMMARY

The conventional calculation of the years of healthy life gained through a health intervention functions best as a health planning device when a one-year intervention is being considered. Its principal problems in this case are

(1) its assumption that all the years of life saved will be healthy years, and

(2) its assumption that all of those saved by the intervention will die at their life expectancy.

Both of these procedures produce an upward bias in estimating years of healthy life gained; the latter bias occurs only when discounting is used.[3]

Most health interventions stretch over periods longer than one year. The index is a poorer planning instrument in these cases. If the aim is to represent the effects of a program on the population alive at the time the program is initiated, then the index produces a severe bias against interventions directed primarily at adults. Health improvements among adults will add healthy years for many cohorts, whereas those directed at children will benefit few. This feature is not represented in the index.

If those unborn at program initiation are to be given equal weight as beneficiaries, then this bias may be largely averted. However, the index typically will still give misleading information about the effects of long-term programs because its values are entirely dependent on the initial age distribution. Because age distributions in most developing countries (apart from Africa) are changing rapidly, important biases can result. In particu-

[3]An upward bias would also result if those saved by the intervention are restored to below-average levels of health in the population, which is particularly likely if interventions are directed at case-fatality rates or at disadvantaged groups.

lar, the index will be biased toward interventions at youthful ages in aging populations.

All of these problems, whether applicable to one-year or multiyear interventions, can be avoided through the use of population projection. Projections also provide a straightforward means of incorporating other dimensions, such as the total gain in production, changes in the balance between production and consumption, or changes in per capita income.

REFERENCES

Barlow, R.
1968 *The Economic Effects of Malaria Eradication.* Economic Research Series No. 15. Ann Arbor: University of Michigan School of Public Health.

Barnum, H.
1987 Evaluating healthy days of life gained from health projects. *Social Science and Medicine* 24(10):833-841.

Coale, A.J.
1972 *The Growth and Structure of Human Populations.* Princeton, N.J.: Princeton University Press.

Coale, A.J., and P. Demeny
1983 *Regional Model Life Tables and Stable Populations.* New York: Academic Press.

Cropper, M.L., S.K. Aydede, and P.R. Portney
1992 Rates of time preference for saving lives. *American Economic Review* 82(2):469-472.

Ghana Health Assessment Project Team
1981 A quantitative method of assessing the health impact of different diseases in less developed countries. *International Journal of Epidemiology* 10(1):73-80.

Jamison, D.T., and W.H. Mosley
1991 Disease control priorities in developing countries. Manuscript, Population, Health, and Nutrition Division, World Bank, Washington, D.C.

Keyfitz, N.
1968 *Introduction to the Mathematics of Population.* Reading, Mass.: Addison-Wesley.

King, M.
1990 Health is a sustainable state. *Lancet* 336:664-667.

Loomes, G., and L. McKenzie
1989 The use of QALY's in health care decision making. *Social Science and Medicine* 28(4):299-308.

Manton, K.G., and E. Stallard
1984 *Recent Trends in Mortality Analysis.* New York: Academic Press.

Mishan, E.J.
1988 *Cost-Benefit Analysis*, 4th ed. London: University Hyman.

Mooney, G., and A. Creese
1990 Cost and cost-effectiveness analysis of health interventions. Health Sector Priorities Review Paper HSPR-23. Population, Health, and Nutrition Division, World Bank, Washington, D.C.

Mosley, W.H., and S. Becker
1991 Demographic models for child survival and implications for health intervention programs. *Health Policy and Planning* 6(3):218-233.

Murray, C.J.L.
1990 Rational approaches to priority setting in international health. *Journal of Tropical Medicine and Hygiene* 93:303-311.

National Research Council
1986 *Population Growth and Economic Development: Policy Questions.* Washington, D.C.: National Academy Press.

Patrick, D.L., and R.A. Deyo
1989 Generic and disease-specific measures in assessing health status and quality of life. *Medical Care* 27(3) supplement:S217-S232.

Preston, S.H.
1976 *Mortality Patterns in National Populations.* New York: Academic Press.

Prost, A., and N. Prescott
1984 Cost-effectiveness of blindness prevention by the Onchocerciasis Control Programme in Upper Volta. *Bulletin of the World Health Organization* 62:795-802.

Rogers, A., R. Rogers, and L. Branch
1989 A multistate analysis of active life expectancy. *Public Health Reports* 104(3):222-226.

Russell, M.
1990 The making of cruel choices. Pp. 15-22 in P.B. Hammond and R. Coppock, eds., *Valuing Health Risks, Costs, and Benefits for Environmental Decision Making.* Washington, D.C.: National Academy Press.

Torrance, G.W.
1986 Measurement of health state utilities for economic appraisal. *Journal of Health Economics* 1-30.

United Nations
1989 *Global Estimates and Projections of Population by Sex and Age: The 1988 Revision.* Population Study No. 93. New York: United Nations.
1991 *World Population Prospects: 1990.* Population Study No. 120. New York: United Nations.

Health Policy Issues in Three Latin American Countries: Implications of the Epidemiological Transition

José Luis Bobadilla and Cristina de A. Possas

Even in middle-income countries, more favorable statistics in the aggregate disguise wide disparities between the conditions, on the one hand, of the rural and peri-urban poor that are typical of low-income countries and the conditions, on the other hand, of more affluent urban dwellers who are better educated and have better access to health services and whose health status closely resembles the profile in industrialized countries.

John Evans et al. (1981)

INTRODUCTION

This paper is concerned with health policy issues in Latin American countries, with emphasis on the changes that health systems need to introduce to meet the health needs resulting from the demographic and epidemiological transitions. To illustrate these policy issues, three country cases are analyzed here: Brazil, Colombia, and Mexico. The population of these

---

J.L. Bobadilla is Health Policy Specialist, Population, Health, and Nutrition Division, The World Bank. C. Possas is with the Department of Administration and Planning, National School of Public Health Oswaldo Cruz Foundation, Brazil. The authors wish to thank Juan Eduardo Cespedes for information and comments on the current health situation in Colombia and Richard Cash, Xavior Coll, Oscar Echeverri, James Gribble, and Samuel Preston for comments.

countries includes about 60 percent of the population of Latin America. These three countries are now facing an important decline in mortality and fertility rates, and new sets of health problems that are related to rapid urbanization and industrialization, such as injuries, accidental intoxications and poisoning, and occupational and noncommunicable diseases affecting an aging population. At the same time, old health problems have not yet been solved; these countries are not yet free of the burden of many infectious and parasitic diseases, although their overall mortality rates for infectious diseases are declining. Analysis of the distribution of both groups of diseases shows wide disparities in health conditions across different regions and social classes.

The coexistence of old and new health problems and the persistence of wide social disparities in these developing Latin American countries have been described before (Evans et al., 1981) and referred to by Frenk et al. (1989) as "epidemiological polarization" and by Possas (1989a) as "structural heterogeneity." These authors have stressed the importance of identifying the main consequences of this complex transitional process in developing countries. The increasing burden of chronic diseases affecting a growing adult population in these Latin American societies will be, in the next decades, an important challenge to their governments because many of their old, unsolved health problems are likely to persist. This epidemiological diversity and the rate of change in the disease profiles make the health transition process in many developing countries much more complex than the situation faced now, or before, by developed societies (Evans et al., 1981). Developing countries are reducing their fertility rates and their mortality rates due to infectious diseases in shorter periods than industrialized countries, leaving a much shorter time to adjust the health system to respond adequately to the needs of adults and the elderly and, at the same time, maintain efforts to reduce the burden of infectious diseases in children and reproductive health problems. Two other factors differ between developing and industrialized countries: first, most developing countries still lack the required health infrastructure to deal with the most pressing health needs of their populations, and to judge from their gross national products and the proportions spent on health, this situation is not likely to improve in the near future; second, most governments of developing countries are being pressed to adopt the therapeutic medical model to deal with the burden of noncommunicable diseases.

The current health care paradigms for developing countries, characterized by the primary health care model, have been effective in dealing with epidemiological scenarios in which infection and reproductive health problems dominate. It is not clear how governments should reorient their health systems to respond to the new challenges posed by population aging and the emergence of noncommunicable diseases. This paper reviews the main policy issues that should be considered in reorienting the health system, in light of the epidemiological transition.

Recent analyses of the epidemiological transition (Caldwell et al., 1989; Laurenti, 1990; Jamison and Mosley, 1991; Frenk et al., 1991; Bell, 1993; Possas, 1991) suggest that the understanding of its policy implications can contribute to highlighting important aspects of the existing theoretical framework related to the health of human populations. Understanding the process of policy formulation in heterogeneous developing societies passing through the epidemiological transition can help to develop new concepts and methodologies for health care planning.

The formulation of policies in the health sector is influenced by various elements that interact with the epidemiological transition. The conceptual model presented in the following section briefly describes the main elements that influence health policy formulation and indicates the most relevant relationships. Next, basic information is presented on the socioeconomic, demographic, and health characteristics of the population and the health system organization in Brazil, Colombia, and Mexico. In the following section, critical policy issues are described and discussed with a focus on how they are affected by the epidemiological transition.

CONCEPTUAL FRAMEWORK FOR EXAMINATION OF POLICY IMPLICATIONS

The underlying causes of long-term changes in epidemiological profiles are not clearly understood. Our limited comprehension of the proximate determinants of health status suggests that changes in the standards of living, lifestyles, access to and quality of health services, and nutrition account for most of the improvements in survival in contemporary societies (Frenk et al., 1991). The technological advances in prevention and treatment of common diseases occurring in the past 50 years have changed the relative importance of these factors. A result is that now some countries with low income per capita ($300) are able to reduce substantially the burden of infectious and parasitic diseases. Thus, health policies in developing countries are addressing an increasingly broader set of issues related to the health status of populations.

Many of the policy issues that governments need to consider when dealing with the consequences of the epidemiological transition are country specific. The factors that determine the health status of the population, and the organization and performance of the health system, need to be taken into account. In this section, we briefly review these factors. Rather than presenting a comprehensive list of these determinants, we highlight those that are likely to play a relevant role in health policy formulation in the three selected countries.

The main determinants of health policy and their interrelationships are summarized in Figure 1. It is essential to understand the population dynamics; size and distribution of the population provide a first idea of the magnitude of health needs. The rate of population growth and the process of population aging are the most important variables to be considered. Within a country, intense rural-urban migration often poses additional burdens on the local health systems of big cities.

The contribution of fertility decline to the aging of populations and changing mortality levels and profiles have been described elsewhere (Bobadilla et al., 1993; Jamison and Mosley, 1991). It is worth mentioning that these demographic factors may play a far more relevant role in the epidemiologi-

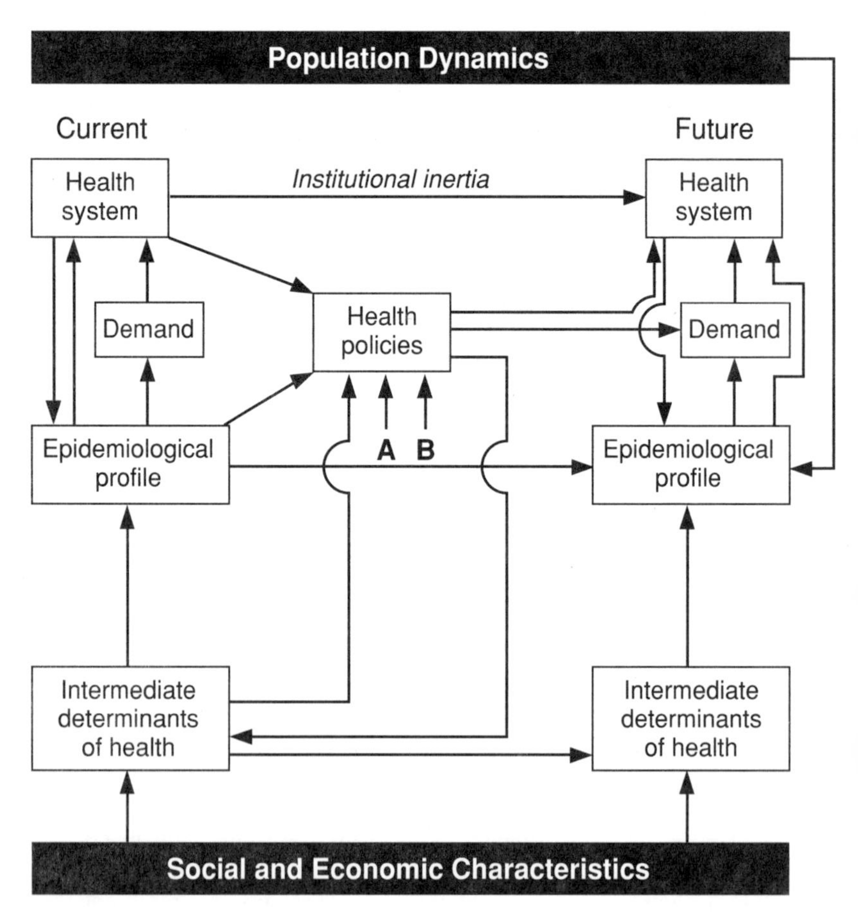

FIGURE 1 Principal determinants of health policy: (A) legal frame, (B) role of the state with regard to social needs.

cal transition than changes in the risk factors for noncommunicable diseases. Nevertheless, the paucity of information on the prevalence and trends of risk factors for noncommunicable diseases in developing countries, including the three analyzed here, precludes any definite statement on their relevance in the forthcoming decades.

The current status of the health system can be described by multiple variables such as number of institutions, coverage of different services, mix of private and public sources and amount of financial resources, efficiency, equity in the distribution of resources, and quality of care. Organizational and performance deficiencies of the health system are common in many countries of the world and obviously need to be corrected before other policies designed to respond to the epidemiological transition can be implemented. Most governments allocate resources in the health sector according to the pattern of expenditure of previous years, creating an institutional inertia to maintain the status quo in their health systems. This inertia reduces the flexibility of the health system to adapt to new challenges, such as those posed by the epidemiological transition.

As Figure 1 illustrates, the current health system is related, in part, to the epidemiological profile, because it is supposed to control, prevent, and treat the main diseases and injuries. However, the health system is also determined by other social and economic factors, such as the market forces of drugs and medical equipment, technological innovation in diagnosis and treatment, the medical labor market, and political interests. Future health policies should ideally be oriented toward improving the capacity of the health system to respond to the changing demand due to the epidemiological transition.

The relationship between the epidemiological profile and the health system is depicted in Figure 1 as occurring directly and mediated through demand. Some health needs of the population elicit direct responses from the health system, as is the case with immunization. Others, such as case management of noncommunicable diseases, are identified through demands from the population. Needs and demands are clearly not synonymous, because demand depends on the health status and the perception of illness by individuals and families. Perceptions are a critical element to consider in health planning because a large proportion of the rise in demand for health care is due to an increase in illness perception and not necessarily to higher prevalence of disease.

Health policy options are also affected by two other factors that are often ignored because they are resistant to change. These are the *legal framework* for health, environment, and health care; and the *ideological standpoint* that governments and leading population groups hold regarding health and the role of the state in the provision of health services. These two factors often limit the options available in the formulation of policies.

They can, of course, be changed and often are objects of policy. Because they are country specific, it is difficult to generalize about the restrictions they impose on health policy alternatives.

HEALTH POLICY IN BRAZIL, COLOMBIA, AND MEXICO

This section describes, for Brazil, Colombia, and Mexico, the most important elements of the conceptual framework described in the previous section.

Social and Economic Characteristics

Wide disparities can be observed in economic factors such as gross national product (GNP) per capita, which ranges from U.S.$1,200 in Colombia to U.S.$2,540 in Brazil, and average annual inflation, which ranges from less than 24 percent in Colombia to more than 200 percent in Brazil, as shown in the appendix. Nevertheless, all three countries share similar patterns of income concentration, with about 40 percent of income in the highest 10 percent income group and from 1 to 4 percent of income in the lowest 20 percent income group.

Social conditions also show similarities and disparities. All three countries share similar proportions of population in poverty ranging from 37 percent in Mexico to 45 percent in Brazil, but other social conditions, such as access to potable water, sanitation facilities, and education, are quite different. In Brazil, there is a very high illiteracy rate (22 percent of adult population), whereas in Colombia and Mexico these rates are 12 and 10 percent, respectively. In Mexico, access to safe water is limited to 69 percent and access to sanitation facilities is 45 percent, whereas in Brazil and Colombia at least 75 percent of the populations have access to piped water and more that 65 percent have access to adequate sanitation facilities.

Finally, it is interesting to note that even though Colombia has the lowest GNP per capita, its social and health indicators are not far below those of Mexico and Brazil. For some indicators, such as under-5 mortality and life expectancy, Colombia is in a better or similar position. Investments in prevention and primary health care in Brazil and Mexico have been relatively small in the past three decades, and only in the mid-1980s did this situation start to change. Colombia, on the contrary, has concentrated national efforts on population-based activities to control communicable diseases.

Population Dynamics

In the past 30 years, the three countries have experienced substantial reductions in their total fertility rate, giving rise to a profound change in the

TABLE 1 Population Dynamics in Brazil, Colombia, and Mexico, Selected Years

					Age Structure (%)			
	1989 Population	Total Fertility Rate			1989		2025	
Country	(millions)	1965	1989	2000	0-14	15-64	0-14	15-64
Brazil	147	5.6	3.3	2.4	36	60	23	67
Colombia	32	6.5	2.9	2.2	36	60	22	68
Mexico	85	6.7	3.4	2.4	38	58	23	68

SOURCE: World Bank (1991:Table 32).

age structure of their populations. Table 1 shows the total fertility rate estimated for the years 1965 and 1989, and projected for the year 2000. From levels between 5.6 and 6.7 children per woman, total fertility dropped to about 3.0 and is estimated to be around 2.2 by the year 2000. This decline has been achieved to a large extent as a consequence of the greater contraceptive use by women of reproductive age, which in 1987 reached levels of 53 percent in Mexico, 63 percent in Colombia, and 65 percent in Brazil. The main change in the population structure is an important growth in the proportion of the population age 15 and over. By the year 2025 almost 70 percent of the population of these countries will be 15 to 64 years old.

Health Status

The health status of the populations of Brazil, Colombia, and Mexico, according to information on mortality levels, has improved considerably over the past 60 years. Currently, life expectancy at birth is 69 years for Mexico and Colombia and 66 years in Brazil. The childhood mortality rates are lower for Colombia and Mexico (50 and 51 per 1,000 children under 5, respectively) than for Brazil (85 per 1,000), as shown in the appendix. Although these indicators show a considerably better health status than many developing countries, they are quite unsatisfactory when compared with countries that have similar or lower annual income per capita such as Costa Rica and Chile.

The epidemiological profile of the three countries shows that according to mortality statistics, infectious and parasitic diseases are no longer responsible for the majority of deaths. Rather cardiovascular disease, cancer, and injury explain between 44 and 59 percent of total deaths, as shown in Table 2. Mexico has a larger share of deaths due to infectious and parasitic diseases and malnutrition, and Colombia has more deaths due to injury.

TABLE 2 Distribution of Deaths by Causes of Death in Brazil, Colombia, and Mexico Around 1986

	Country (%)		
Causes of Death	Brazil (1985)[a,b]	Colombia (1986)[c]	Mexico (1986)[b]
Infectious and parasitic diseases, and malnutrition	12	12	20
Perinatal and maternal causes	7	6	7
Injury and violence	11	19	16
Cardiovascular disease	28	27	19
Cancer	9	13	9
Other	12	19	26
Ill defined and senility	21	4[d]	3
Total	100	100	100
Total of registered deaths	(787,341)	(146,400)	(396,565)

[a]Data for Brazil include only some reporting areas that concentrate on the more developed parts of the country. Therefore, figures underestimate the share of deaths due to infectious diseases and overestimate the deaths due to noncommunicable diseases.

[b]World Health Organization (1990).

[c]Ministerio de Salud (1990).

[d]Only ill defined.

The coverage of mortality statistics in Brazil is less than in the other two countries; thus the information in Table 2 probably underestimates the number of deaths due to infectious and parasitic diseases in Brazil.

To understand better the heterogeneity in epidemiological profiles, health status indicators at the national level need to be stratified by socioeconomic variables. Table 3 shows childhood mortality rates according to different levels of the mother's education. The childhood mortality rates among children whose mothers are less educated are between three and four times greater than those for children whose mothers have the highest educational level.

Main Characteristics of Health Systems

Organizational Structure

Health systems in the three countries have different organizational structures. In Brazil, government and social security agencies have been integrated into the Unified Health System, but in Mexico and Colombia, there is a clear division of responsibilities between the ministries of health and the social security agencies. The responsibilities differ in the two countries: in Colombia, the Ministry of Health provides the majority of health services to

TABLE 3 Mortality Rates (per 1,000 population) for Children Under 5, According to Formal Education of Mother—Brazil, Colombia, and Mexico

	Country		
Mother's Education	Brazil (1978-1986)	Colombia (1978-1986)	Mexico (1979-1987)
None	136	78	112
1 - 3 years	137	65	91
4 - 6 years	70	40	54
7-11 years	40	25	29
Ratio of highest to lowest rate	3.4	3.1	3.9

SOURCE: Rutstein (1992:Table 3).

the population and the Social Security Institute covers only a small proportion of the population active in the labor force. In contrast, in Mexico, the Ministry of Health concentrates its services on the poor, and social security agencies cover about 60 percent of the total population.

The size and role of the private sector are also quite different in the three countries. In Brazil the private sector is very large and provides services to the unified public system. Private insurance plans are also growing very fast. In Colombia and Mexico the private sector also plays an important role, but there is no significant provision of private services funded by the public system. The insurance plans in these countries are also growing, but their sizes are very small.

Source of Finance

The sources of finance follow the organizational structures in the three countries. In Mexico and Colombia, where a clear division between the social security institutes and the ministries of health exists, the services of the former are financed through contributions from employers and employees, and of the latter through general taxation and fees. Colombia also obtains funds through earmarked taxation of specific products (such as beer or tobacco) to finance specific components of the health services. Brazil, on the other hand, integrates these different sources into a single health fund to finance its Unified Health System.

Coverage

Despite the relatively high income per capita of these three countries (within the context of developing countries), there is evidence to suggest that 20-30 percent of the population have not access to basic health services. The coverage of deliveries attended by health professionals range from 70 percent in Mexico to 81 percent in Brazil, and immunization of children receiving the third dose of the diphtheria-pertussis-tetanus vaccine varies from 66 percent in Mexico to 87 percent in Colombia (United Nations Children's Fund, 1992).

Distribution of Resources

Health conditions in Brazil, Colombia, and Mexico have improved considerably for the majority of their populations during the recent decades. Unfortunately, the uneven distribution of social benefits derived from development has accentuated health inequalities. The current organization of health services widens existing health inequalities in the three countries analyzed here, mainly because the distribution of resources is biased toward the middle and upper classes, and the quality of care, for those who have access, is generally inversely related to socioeconomic status (Bobadilla, 1988).

Decentralization of Health Services

The three countries analyzed here underwent a very intense decentralization process in their health systems during the 1980s. This process was a consequence of two main determinants: the growing political pressure for the empowerment of local levels and the need to increase the flexibility of the health systems, making them more adequate to the growing diversity in epidemiological profiles and local realities (Rondinelli and Cheema, 1983). Analysis of the decentralization experiences in these countries indicates that this process seems, in general, to constitute a positive response to the social changes and increasing epidemiological diversity. However, a major problem for local governments and communities in this process, especially in poorer areas and regions, has been the lack of managerial capacity and instruments at the local level to deal with the new duties and attributions transferred in decentralization (Vianna et al., 1990).

The information presented in this section indicates that the three countries analyzed are relatively similar in their demographic and health profiles, but exhibit large disparities in the organization and delivery of health services. The reforms, still in process in the three countries, are all oriented in the same general directions: greater unification of health institutions, more decentralization of operations, greater responsibility of the government to finance health care, and sustained commitment to expand the coverage of services and strengthen the primary level of care. It is also difficult to assess the effectiveness of health policies that are implemented by other sectors of the economy: water and sanitation, pollution control, food distribution and safety, tobacco taxation, road safety, etc. Ministries of health in these countries express concern over these intersectoral policies but generally assign lower priority to these issues compared to the provision of health services. Even health programs that fall into their domain, but are not related to health care, such as sanitary regulation or health education, tend to receive lower priority. This outcome is due in part to the low level of expenditure in social sectors and the relative weakness of the ministries of health to enforce laws and regulations, and to lead other ministries to undertake intersectoral policies.

HEALTH POLICY ISSUES AND OPTIONS

Analysis of the complex epidemiological transition process in these three Latin American countries suggests that *it is not possible to formulate a homogeneous health policy agenda* for developing countries. The health problems faced by the middle-income countries need to be addressed differently from those of low-income countries where infectious diseases and undernutrition still clearly predominate. In spite of this need for specificity in the analysis of each country case, we have identified a set of issues that should orient health planning strategy. The discussion of each issue illustrates the complexities involved in reshaping the health system so that it is more responsive to demographic and epidemiological changes, and also serves as a guide to analyzing policy options in other developing countries.

Provision of Health Services as a Means to Redistribute Welfare

Inequalities in health status are the consequence, in large part, of concentration of income and other goods and services. According to the social justice objectives declared by the governments of the three countries studied here, social services, including health services, should contribute to the redistribution of the benefits of development. In these three countries, the health system fails to do so and, in some situations, exacerbates inequalities (Médici, 1989; Bobadilla et al., 1988). Five systemic policies are proposed to achieve greater equity in the distribution of health services.

Change in Eligibility Criteria for Access to Health Services

The partial coverage of social security in Colombia and Mexico shows regressive effects in the distribution of welfare because the financing of the system is supported by the whole society, but the benefits are restricted to the middle and lower-middle classes. By eliminating the barrier to social security for the unemployed, peasants, and workers in the informal sector (largely self-employed), greater equity in the distribution of resources by socioeconomic groups could be achieved. Incorporation into the Brazilian Constitution of the notion that social security should be universally accessible and distinguished from the more restricted notion of *seguro social*, which limits access on the basis of employment, is an example of the legal steps that can be taken toward this policy.

Tax Reform

A tax reform that eliminates differential health subsidies for the middle and upper classes could contribute to greater equity in health services. Medical expenses and drugs are tax deductible in the three countries. The net result is that the middle and upper classes benefit because they are more likely to earn enough to pay taxes, and they consume the vast majority of private health services (Cruz et al., 1991). The lower-middle class and some groups of the poor live with low cash income and also utilize private health services, but have no means of recovering their expenditure. In addition, most of the population groups that have no access to health care are in extreme poverty. This type of tax policy, intended to provide incentives for the utilization of health services, produces a regressive effect in the distribution of welfare.

Ration or Eliminate Health Interventions of Low Cost-Effectiveness

Implementing a policy in the public sector to limit health interventions that are not cost-effective is justified in all circumstances because health needs are infinite and resources are not. Its importance should be stressed now because the current trend in Brazil, Colombia, and Mexico is to reproduce the therapeutic component of the health care model for noncommunicable diseases, as is done in industrialized countries. Most of the technologies and interventions available to treat the most common chronic and degenerative diseases are extremely expensive and relatively ineffective (Jamison and Mosley, 1991). The proposed policy would free scarce resources that can be used to finance the next two proposed policies, which require additional investment.

Expand Coverage of Public Health Services for the Poor

Expansion of public health services for the poor is already a policy in the three countries analyzed here. The problem is that the poorest segments of the population have not been reached. Brazil and Mexico face serious difficulties in reaching rural areas due to long distances and lack of transport and of other goods and services in these communities. Many rural communities are very small (Mexico has more than 100,000 communities with fewer than 500 inhabitants), making investment in these communities not very cost-effective. On the other hand, in communities where transportation is readily available, potential still exists for increasing coverage. Successful models that use community health workers to reach the rural communities in the three countries should be replicated and the scope of their activities reviewed to assess their abilities to prevent noncommunicable diseases.

The financial feasibility of extending coverage to all the poor who lack access to health care needs to be carefully reviewed. If the current allocation of resources (by health programs) is maintained and extension depends exclusively on new funds, this proposal is not feasible in the next decade or so. As mentioned earlier, waste derives from inefficiencies and application of non-cost-effective interventions. There is evidence to suggest that the current human and financial resources in Brazil and Mexico would clearly be sufficient to extend coverage to all the poor unserved communities just by improving the efficiency and rationalizing the allocation of resources for health programs. The political and technical feasibility of designing and implementing these reforms is difficult to assess, but given the major macroreforms already implemented in Mexico and Brazil, this policy seems to be feasible.

Reduce Differences in Quality of Care between Health Agencies

Equalizing quality of care is necessary regardless of the implications of the epidemiological transition, because of the low standards of care prevailing in many health institutions in these countries (Gish, 1988). The equity objective reinforces the need for quality and overcoming the uneven distribution that exists among institutions that serve different socioeconomic groups. A large study of the quality of perinatal health services in Mexico City demonstrated that neonatal mortality rates (standardized for obstetric risk) were higher in Ministry of Health hospitals, which serve mainly the poor, compared to social security hospitals (Bobadilla and Walker, 1991).

Reform of the Health Care Model

The current health care model of the three countries is inadequate to deal with the increasing complexity of the epidemiological profile. As in many other countries, in these three countries, primary care is weak and underutilized, and most of the public hospitals are overcrowded and used for conditions that could be treated at lower levels of care. Three interrelated changes in the current health care model are proposed to correct these problems.

Increase the Technological Complexity of the Primary Level of Care

The increasing demand for health services that results from a rise in the absolute number of noncommunicable disease cases will not be met adequately with the limited health personnel and restricted technology available at the primary level of care. Common conditions, such as hypertension, ischemic heart disease, cervical dysplasia, cataracts, and varicose veins, can currently be treated with inexpensive treatments. Early detection of many chronic conditions can save resources by reducing the number of cases that advance to more severe stages and require hospitalization. Diagnostic and screening procedures and cost-effective ambulatory therapies should be selected and made available at the primary level of care. This policy should not be implemented, however, if resources are going to be taken from services for maternal and child health, which should still be the priority in poor areas.

Restrict Hospital Care

A second proposed change is to restrict hospital care to the most severe conditions and give priority to conditions amenable to treatment with cost-effective interventions. Low-risk deliveries, sterilizations, and minor surgery are examples of services that can be provided at a lower-level health facility. The next policy proposal defines such a facility.

Create or Strengthen Advanced Primary Health Care Centers

With different names and slight changes in the content, the three countries analyzed here have already recognized the need for a new level of care that would deal with the health problems mentioned previously: low-risk delivery, ambulatory surgery, common diseases, and conditions that require a specialist. This proposal for a more complex intermediate level of care is feasible only for urban areas that have a population base large enough to support such an institution. For this reason, it is important to note that this policy—without the preceding one—could aggravate current inequalities between the urban and rural populations. It is an extremely important strategy to face the fast-growing health problems of urban areas, and defining mechanisms of cooperation between public and private sectors can be very effective because both are already providing care for these conditions. Perhaps the most successful experience that has applied these reforms to the health care model comes from Cali, Colombia. Several reports have shown that with limited investment, these policies led to improved efficiency and effectiveness at the hospital level, greater coverage of delivery care and other conditions, improvements in the satisfaction of patients, and lower (direct and indirect) costs (Vélez and de Vélez, 1984; Guerrero, 1990).

Improved Efficiency and Quality of Care

The evidence for inefficiency in the use of resources abounds in the health sectors of developing countries (Akin et al., 1987). The most common example is given by the low output of facilities and health personnel at the primary and secondary levels of care. Occupancy rates of less than 40 percent are common in district- and other second-level hospitals, mainly in the public sector. The reasons for this underutilization of resources are related to poor organization of the health centers, lack of resources (drugs, equipment, and other), and poor quality of care. Potential users perceive these services as inadequate to meet their health needs and resort to alternative options, such as private doctors and hospitals or tertiary level of care public hospitals. As a consequence, tertiary-level hospitals are typically overloaded with patients having trivial or nonsevere conditions. Occupancy rates of these hospitals range from 80 to more than 100 percent, depending on the ward. Moreover, many admissions and lengths of stay are not medically justified, adding to the misuse of scarce resources in these hospitals.

The services provided by the ministries of health of Brazil, Colombia, and Mexico all share these characteristics. In Colombia and Mexico, however, the social security and private schemes are more efficient, with higher output per health personnel and health facility. On the other hand, inefficiency in Brazil is high because the National Institute for Medical Care (INAMPS), which originated from the social security system and is now linked with the Ministry of Health, is the largest health scheme in the country and buys most of the hospital services from the private sector. With INAMPS the excess of intervention and the problems of quality are further exacerbated because the control over private practice is very limited (Mello, 1981; McGreevey, 1989; Possas, 1989b).

Suboptimal quality of health care in developing countries is, to a large extent, due to scarcity of resources and administrative inability to deliver the required inputs on time, but more money and resources alone will not improve the standards of care. Unnecessary interventions, which are a reflection of poor quality, occur more often in institutions and facilities where the supply of resources is adequate. Hysterectomies, caesarean sections, tonsillectomies, and appendectomies are only a few of the interventions that are provided excessively in some health institutions of developing and industrialized countries. Brazil and Mexico experience some of the highest levels of caesarean deliveries in the world (Bobadilla, 1988), but paradoxically, in the rural areas of these countries, between 20 and 30 percent of births are not attended by a health professional. Excessive medical intervention wastes money, produces morbidity and mortality (sometimes offsetting its health benefits at the population level), and entails a high opportunity cost for the health care of the poor.

The problems of the quality of hospital-based services are more difficult to solve and have more severe consequences than those of the health centers or doctors' offices. It has been documented that cuts in the health budgets of many Latin American countries affected the purchase of drugs and supplies, as well as salary levels, but left the scope, number, and content of existing health programs largely untouched (Cruz et al., 1991). Less money for medical supplies and for equipment, maintenance, supervision, administration, and salaries has produced two effects: an improvement in the efficiency when there was a margin to do so, and a deterioration in the quality of care (Ayala and Schaffer, 1991). Public hospitals have been more severely affected because of the increased demand from the population group that had previously sought attention through private hospitals.

Three policies deserve serious consideration to improve the quality of care and the efficiency of service delivery:

Certification of Hospitals

The diversity of institutions engaged in the provision of services in these three countries suggests that a single nationally recognized commission or office should perform regular evaluations of hospitals. Such a commission ought to be independent of the interested parties and probably separate from the government. Failing to pass the certification a predetermined number of times should lead to closure of a facility. Obviously new laws would be required to make hospitals comply and to settle disputes. This policy has already been suggested for Mexico (Ruelas, 1990).

Certification of Physicians and Other Health Professionals

A system similar to that proposed above would ensure that health professionals update their knowledge and improve their practice over time.

Quality Assurance Systems

Good administration of health facilities is not enough to achieve optimal quality of care. It is necessary to develop information systems on process and outcome that facilitate monitoring the performance of health facilities, particularly hospitals. Peer review systems should be formed with authority to introduce the necessary changes in the organization of an institution and to modify the incentives that guide the behavior of health personnel. The development of techniques and methods for quality assurance has been substantial over the last decade in industrialized countries. There is an urgent need to adapt these techniques and methods, and to train health professionals in this relatively new area of health management (Ruelas, 1990).

The relative rise in noncommunicable diseases will pose additional problems to health institutions that are currently not prepared to deal adequately with complex services. These policies to improve quality are more justified today by the epidemiological transition as the demand for hospital care increases while resources remain the same or decrease.

National Capacity Building for Strategic Health Planning

Debate on the policies for human resource development in these countries has often been polarized around two alternative approaches: (1) comprehensive health care and (2) vertical programs that focus on preventive and/or curative services. The short-term concerns, together with other social and cultural factors, have led governments to neglect investment in analytical-capacity building in fields such as health policy, epidemiology, and health economics. Until this gap is filled, the application of modern methodologies and conceptual frameworks to the analysis of health needs may be seriously jeopardized.

The development of more adequate institutional and management structures to deal with the consequences of the epidemiological transition will require multisectoral activities and multidisciplinary inputs that exceed the limited, medically oriented approach commonly used in the ministries of health and the social security institutes of these countries (Marques, 1989). To face this challenge, countries will need to invest in four critical areas:

Development of Human Resources in Planning and Management

The strengthening of planning and management activities at all levels will require new priorities for health personnel training. The relationships among universities, technical schools, and health institutions will need to be reinforced (Soberón et al., 1988a,b) in a few key areas where collaboration is critical: evaluation of services, cost-effectiveness analysis of alternative interventions, and updating of the curricula and health personnel knowledge.

Better Quality of Health Information Systems

Large amounts of health information are available in middle-income countries, but only a fraction of this is used in decision making (Cordeiro et al., 1990). Even if all the available information were processed and adequately presented for decision making, critical pieces of information would usually still be missing. Finally, the information on births and mortality, collected through vital statistics, is essential for health planning, but the coverage and quality of the data are still deficient in most Latin American countries (Chackiel, 1987).

Development and Strengthening of Essential National Health Research

Essential National Health Research has been proposed (Commission on Health Research for Development, 1990) as one of the most effective means to overcome the heavy burden of disease in developing countries and to reduce the health status inequalities within and among them. This idea refers to the capacity to undertake research on health problems primarily relevant for the developing countries and to advance knowledge on global health issues. It is a system in which the main actors serve both as research-oriented universities, schools of public health, and research centers, and as the providers of health services, and it embodies substantial political commitment, adequate financial support, and the demand for research. Currently, the strength of Brazil, Colombia, and Mexico is in biomedical research, and less so in clinical and public health research (Bobadilla et al., 1988; Cordeiro et al., 1990). The epidemiological transition and the challenges posed to the health system will require a substantial growth in the quantity, relevance, and quality of epidemiological and health systems research.

Capacity Building in Health Technology Assessment

New technologies in clinical medicine are typically additive, inducing more diagnostic and therapeutic procedures—not replacing existing ones (Possas, 1991). This additivity, coupled with rapid technological innovation, has resulted in profound effects on health care costs, with as much as 50 percent of the marginal increments in health care costs being due to new technologies (Panerai and Mohr, 1989). The introduction of new technologies and drugs should be preceded by a thorough assessment of their likely effect on different parts of the health system (cost and effectiveness among other aspects) and on the health of the population (ethical and cultural issues). Such an evaluation requires a critical mass of professionals trained in epidemiology, engineering, health economics, behavioral sciences, and health management. A broad range of modern technologies is already available in these middle-income countries, but limited information and research on the consequences of their incorporation into the health system have been used to approve their purchase and diffusion (Marques, 1989).

CONCLUSION

Since the mid-1980s many developing countries and most of the international agencies that work in the health field have become increasingly aware of the importance of the epidemiological transition. The policy implications of the transition have attracted the attention of scholars and health specialists from a wide variety of disciplines. As a consequence of this renewed interest in the transition, four major positive changes in the conceptual model of health can be identified: (1) health policies are examined through a multidisciplinary approach; (2) health policies deal more with increasing overall health status of populations, and evaluations of the health system are more often linking resources with health improvements; (3) inclusion of health problems of all age groups and not only children in the analysis of the burden of disease, and inclusion of noncommunicable diseases and injury in the spectrum of preventable causes of ill-health; and (4) broadening of health interventions to encompass social policies aimed at reducing environmental risk factors and modifying negative lifestyles.

Examination of the health policies in Brazil, Colombia, and Mexico has led us to conclude that there are five main implications of the epidemiological transition for health policy in developing countries. First, the transition offers an empirical framework for strategic planning of the health system, because it allows anticipation of future trends of mortality and its causes, and suggests some of the future scenarios in the burden of disease. Second, because the transition anticipates a greater burden of disease in the adult and elderly populations, the mission of the health system needs to be revised, giving more emphasis to disease prevention and control, and less to demand satisfaction. Third, the current deficiencies of the health system, both organizational and operational, must urgently be corrected because they would be major obstacles in the implementation of other policies intended to improve the health status of the population. Fourth, explicit criteria to set priorities in the health sector need to be defined, so that resources can be distributed among competing socioeconomic groups and health needs. Fifth, the capacity to analyze the health status of populations, evaluate the performance of the health system, and design cost-effective interventions to deal with noncommunicable diseases needs to be strengthened.

Most of the policy issues identified in this paper deal with current deficiencies of the health system and propose ways in which they can be corrected within the legal and financial constraints existing in these countries. A second group of issues suggests ways to deal with the growing burden due to noncommunicable diseases and injury. Most of the suggestions can be implemented without extra financial resources, but call for a substantial reallocation of the available resources.

Only the national level has been analyzed, and this clearly leads to some generalizations that cannot be sustained when provinces or districts are examined. The intracountry variations in health profiles, and the performance and organization of health systems are substantial in the three countries and warrant more detailed analysis of the issues and recommendations made in this paper. Finally, it is worth remembering that immediate political interests have not been considered because they are beyond the scope of this analysis.

The challenge facing all developing countries in the next century will be to define realistic and feasible strategies able to avoid the increasing burden of noncommunicable diseases and injuries before they reach the levels observed in developed countries and, at the same time, to maintain the efforts to reduce the "unfinished agenda." More than a decade ago, John Evans and colleagues (1981:1126) said that "no satisfactory strategy has been developed to meet the health needs of older children and adults within the financial means of most developing countries" and that "the search for health technology appropriate to the financial and organizational circumstances of developing countries must be seen as a high priority for the research and development community of the entire world." Research, innovation, creativity, and imagination are readily available for many social problems worldwide. The most rational policy for future health problems in developing countries is to apply our best resources to search for appropriate answers to fill this gap identified more than a decade ago.

REFERENCES

Akin, J., N. Birdsall, and D. de Ferranti
1987 *Financing Health Services in Developing Countries: An Agenda for Reform.* World Bank Policy Study. Washington, D.C.: World Bank.

Ayala, R., and C. Schaffer
1991 *Salud y Seguridad Social. Crisis, Ajuste y Grupos Vulnerables.* Perspectivas en Salud Publica No. 12. Mexico: Instituto Nacional de Salud Publica.

Bell, D.
1993 Some implications of the health transition for policy and research. In L. Chen, A. Kleinman, and N. Ware, eds., *Health and Social Change: An International Perspective.* Cambridge, Mass.: Harvard School of Public Health.

Bobadilla, J.L.
1988 *Quality of Perinatal Medical Care in Mexico City.* Perspectivas en Salud Pública No. 3. Mexico: Instituto Nacional de Salud Pública.

Bobadilla, J.L., and G. Walker
1991 Early neonatal mortality and cesarean delivery in Mexico City. *American Journal of Obstetrics and Gynecology* 164:22-28.

Bobadilla, J.L., J. Frenk, and J. Sepúlveda
1988 Health research in Mexico: Strengths, weaknesses and gaps. Background paper prepared for the Commission on Health Research for Development, Mexico City.

Bobadilla, J.L., J. Frenk, T. Frejka, R. Lozano, and C. Stern
1993 The epidemiological transition and health priorities. In D. Jamison and H. Mosley, eds., *Disease Control Priorities in Developing Countries*. New York: Oxford University Press for the World Bank.

Caldwell, J., S. Findley, P. Caldwell, G. Santow, W. Cosford, J. Braid, and D. Broers-Freeman, eds.
1989 What we know about health transition: The cultural, social and behavioural determinant of health. Proceedings of an International Workshop, Australian National University, Canberra, May.

Chackiel, J.
1987 La investigación sobre causas de muerte en America Latina. *Notas de Poblacion* 44:9-30. Santiago de Chile: Celade.

Comision Economica para American Latina y el Caribe
1990 *Magnitud de la Pobreza en America Latina en Los Anos Ochenta*. Santiago de Chile: CEPAL.

Commission on Health Research for Development.
1990 *Health Research: Essential Link to Equity in Development*. New York: Oxford University Press.

Consejo Consultivo del Programa Nacional de Solidaridad
1990 *El Combate a la Pobreza: Lineamientos Programaticos*. Mexico: El Nacional, S.A. de C.V.

Cordeiro, H.A. (Coord.), M.B. Marques, C.A. Possas, and P.M. Buss
1990 Prioridades Nacionais, Pesquisa Essencial e Desenvolvimento em Saude. Serie Politica de Saude No. 10, Fundacão Oswaldo Cruz, Rio de Janeiro, 1990. Paper prepared for the workshop held in the Oswaldo Cruz Foundation with the Commision on Health Research for Development, Rio de Janeiro, October.

Cruz, C., R. Lozano, and J. Querol
1991 *The Impact of Economic Crisis and Adjustment on Health Care in México*. Innocenti Ocassional Papers Number 13. Florence: International Child Development Centre (UNICEF).

Evans, J., K. Lashman Hall, and J. Warford
1981 Shattuck lecture—Health care in the developing world: Problems of scarcity and choice. *New England Journal of Medicine* 305:1117-1127.

Frenk, J., J.L. Bobadilla, J. Sepúlveda, and M. López-Cervantes
1989 Health transition in middle-income countries: New challenges for health care. *Health Policy and Planning* 4:29-39.

Frenk, J., J.L. Bobadilla, C. Stern, T. Frejka, and R. Lozano
1991 Elements for a theory of the health transition. *Health Transition Review* 1:21-38.

Gish, O.
1988 Intervenciones minimas de atencion primaria a la salud para la sobrevivencia en la infancia. *Salud Pública de México* 30:432-446.

Guerrero, R.
1990 Regionalizacion de la atencion quirurgica: Un ejemplo de investigacion aplicada. In J. Frenk, ed., *Salud: de la Investigación a la Acción*. Mexico: Fondo de Cultura Economica.

Jamison, D., and H. Mosley
1991 Disease control priorities in the developing countries: Health policy responses to epidemiological change. *American Journal of Public Health* 81:15-22.

Laurenti, R.
1990 Transicáo Demográfica e Transicáo Epidemiológica. *Anais, 1o. Congresso Brasileiro*

de Epidemiologia. Epidemiologia e Desigualdade Social: Os Desafios do Final do Século. Campinas: UNICAMP.

Marques, M.B.

1989 *A Reforma Sanitária Brasileira e a Política Científica e Tecnológica Necessaria*, Serie Política de Saúde No. 8. Rio de Janeiro: FIOCRUZ/NEP.

McGreevey, W.P.

1989 Los altos costos de la atencion de salud en el Brasil. In *Economia de la Salud: Perspectivas para America Latina.* Organización Panamericana de la Salud, Publicación Cientifica No. 517. Washington, D.C.

Médici, A.C.

1989 Financiamento das políticas de saúde no Brasil. In *Economia de la Salud: Perspectivas para America Latina.* Organización Panamericana de la Salud, Publicación Cientifica No. 517. Washington, D.C.

Mello, C.G.

1981 *O sistema de saude em crise.* CEBES-HUCITEC. Sáo Paulo: Colecáo Saude em Debate.

Ministerio de Salud

1990 *La Salud en Colombia, Tomo 1.* Bogota.

Panerai, R.B., and J.P. Mohr

1989 *Health Technology Assessment Methodologies for Developing Countries.* Washington, D.C.: Pan American Health Organization.

Possas, C.

1989a *Epidemiologia e Sociedade: Heterogeneidade Estrutural e Saúde no Brazil.* São Paulo: HUCITEC.

1989b *Saude e Trabalho: a Crise da Previdencia Social.* Prefácio a 2a edicao. São Paulo: HUCITEC.

1991 Fiscal crisis, social changes and health policy strategies in Brazil. Background paper to the discussion of the Takemi Research Proposal, Takemi Program in International Health, Harvard School of Public Health, Boston, October.

Rondinelli, D.A., and G. S. Cheema

1983 Implementing decentralization policies: An introduction. In G.S. Cheema and D.D. Rondinelli, eds., *Decentralization and Development Policy Implementation in Developing Countries.* Beverly Hills, Calif.: Sage Publications.

Ruelas, E.

1990 Transiciones indispensables: De la cantidad a la calidad y de la evaluacion a la garantia. *Salud Pública de México* 2:108-110.

Rutstein, S.O.

1992 Levels, trends and differentials in infant and child mortality in the less developed countries. Pp. 17-42 in K. Hill, ed., *Child Survival Priorities for the 1990s.* Baltimore, Md.: Johns Hopkins University Institute for International Programs.

Soberón, G., J. Kumate, and J. Laguna

1988a *La Salud en México: Testimonios 1988. I. Fundamentos del Cambio Estructural.* Mexico: Fondo de Cultura Económica.

Soberón, G., J. Frenk, and A. Langer

1988b Requerimientos del paradigma de la atención primaria a la salud en los albores del siglo XXI. *Salud Pública de México* 30:791-803.

United Nations Children's Fund

1992 *The State of the World's Children 1992.* New York: Oxford University Press.

Vélez, A., and G. de Vélez

1984 Investigación de modelos de atención en cirugia: Programa sistema de cirugia simplificada. *Educacion Médica y Salud* 8.

Vianna, S.M., S.F. Piola, A.J.E. Guerra, and S.F. Camargo
1990 *O Financiamento da Descentralizacáo dos Servicos de Saúde: Criterios para transferencias de Recursos Federais para Estados e Municipios.* Série Economia e Financiamento No. 1. Brasília: OPAS, Representacáo.
World Bank
1991 *World Development Report 1991: The Challenge of Development.* Washington, D.C.
1992 Global Health Statistics. Unpublished tables. World Health Organization, Washington, D.C.
World Health Organization
1990 *1989 World Health Statistics Annual.* Geneva: World Health Organization.

APPENDIX

Economic, Social, and Health Status Characteristics of Brazil, Colombia, and Mexico

BRAZIL

Economic

Per capita GDP (1989): U.S.$2,540.[a]
Average annual inflation (1980-1989): >200%.[a]
Very high income concentration (1983): highest 10% with 46% of income, and lowest 20% with 2.4% of income.[a]

Social[b]

Population in poverty (1987): 45%.[c]
Access to safe water (1983-1986): 75%.[d]
Access to sanitation facilities (1983-1986): 78%.[d]
Illiteracy rate in adult population (1985): 22%.[a]

Heath Status

Life expectancy at birth (1984): 66 years.[a]
Mortality under 5 (1989): 8.5%.[a]
Percentage of deaths due to infectious diseases (1985): 12%.[e]
Malaria, tuberculosis, and AIDS are rising very fast.
Cholera is spreading fast from the north and northeast.
Life expectancy is 16 years lower in the northeast than in the south.[f]

COLOMBIA

Economic

Per capita GDP (1989): U.S.$1,200.[a]
Average annual inflation (1980-1989): 24%.[a]
Very high income concentration (1988): highest 10% with 37% income and lowest 20% with 4% income.[a]

Social[b]

Population in poverty (1986): 42%.[c]
Access to safe water (1985): 88%.[d]
Access to sanitation facilities (1985): 65%.[d]
Illiteracy rate in adult population (1985): 12%.[a]

Health Status

Life expectancy at birth (1989): 69 years.[a]
Mortality under 5 (1989): 5.0%.[d]
Percentage of deaths due to infectious diseases (1986): 10%.[e]
Violence and other cause of injury are probably the major cause of premature mortality.
Malaria and cholera are resurging.

MEXICO

Economic

Per capita GDP (1989): U.S.$2,010.[a]
Average annual inflation (1980-1989): 72%.[a]
Very high income concentration (1983): highest 10% with 40% of income and lowest 20% with 1.3% of income.[g]

MEXICO—continued

Social[b]

Population in poverty (1984): 37%.[c]

Access to safe water (1983-1985): 69%.[d]

Access to sanitation facilities (1983-1985): 45%.[d]

Illiteracy rate in adult population (1985): 10%.[a]

Health Status

Life expectancy at birth (1989): 69 years.[a]

Mortality under 5 (1989): 5.1%.[d]

Percentage of deaths due to infectious diseases (1986): 20%.[e]

Malnutrition in rural areas is still a high public health priority; inequalities of health status between population groups are very wide.

Oaxaca has a life expectancy 12 years less than Nuevo Léon.

NOTE: GDP = gross domestic product.

[a]World Bank (1991).

[b]Population in poverty is defined as those who earn an income less than two times the required amount to purchase the basic food basket.

[c]Comision Economica para America Latina y el Caribe (1990).

[d]World Bank (1992).

[e]See Table 2 footnotes for sources.

[f]Instituto Brasileiro de Geografia e Estadistica (1984).

[g]Consejo Consultivo del Programma Nacional de Solidaridad (1990).

Goals of the World Summit for Children and Their Implications for Health Policy in the 1990s

Anne R. Pebley

INTRODUCTION

With great fanfare and major media coverage, the World Summit for Children was held at the United Nations on September 29-30, 1990. The summit was initially proposed by UNICEF in its *State of the World's Children* report published in December 1988. At the invitation of United Nations Secretary General Javier Perez de Cuellar, heads of state from 72 countries and representatives from 88 others attended.

The underlying objective of the summit was to focus the attention of international political leaders on the problems of children, particularly children's health, at a time when international political alignments and priorities were changing rapidly. The summit was also intended as a public endorsement of and a renewed commitment to a specific approach to health policy in developing countries—the "child survival strategy"—which has been a central component of health programs implemented by UNICEF, the World Health Organization (WHO), private nongovernmental organizations (NGOs), and many developing countries, and funded by many donor countries during the 1980s. The statement in which the summit was announced (UNICEF, 1990b:2) by the six initiating governments explained that

---

Anne R. Pebley is at the Woodrow Wilson School and Office of Population Research, Princeton University. The author is grateful to Noreen Goldman, James Gribble, and Barry Wolf for their comments and suggestions.

> the purpose of the World Summit for Children is to bring attention and promote commitment, at the highest political level, to goals and strategies for ensuring the survival, protection, and development of children as key elements in the socio-economic development of all countries and human society. . . . Experience in recent years with the approaches known generally as the Child Survival and Development Revolution has demonstrated that dramatic progress can be achieved in reducing child deaths and improving child health and well-being. The necessary mobilization of multiple sectors of government and society to achieve this progress invariably requires the personal and active involvement of national leaders. It has also been demonstrated that this improvement in the survival of children through the involvement of parents contributes to a subsequent voluntary reduction in births.

The summit issued a "World Declaration on the Survival, Protection and Development of Children," which included specific goals that the summiteers endorsed "for implementation by all countries where they are applicable . . ." prior to the year 2000. Because some of the wording used in the original text is open to varying interpretation, I have reproduced the goals as they are stated in the declaration in the appendix to this paper. They are summarized in Table 1 according to the type of outcome sought through each goal.

I have intentionally placed mortality reduction goals first because they are the principal subjects of this paper. Nonetheless, it is important to recognize that the summit goals themselves are *not* limited to mortality reduction, but include substantial reductions in morbidity and improvements in health-related conditions (such as nutritional status and dietary deficiency diseases) and health-related services (such as access to safe drinking water and to prenatal care). The summit goals address most of the major health problems afflicting children in developing countries, and many of these conditions have a far greater effect numerically on children's morbidity than they do on mortality. As Mosley and Gray (this volume) have shown, reduction in childhood morbidity or malnutrition may also improve the health and survival chances of adults later in life.

Despite the broad reach of the summit goals, they may or may not constitute the optimal and most realistic approach for all developing countries to improving children's health in the next decade, for a variety of other reasons. This paper is a brief assessment of the implications and consequences of pursuing and/or achieving the goals of the summit. In the first section of the paper, I consider whether the magnitude of the mortality reduction goals proposed seems feasible in light of past experience and whether achievement of these goals is likely to lead to substantial additional population growth. The second section of the paper is a discussion of the methods proposed in the summit document for implementing the goals, and the implications of governments and donors pursuing some goals but not others.

MAGNITUDE OF THE SUMMIT GOALS

Proposed Mortality Reductions in Light of Past Experience

One striking characteristic of the summit goals is that most are very specific with regard to desired numerical targets, and the targets chosen are often quite ambitious. There are at least two advantages of clear numerical targets. First, the success (or lack of success) that programs make toward achievement of the goals can be evaluated more effectively. Second, as those involved in business and program development have known for years, the target number itself provides a strong motivational force for fund raising, program planning, and program implementation. Some of the goals appear to be intended more as motivational targets—in the sense of what can be accomplished under ideal conditions—than as realistic goals that are likely to be accomplished. As a UNICEF (1990b:4) publication issued on the eve of the summit explains:

> The goal of 80% child immunization by the end of 1990 has undoubtedly helped to lift coverage from 10% in the late 1970s to over 70% at the time of writing. It may therefore now be useful to adopt specific goals for the year 2000 . . . . The following list of child-related goals are considered to be both technically feasible and financially affordable over the course of the next decade.

A potential disadvantage of specific numerical targets is that the attention of public health workers, government officials, and the donor community may be so strongly focused on achieving the targets themselves that they lose sight of the general objectives of improving children's health, sustaining health improvements, and strengthening public health care systems (Unger, 1991). There is also the potential for considerable frustration on the part of government officials and donors if the goals are not achieved.

How realistic are the child mortality goals in light of the experience of the last several decades? The goals adopted at the summit for infant and child mortality (see Table 1) for individual countries depend on the level of those mortality rates in 1990. It is not clear from the language used in the declaration whether infant mortality, for example, is to be reduced either by one-third or to 50 per 1,000 live births, whichever produces the *lower mortality rate* in the year 2000, or whether the reference is to whichever *reduction* is less. The difference between these two interpretations is substantial: if the objective is to achieve the lowest rate, then the proposed mortality reductions, particularly in those parts of the world in which mortality is very high such as sub-Saharan Africa, will be considerably more than one-third. If, for simplicity, we assume that the goal is to reduce both under-5 mortality rates and infant mortality rates by one-third in the 10 years

TABLE 1 Summary of Specific Goals of the World Summit for Children by 2000 (except as noted)

Mortality Reduction Goals
- *Infant mortality rates* reduced by one-third or to 50 per 1,000 live births, whichever is less;
- *Under-5 mortality rates* reduced by one-third or to 70 per 1,000 live births, whichever is less;
- *Maternal mortality rate* reduced by half;
- *Deaths due to measles* reduced by 95 percent compared to preimmunization levels by 1995;
- *Deaths due to diarrhea* reduced by half;
- *Deaths due to acute respiratory infections* reduced by one-third.

Disease[a] Elimination or Eradication
- *Poliomyelitis* eradication;
- *Neonatal tetanus* elimination by 1995;
- *Iodine deficiency* (virtual) elimination;[b]
- *Vitamin A deficiency* (virtual) elimination;[b]
- *Guinea-worm disease (dracunculiasis)* elimination.

Disease Condition Reduction
- *Severe and moderate malnutrition* among children under-5 reduced by half of 1990 levels;
- *Low birthweight (2.5 kilograms or less)* reduced to less than 10 percent;
- *Iron deficiency anemia in women* reduced by one-third of 1990 levels;
- *Measles* cases reduced by 90 percent compared to preimmunization levels;
- *Diarrhea incidence* rate reduced by 25 percent;

Health Service Provision-Related Goals
- Universal access to *safe drinking water* and to *sanitary means of excreta disposal*;
- Access to *contraceptive information* and *contraception* for spacing, delaying, and terminating childbearing;
- Access to *prenatal care* and *trained childbirth attendants*;
- Institutionalization of *growth promotion* and *regular monitoring*.

Other Goals
- Universal access to *basic education* and completion of primary school by at least 80 percent of primary school-age children;
- Reduction of *adult illiteracy* and emphasis on female literacy;
- Dissemination of knowledge and supporting services to *increase food production* to ensure household food security;
- Use of mass media and social action to impart *skills for better living* to families and individuals;
- *Protection of children* in especially difficult circumstances.

NOTES:

[a]As used here, "disease" includes nutritional deficiency diseases.

[b]The goals do not give a specific year by which iodine deficiency and vitamin A deficiency are to be eliminated. The year 2000 is assumed because these goals are intended to be accomplished during the 1990s.

between 1990 and 2000, we can compare this goal with previous experience in mortality reduction in developing countries.

Table 2 presents estimates of the percentage decline in under-5 mortality rates ($_5q_0$) (i.e., deaths of children less than 5 years of age per 1,000 live births) for 10-year periods since the 1960s from an article by Hill and Pebley (1989), updated with more recent data from Sullivan (1991). Table 2 includes only countries that have data judged to be reliable for at least two periods of time 10 years apart. Nonetheless, caution should be exercised in interpreting the magnitude of the changes because of remaining problems with data quality. In Latin America, Asia, and the Middle East, many countries have been able to achieve reductions in under-5 mortality of at least one-third in at least one decade since 1960-1965. In four Latin American countries (Chile, Colombia, Costa Rica, and Cuba), Puerto Rico, three Asian countries (Hong Kong, Singapore, and Thailand), and one Middle Eastern country (Kuwait), mortality declined by 33 percent or more in at least three of the four decades. Such reduction was most likely also the case for China and Korea, and may also have been true for Jamaica, although data for the last time period are unavailable.

However, there are also a number of countries outside of sub-Saharan Africa in which estimates are available for three or four decades but in which declines of 33 percent or more were not achieved in any of these decade-long periods, including Brazil, Guatemala, Mexico, Peru, Indonesia, the Philippines, and Turkey. Several of the poorest countries in each region, with data available for only one or two decades, also failed to achieve declines of 33 percent in under-5 mortality in any of the decades for which data are available. This group includes Bangladesh, Haiti, Nepal, and Pakistan.

The case of Africa is much harder to assess because of the lack of data for many countries and time periods. To the extent that there is a correlation between the availability of reliable mortality data and the likelihood of major mortality declines on the order of those experienced by China, Chile, or Costa Rica, it is less likely that especially large declines occurred in many of the countries for which data are unavailable. Despite the relative lack of data on under-5 mortality change for African countries, the data that are available make it clear that declines of 33 percent or more were rare: only Botswana, Kenya, and Zimbabwe experienced under-5 mortality declines of this magnitude, in at least one of the decades shown. It is important to note that several major public health programs, such as WHO's Expanded Programme of Immunizations (EPI), were initiated in sub-Saharan Africa in the early 1980s. These efforts are likely to have had their greatest effect on under-5 mortality by the late 1980s and early 1990s, the period for which the least information is currently available. Unfortunately, the effects of these programs on child mortality may have been reduced by the economic crises suffered by African economies during this period.

TABLE 2 Decline in Under-5 Mortality Rates ($_5q_0$) in Developing Countries with Reliable Data by Country, Region and Time Period (percent)

Country	1960-1965 to 1970-1975	1965-1970 to 1975-1980	1970-1975 to 1980-1985	1975-1980 to 1985-1990
Latin America				
Argentina	19.4	29.4	27.6	—
Bolivia	—	—	34.8	—
Brazil	17.8	23.0	31.2	—
Chile	41.9	53.6	64.5	—
Colombia	34.1	46.2	52.8	—
Costa Rica	42.9	60.2	62.5	—
Cuba	41.6	54.1	53.3	—
Dominican Republic	—	—	33.3	—
Ecuador	22.3	25.6	33.8	29.3
Guatemala	—	28.0	27.2	20.9
Haiti	—	—	18.5	—
Jamaica	37.7	48.4	—	—
Mexico	21.3	23.0	23.0	29.9
Panama	29.9	42.7	45.6	—
Peru	27.1	24.2	29.6	—
Puerto Rico	46.3	43.6	34.5	—
Trinidad and Tobago	30.2	36.0	24.3	—
Uruguay	1.9	9.3	34.6	—
Asia				
Bangladesh	—	3.1	5.7	—
China	48.8	48.7	—	—
Hong Kong	55.3	50.0	42.9	—
Indonesia	22.2	27.4	30.3	30.8
Republic of Korea	38.4	36.8	—	—
Malaysia	31.9	36.1	33.9	—
Nepal	17.2	—	—	—
Pakistan	—	16.3	—	—
Philippines	21.1	21.9	17.8	—
Singapore	45.2	48.4	47.8	—
Sri Lanka	21.8	24.1	—	47.0
Thailand	33.1	40.7	39.6	35.7
Middle East				
Egypt	—	32.1	35.4	46.3
Jordan	38.7	30.3	—	—
Kuwait	48.6	42.5	50.9	—
Syria	—	39.3	—	—
Tunisia	26.5	38.1	—	50.0
Turkey	23.0	22.8	23.4	—

continued

TABLE 2 *Continued*

Country	1960-1965 to 1970-1975	1965-1970 to 1975-1980	1970-1975 to 1980-1985	1975-1980 to 1985-1990
Africa				
Benin	—	15.7	—	—
Botswana	19.4	32.3	47.4	49.5
Burkina Faso	5.0	—	—	—
Burundi	8.2	—	—	—
Cameroon	19.7	—	—	—
Central African Republic	24.9	—	—	—
Ghana	20.2	23.5	8.1	-3.3
Kenya	20.6	39.6	—	16.8
Lesotho	7.1	—	—	—
Liberia	6.5	12.9	20.0	—
Malawi	6.2	—	—	—
Mali	—	—	16.3	17.2
Nigeria	17.9	11.5	—	—
Rwanda	-2.2	-3.6	—	—
Senegal	2.5	14.2	23.6	21.1
Sudan	—	25.5	—	14.0
Tanzania	7.6	—	—	—
Togo	—	10.6	—	22.2
Uganda	15.6	11.5	-3.6	-5.3
Zimbabwe	6.5	10.5	—	45.3

SOURCE: Hill and Pebley (1989:Table A-1); Sullivan (1991).

Achievement of a specific *percentage* of mortality reduction may be considerably easier for countries with lower initial mortality rates. This observation may account for part of the difference in size of the percentage change between African countries and those in other parts of the world. For example, a reduction of one-third in a relatively low-mortality country with an initial infant mortality rate of 30 per 1,000 live births means preventing 10 additional deaths per 1,000 live births each year. However, in a country with an initial infant mortality rate of 90, a one-third reduction in infant mortality would require the prevention of 30 additional deaths per 1,000 live births[1] each year, three times as many deaths as in the low-mortality country.

[1]On the other hand, it may be easier to bring about large mortality declines in high-mortality countries because the causes of childhood death that predominate in these countries (e.g., infectious diseases) are easier to prevent and treat than the causes of death that predominate in lower-mortality countries (e.g., perinatal problems). Previous experience shown in Table 2, however, suggests that high-mortality countries have not generally experienced the greatest mortality declines in the past several decades.

The pattern of changes in infant mortality rates (not shown) during decades between 1960-1965 and 1985-1990 is very similar to that shown in Table 2 for under-5 mortality. This is not surprising because deaths in infancy constitute a substantial part of all deaths before the fifth birthday.[2]

In summary, a number of countries have been able to achieve reductions in under-5 and infant mortality of 33 percent or more over a 10-year period. Thus, the goal of a one-third reduction in mortality rates for children seems plausible in light of previous experience. However, it is important to recognize that many of the countries that have been most successful at achieving declines of this magnitude either have unusually well-organized health care systems (e.g., Cuba and China, and perhaps Costa Rica), and/or are economically well-off relative to other countries in their region (e.g., Chile, Korea, Hong Kong, Singapore, Thailand, Kuwait, Zimbabwe, Kenya, and Botswana). The evidence is not in yet on whether infant and child mortality can be reduced by as much as one-third in a 10-year period in poorer, high-mortality countries, with less well-organized health systems, through the type of program adopted at the summit.

The summit goals also include the reduction of maternal mortality rates by half. Reliable data on past reductions in maternal mortality on a national basis over a 10-year period are even more scarce than information on childhood mortality reductions. Thus, it is difficult to determine whether reductions of 50 percent appear feasible in light of previous experience, and I have not attempted to do so here. Compared with deaths in infancy, deaths due to maternal mortality are relatively uncommon even in countries that have high maternal mortality rates by international standards. Nonetheless, reduction in maternal mortality rates is an important goal because the institution of practices to reduce these rates will also reduce the incidence of nonlethal maternal injury, illness, and infection connected with pregnancy, which affect a substantially larger number of women in developing countries. Reductions in maternal mortality and morbidity are also an essential part of programs designed to improve the health of children. In most developing countries, mothers continue to play the key role in care for children, and children whose mothers have died have much lower survival rates and are also likely to be sicker. Mothers who have suffered serious but nonfatal birth injuries are also likely to be considerably less effective in caring for their newborn children.

---

[2]In fact, from a demographer's point of view, it would make considerably more sense to specify goals for infant mortality and for 1- to 5-year-old mortality. Focusing on both infant and under-5 mortality seems like a form of double counting because infant mortality is included in rates for both age groups. However, "1- to 5-year-old mortality" is not a particularly memorable phrase for purposes of publicity and promotion, and the term "childhood mortality" is presumably too vague.

Despite the importance of reducing maternal morbidity and mortality, this goal may be considerably more difficult to achieve than some of the others because of the nature of measures required. Unlike measles immunization, for example, which requires one contact for each child, the provision of adequate prenatal care (even if it is limited to one prenatal visit), safe delivery, and postpartum care for each pregnancy, or contraceptive services to prevent unsafe abortions to all women, is a monumental task in many poor countries.

Potential Demographic Consequences

During the 1960s and 1970s, there was considerable debate in the public health community about whether reducing infant and child mortality rates, in the absence of strong fertility reduction efforts, would add to the rapid population growth already being experienced by many countries in the world. The controversy has recently been raised again (see Kalish, 1992). Would implementing the goals of the summit dramatically increase population growth rates?

In the absence of other demographic changes, mortality declines generally have three demographic consequences: (1) an increase in population growth rates, (2) a change in the age structure, and (3) a change in the relative importance of different causes of death. A 33 percent reduction in infant and child mortality rates in developing countries between 1990 and 2000 would increase population size (particularly the size of the population under age 10). However, it would clearly not affect the annual number of births (at least directly) until after the year 2000, because the additional children who survived because of the mortality reduction would generally not yet have reached their childbearing years by 2000. If mortality rates for children under 5 decreased faster than rates at other ages, the population would be "younger" on average than it would be otherwise—an effect that would subsequently be compounded when additional surviving children reached childbearing ages and gave birth to a larger total number of children. The cause-of-death structure would obviously also change to some degree as well because of the reduction of mortality for diseases that specifically affect children.

The amount of increased population growth that might actually be produced by a one-third reduction in infant and child mortality in a particular population between 1990 and 2000 will depend on three factors: (1) demographic trends in 1990 (including fertility and infant and child mortality rates), (2) the timing of the mortality decline, and (3) the level of fertility rates between 1990 and 2000. The initial level of infant and child mortality is important because a one-third decline from a lower mortality rate adds fewer survivors to the population. For example, if the infant mortality rate is 21 per 1,000, a one-third reduction will mean an additional 7 survivors per 1,000 live births. A one-third reduction in an initial rate of 210, however, implies an additional 70 survivors per 1,000 live births. This effect is compounded by the fact that fertility would likely remain high in many high-mortality countries; thus the number of live births annually (the denominator of the infant mortality rate) per size of the population is much larger than in the lower-mortality countries.[3] Thus, if the summit's goal of reducing all infant and child mortality rates by one-third were achieved, the potential for increased population growth would be greatest in high-mortality countries. However, note that these are exactly the countries in which, as I argued earlier, complete achievement of the summit's mortality reduction goals over the next several years is likely to be the most difficult.

The second factor, the timing of the reduction, would also help to determine the extent of the actual increase in population growth. If, for example, all the efforts proposed as part of the summit declaration were introduced immediately and effectively in 1990, the potential effect on population growth would be greater than if the efforts were phased in over 10 years. Although many countries began EPI, oral rehydration salts (ORS), and related programs during the 1980s, it seems doubtful that all of the proposed interventions would be in place until the end of the decade, at earliest, in many countries. Even in those countries that do achieve infant and child mortality rates in 2000 of one-third less than their 1990 rates, the change is likely to be a gradual one. In some countries, it may even be true that much of the change achieved occurs at the end of the decade as governments and NGOs increase their efforts to achieve the goals by 2000.

The third factor, the trend in fertility rates between 1990 and 2000, is especially important to any estimate of potential population growth rates. Clearly, if fertility rates decline quickly enough, this change can outweigh any increase in population growth rates due to mortality reductions.

Even in countries with currently high levels of fertility and mortality, however, a reduction by one-third in under-5 mortality that occurs evenly over 1990-2000 would not bring about a great change in population growth rates by the year 2000. Take, for example, the case of Senegal. The 1988 United Nations projection for Senegal for 1990-2000 was that infant mortal-

[3]For example, in a population with 1,810 births annually and an under-5 mortality rate of 210 deaths per 1000 live births, a one-third reduction in this rate would mean 70 additional survivors per 1,000 live births, or about 127 additional survivors every year. As the text indicates, another population with an initial rate of 21 deaths per 1,000 live births would have 7 additional survivors per 1,000 live births if mortality rates were reduced by one-third. If the annual number of births were the same as in the first population, this would mean an addition of only about 13 survivors annually. If the annual number of births were halved in each of the populations, the total number of additional survivors from a one-third reduction in under-5 mortality would be about 63 and 6, respectively.

ity would decline by about 16 percent, under-5 mortality by about the same amount, and the annual population growth rate during this period would be about 2.80 percent. If we assume that fertility rates remain constant[4] and that both infant and age 1-4 mortality rates decline by 33 percent—instead of 16 percent—between 1990 and 2000, the annual population growth rate for this period would increase only about 2.9 or 3.0 percent, depending on how the decline occurred.[5]

The longer-term consequences of the proposed reduction in under-5 mortality for population growth will be somewhat greater as additional survivors move into the childbearing years. However, fertility rates in high-fertility countries are also more likely to fall in the long term than in the next decade.

Child Mortality Decline and Fertility Decline

Many in the public health community—including UNICEF in its materials prepared for the summit—have argued that increased child survival itself will motivate parents to reduce their fertility. The logic of this argument is twofold: (1) that parents in high-mortality settings feel they must have as many children as possible (or perhaps simply a large number of children) to minimize the risk of ending up with very few or no children surviving to adulthood, and (2) that, for the same reason, parents try to replace children who have died as rapidly as possible. Among demographers, the former hypothesis has been known as the "insurance effect" and the latter as the "replacement effect."

These ideas originated with demographers studying the "demographic transition" in the 1930s through 1950s. Early demographers, including Walter Willcox and especially Frank Notestein argued that fertility change would not occur until mortality was reduced. Notestein explained that "any society having to face the heavy mortality characteristics of the premodern era must have high fertility to survive" (Notestein, 1945:39, as quoted in Caldwell, 1986:32) and hence had in place social incentives for families to maintain high fertility. In the 1970s, renewed interest was focused on the more specific issue of whether parents changed their fertility behavior based on their perceptions of child mortality levels. The basic conclusion of many studies is that there is a significant biological effect, especially in popula-

[4]That is, fertility rates decline gradually as in the United Nations projection from a crude birth rate of 45.7 in 1990-1995 to 44.5 in 1995-2000.

[5]The growth rate by assuming zero decline in mortality rates between 1990 and 2000 (i.e., assuming that the 1985-1990 rate would prevail for the entire period) would be 2.6 percent. The comparison is made in the text with the United Nations assumption of a 16 percent decline in under-5 mortality because a decline in mortality rates would be expected even in the absence of effective implementation of the summit goals.

tions where breastfeeding is common, whereby the death of a breastfeeding child leads to an earlier return to ovulation and thus a greater likelihood of becoming pregnant again quickly. There is also some evidence from societies in which fertility control is practiced that there may be a behavioral effect as well, that is, parents may try to become pregnant more quickly after a child dies (Mensch, 1985; Knodel, 1982). There is less evidence in favor of the "insurance effect," that is, that parents make their decisions about how many children to have based on their perceptions of childhood mortality rates.

It is true that very few countries in Latin America, Asia, and Africa have undergone a significant fertility decline without having previously experienced a reduction in mortality. However, this observation does not imply that once a certain level of mortality reduction has been achieved fertility will automatically decline. This kind of mechanistic model of demographic change is as oversimplified and potentially misleading for the international health community as W.W. Rostow's model of economic development was for the international development community in the 1960s. Although it is less simple and thus less satisfying, I think John C. Caldwell's conclusion is more realistic. He says that the consensus that has developed out of previous research is the following: major social and economic change produces both mortality and fertility declines, with the fact of mortality decline perhaps bringing the onset of fertility decline forward in time and certainly deepening it (Caldwell, 1986:38).

So what is the bottom line of the relationship between achieving the summit's infant and child mortality goals and the potential for substantial increases in population growth? Without any change in fertility rates a one-third reduction in under-5 mortality rates will certainly cause some additional population growth. However, as demonstrated above, the effect in the short run is likely to be small even if fertility does not decline. In the longer run, the increase in population growth may be partly or entirely swamped by the effects of fertility declines in most countries, but the outcome clearly will depend on how quickly fertility declines occur.

METHODS FOR IMPLEMENTING SUMMIT GOALS

Interventions That Are Most Likely to Reduce Child Mortality and Morbidity

The goals of the summit are an outgrowth of a specific approach to child mortality and morbidity reduction, which has been part of the programs of international donors during the 1980s, particularly UNICEF's child survival and development revolution, and U.S. Agency for International Development (U.S.A.I.D.) child survival program. In this section, I will attempt to address briefly two related issues: (1) the advantages and disadvantages of this approach, and (2) the experience with this approach during the 1980s.

The 1978 Alma-Ata conference, which proclaimed the goal of health for all by the year 2000 and strongly promoted the idea of "primary health care," generated a debate that continues today (see, for example, Rifkin and Walt, 1986; Unger and Killingsworth, 1986; Grodos and de Bethune, 1988; Warren, 1988; Mosley, 1985, 1988; Newell, 1988; Taylor and Jolly, 1988; Unger, 1991; Morgan, 1990). The basic idea of primary health care, as discussed at the Alma-Ata conference, was to provide widely available, comprehensive, equitably distributed, first-line health care based on appropriate technology. Primary health care was also intended to include three elements that have subsequently proved difficult to implement: active community participation, social relevance, and intersectoral involvement (Mosley, 1985).

In 1979, Walsh and Warren published an influential paper in which they argued that the primary health care approach, while laudable in its objectives, was not feasible for most governments in developing countries to implement all at once. They argued that it was more realistic to target scarce resources toward diseases that could be controlled or treated with low-cost technologies, an approach that has come to be known as "selective primary health care" (SPHC). As the title of the Walsh and Warren article indicated, this approach was intended as an "interim strategy" while governments were developing the resources, infrastructure, and experience to implement comprehensive primary health care (CPHC). The specific interventions proposed were immunization, oral rehydration, breastfeeding, and use of antimalarial drugs. Many agencies, donors, and governments subsequently adopted the selective primary health care approach, including WHO's Expanded Program of Immunization, UNICEF's program based on growth monitoring, oral rehydration therapy, breastfeeding, and immunizations (GOBI), and U.S.A.I.D.'s Control of Childhood Communicable Diseases program. The programs generally include some combination of immunization (against measles, tetanus, diphtheria, polio, pertussis, and tuberculosis), oral rehydration therapy, diarrheal disease control, malaria control, acute respiratory disease control, and nutritional programs (especially growth monitoring and nutrition education).

These programs have had several distinct advantages for donors, for international agencies, and also, to some degree, for national governments. A significant advantage has been the ability to circumvent the cumbersome public health bureaucracies, political battles, and sometimes corrupt hierarchies that are unfortunately common in many parts of the world, and to reach the target population directly. Because donors and international agencies must continuously demonstrate progress either to their national governments or to their own donors, they are generally not in a position to be patient with what is often the long process of institutional change. From a more altruistic point of view, donors, international agencies, and national governments have also argued that if children's health can be improved immediately with available know-how, we ought to be trying to do so at the same time as undertaking institutional change.

Critics of selective primary health care (e.g., Habicht and Berman, 1980; Rifkin and Walt, 1986; Grodos and de Bethune, 1988; Newell, 1988) have argued, however, that what many perceive as an advantage of SPHC (i.e., its ability to circumvent the bureaucracy) is really a major disadvantage because it directs attention, effort, and money away from the very institution building that is essential to bring about and sustain long-term improvements in health. Furthermore, narrowly focused programs, although easier to implement, place the control of, and decision making about, public health policy more firmly in the hands of donors and international agencies. The consequence is increased dependency of countries, and especially of local communities, on external funds and on decisions made abroad.

Although Taylor and Jolly (1988) warn that the debate about the merits of the SPHC approach "diverts time and attention from more substantive action," it seems to me that it has been a useful and important discussion about conflicting goals. The debate, along with practical experience in implementing both CPHC and SPHC programs, has brought significant change in both approaches. For the most part, advocates of "interim approaches" now acknowledge "that the greatest weakness of current CSDR [UNICEF's child survival and development revolution] efforts has been that generally insufficient attention has been paid to long-range objectives in the pressure to get something/anything started fast" and that "overly circumscribed activities have tended to leave countries with entrenched bureaucracies that resist eventual integration into PHC [primary health care]" (Taylor and Jolly, 1988:973, 975, respectively). Advocates of comprehensive primary health care have also acknowledged the difficulties of implementing all aspects of CPHC immediately and have proposed more prioritized approaches (see, for example, Van Lerberghe and Pangu, 1988; Unger, 1991). Nonetheless, considerable work remains to be done on the development of practical approaches to implementation of CPHC (especially in countries with poor central control or weak administrative capabilities) and on the longer-term sustainability of programs implemented by using an SPHC approach.

As Mosley (1985, 1988) points out, the debate has had at least one other very important effect. It has moved the focus of the discussion about national health care policy away from the construction or maintenance of hospital-based and high-technology-intensive systems, which were the norm before the Alma-Ata conference. Although many countries still maintain health care systems whose priority is hospital-based medicine, it has become increasingly difficult for governments and the medical profession to justify this type of system either to donors or to the populations they serve.

The goals of the World Summit for Children are derived from UNICEF's GOBI-female education, family spacing, and food supplements (FFF) and child survival and development revolution—strategies that are clearly derived from the SPHC approach. The proposed program has been broadened by a greater emphasis on providing prenatal and delivery services to pregnant women and on eradication or elimination of certain diseases and nutritional deficiencies. The emphasis is also greater on intersectoral efforts including the provision of safe water and latrines, and on the dissemination of information about improved agricultural techniques for increasing food production.

The crucial question is how the goals will be achieved. Achievement of many of the goals, particularly those that have received less emphasis in the EPI and CSDR programs, will require a substantial amount of institution building in many countries.[6] These goals include some that are specifically health related, such as improvements in prenatal and delivery care, and others that are more indirectly (but very significantly) related to health such as increases in education and improvements in agricultural production to reduce the incidence of malnutrition. There are also several goals toward which SPHC programs have been directed in the past that are likely to be implemented more successfully in a primary health care setting, such as reduction in the incidence of and case-fatality rates from acute respiratory infections and diarrheal diseases.

However, the summit document says little about institution building.[7] To be fair, it is intended to be a political document and not a detailed plan of action for international agencies and national ministries. Nonetheless, the tone of the document clearly suggests that the emphasis is on a continuation of the approach currently employed by UNICEF and others. However, many donors, including U.S.A.I.D. in at least some countries, and some national governments are moving toward an approach that concentrates primarily on building institutional and administrative capacity. Thus, it seems likely that compared to the 1980s, the 1990s will be characterized by a greater diversity of approaches toward improving children's health.

How successful has the SPHC approach been in reducing morbidity and mortality? A summary of the evidence by Gadomski and Black (1990) concludes that although some of the SPHC interventions have been quite successful, the effectiveness of all of the interventions could be improved in

[6]Measurement of progress toward achieving the goals will also be improved by institutional strengthening.

[7]Although governments are urged to pursue child-specific actions "as part of strengthening overall broader national development programmes" (UNICEF, 1990a:24).

the future if primary health care services are strengthened and if other modifications in each specific program are implemented.

In particular, they show that the EPI program has been quite successful in achieving relatively high immunization coverage rates in many countries, as measured by coverage surveys. Furthermore, Gareaballah and Loevinsohn's (1989) results and my own work (Goldman and Pebley, 1992) indicate that some of these vaccination coverage figures may be underestimated. Nonetheless, Unger's study (1991:254) of the Senegal immunization program provides a cautionary tale about the "ephemeral nature of coverage rates" achieved in intensive immunization campaigns and about the potentially disruptive effect of immunization campaigns on the provision of other types of health service.

Gadomski and Black (1990) also indicate that several other programs in the SPHC package have been less successful. Data from the Demographic and Health Surveys (Gadomski and Black, 1990:Table 2) show that oral rehydration therapy (ORT) use rates are low for most countries included, and Gadomski and Black report significant implementation problems that have limited the effects of diarrheal disease control programs. Nonetheless, the development of ORT salts that can be administered by family members is a significant improvement over previous methods of treating dehydrated patients, and has the potential to reduce mortality once its use is understood.[8]

Despite the initial dramatic success of vertical antimalarial programs (Molineaux, 1985), subsequent efforts have been less successful for reasons including vector resistance to insecticide, parasite resistance to chemotherapy, the difficulty of maintaining a regular spraying program, and problems in distribution and acceptability of chemoprophylaxis (Gadomski and Black, 1990). Efforts to control acute respiratory infections (ARI) are relatively recent but have suffered from similar implementation problems. As Gadomski and Black (1990:93) note in the case of acute respiratory infection control in particular, "it will be difficult to implement case management in areas where this infrastructure is poor or lacking, since effective case management depends on a reliable supply of antibiotics, adequate training and supervision of CHWs [community health workers] and on an operative referral network."

Growth monitoring, which has been an important feature of UNICEF's

---

[8]Ironically, the cholera epidemic in several Latin American countries may significantly increase awareness of ORT and its use among the general public in these countries. Casual observation in Guatemala, for example, indicates that the potential cholera epidemic and what measures the public should take have received considerably more publicity than diarrheal diseases ever have in the past (despite the greater role of diarrheal diseases other than cholera in causing morbidity and mortality).

GOBI and CSDR programs, is also included in the summit goals as one of the program strategies. However, experience with growth monitoring as a diagnostic and educational tool has been mixed (Gadomski and Black, 1990; Ruel, in press). Gadomski and Black (1990:106) conclude that even if the interaction in the growth monitoring session "is a positive one, the returns on implementing nutritional advice are slow to materialize and therefore less tangible, and involve more of a leap of faith for the individual mother. Additionally, the other constraints on a mother's time and resources may limit her ability to implement the advice she receives." Based on their observational study in Zaire, Gerein and Ross (1991:667) conclude that "the case for including growth monitoring in child health programmes remains unproven either on theoretical grounds or in practice."

In summary, among the components of SPHC programs implemented during the 1980s, immunization programs appear to have had the most success, at least in achieving relatively high coverage levels. Experience has shown that the difficult task in the case of immunization is to sustain the high level of social mobilization and high coverage levels that are often achieved in the initial campaign, while not absorbing all available health care resources in the process (Unger, 1991). Other programs, such as diarrheal disease control, malaria control, and ARI control, have had more mixed results and at least in some settings, may be limited in their effectiveness in the future if they are not implemented as part of a more comprehensive primary health care program. Finally, experience with other SPHC components, such as growth monitoring (as distinguished from other nutritional programs), has led to doubts about their cost-effectiveness.

Implications of Pursuing Some Goals and Not Others

What are the implications for child health of pursuing some of the summit goals and not others? The answer to this question is clearly related to the debate outlined above about the relative merits of the SPHC and the CPHC approaches. To use its resources most effectively, even a CPHC program must make choices about which causes of morbidity are and are not most important in its population. However, unlike a package of programs aimed at specific diseases (or based on a particular set of medical technologies), the potential advantage of an effective CPHC system is its ability to attend to patients with other health problems that are not part of its main objectives, as well as to adapt to changes in the causes of morbidity.[9] An SPHC-type program that concentrates on immunization and ORT distribution, for example, clearly offers nothing to patients with respiratory

---

[9]Of course, the potential disadvantage of a CPHC program is that its goals are so general that effective implementation is impossible.

infections or to their family members who are trying to avoid contracting ARI themselves. The point here is that any health program must choose a limited set of goals, but the choice of a subset of summit goals is likely to have quite different and perhaps more serious implications in "child survival" programs (as they were implemented during the 1980s) than in an effective CPHC program.

In terms of criteria for choosing among health interventions, Ewbank and Zimicki (1990:142) have argued persuasively that it is time to move beyond the "very focused, short-term and generalized approach" that characterized SPHC programs during the 1980s, and move on to "successor programs" that are considerably less generalized and are based on the major health problems of each country or region. Specifically, they propose that these programs should be based on a "more careful consideration of local cause structures of mortality, that is, the relative importance of causes of death." The thrust of their argument is that to use the limited funds available for health during the 1990s, developing countries and, especially, donor and international agencies will have to move away from fairly uniform intervention packages, which are implemented in all parts of the world, toward a much greater diversity in programs. For example, they argue that in West Africa, the most effective use of additional funds would be "substantially increased efforts to vaccinate children against measles." In many poor Latin American countries, on the other hand, measles are comparatively less important than in West Africa, and diarrheal diseases and ARI are relatively more important. Thus, the most cost-effective use of funds in these countries might be prevention and treatment of these two groups of diseases.

Ewbank and Zimicki argue that the basis for determining what health conditions should be the focus of a program in a given country or region is an analysis of causes of death, not because health programs should concentrate primarily on reducing mortality, but because death and its causes are somewhat easier to measure accurately than morbidity. Although reliable measurement of cause of death is unavailable from the vital statistics systems in many countries, Zimicki (1988), Garenne and Fontaine (1988), and others have been developing and testing new methods of assessing causes of death, which provide much more useful information for setting priorities in health programs.

A topic of considerable concern to health personnel, especially those involved in SPHC programs, has been that attacking some diseases and not others may be a waste of time and money because children saved from one disease may go on to die of another shortly thereafter. A large body of previous research has shown that there are important interactions among infectious diseases, and between these diseases and malnutrition. In general, an intervention targeted at a particular disease has one of three possible effects, if it is at least minimally effective (Foster, 1984:124). It may (1) reduce mortality from the specific disease and from other related diseases, so that overall mortality declines more than would be expected from cause-specific mortality alone; (2) reduce mortality from the disease alone and therefore lower that cause-specific mortality and overall mortality by a corresponding amount; and (3) save weaker children from dying only to have them die later on from the same or other causes (i.e, reduce mortality by less than would be expected). The third outcome would presumably be avoided by an effective CPHC program because it would provide prevention or treatment for a wide range of illnesses. But is the effectiveness of single intervention programs diminished by this "negative synergism" or "replacement mortality"?

Mosley and Becker (1990) suggest that the answer depends on the type of intervention. If the intervention prevents the *incidence* of disease, such as immunization against measles and other childhood diseases, it is likely to reduce mortality not only from that disease but also from other diseases as well. However, the effect of interventions that are "curative," such as ORT treatment for diarrhea, may be diminished somewhat because children who survive are left weakened by the effects of the disease. Mosley and Becker also indicate that "broad based preventive measures like water programs, personal hygiene, and breastfeeding promotion which reduce the incidence of multiple diseases simultaneously will show a substantial demographic impact on overall survival, even if the direct effects on individual diseases are modest" (Mosley and Becker, 1990:172).

Empirical research on the effects of measles immunization supports Mosley and Becker's conclusions about interventions that reduce the incidence of a specific disease. A study in eastern Zaire in the 1970s (Kasongo Project Team, 1981) suggested that immunization against measles would save the lives of both strong children (most of whom would have survived measles anyway) and weak children, but that many of the weak children would die quickly of other diseases (known as "replacement mortality"). However, this study has been severely criticized by others (Aaby et al., 1981; Manshande and De Caluwe, 1981) because the results were ambiguous and did not appear to support the authors' conclusions. More recent work (Stephens, 1984; Hull et al., 1983; Holt et al., 1990; World Health Organization, 1987) indicates that measles immunization seems to reduce child mortality by a greater amount than might be expected from reducing measles-related mortality alone. The evidence in the case of malaria—a very different disease requiring a very different control approach—is similar (Hill and Pebley, 1989).

Mosley and Becker's conclusion about programs designed to *treat* infections makes sense in terms of previous research (see, for example, Mata, 1978; Martorell and Ho, 1984), but there is less clear-cut evidence on the extent of the diminished effectiveness of these intervention programs because of subsequent "replacement mortality." Gadomski and Black (1990) report, for example, that several of the studies of ARI interventions that they reviewed "demonstrate a reduction in total mortality, a reduction that is sometimes larger than that due to ARI alone. The reduction in overall mortality is surprising because it implies that replacement mortality is not overriding the impact of this particular intervention."

SUMMARY AND CONCLUSIONS

The World Summit for Children played an important role in focusing media and political attention on the continuing high mortality and morbidity rates for young children in developing countries, and on the availability of measures to improve child health. The increased attention in and of itself was a significant accomplishment in a rapidly changing international political and economic climate. Rather than assessing political consequences of the summit, this paper has concentrated on the specific goals approved by the Summit as a guide for international- and national-level health programs directed toward children during the 1990s. There are four general characteristics of these goals: (1) many of them include very specific numerical targets; (2) taken as a whole, they are very ambitious; (3) they are pragmatic in the sense that many are based on existing public health technology and at least a decade of experience with implementation; and (4) they are philosophically grounded in the ideas underlying what has come to be known as "selective primary health care." The goals include mortality reduction, reduction of mortality from specific diseases, eradication of certain diseases, and reduction in the incidence of specific health conditions, as well as improved public services such as water, sewage disposal, and education. In this paper, I have concentrated primarily on mortality reduction-related goals.

An examination of previous mortality declines in developing countries since the 1960s shows that the goal of a one-third reduction in mortality rates for children seems plausible in light of previous experience. However, many of the countries that have been most successful at achieving declines of this magnitude either have unusually well-organized health care systems (e.g., Cuba, China, and perhaps Costa Rica) or are relatively well-off for their region (e.g., Chile, Korea, Hong Kong, Singapore, Thailand, Kuwait, and Botswana).

Results presented in this paper also show that although population growth rates would be increased slightly, especially in high-fertility and high-mortality countries, by a one-third reduction in infant and child mortality, the increases over the next decade would be very small and could well be wiped out by fertility declines. Thus, concern that implementation of the summit goals would bring about a significant increase in population growth is not well justified. To my mind, more well-founded concerns about specific summit goals include (1) whether pursuit of these particular numerical targets will lead public health workers, government officials, and the donor community to lose sight of the general objectives of improving children's health, sustaining health improvements, and strengthening public health care systems; (2) whether a continuation of the "child survival" approach, which was important and effective during the 1980s (and is implicit in the summit goals), is the best strategy for improving children's health in the 1990s; and (3) whether some of the goals (e.g., prenatal and delivery assistance, ARI and malaria prevention and treatment, and diarrheal disease prevention and control) can be implemented effectively without major, long-term work on strengthening the health care infrastructure.

Child health programs in developing countries during the 1990s, and more specifically efforts to implement the summit goals, will face at least two major challenges if they are to be successful. First, greater diversity in the focus of health programs among countries will be required if funds and human resources are to be used most effectively. Experience with health interventions and data collected in the past 10 years makes it clear that there is considerable variation in the types of health problems faced by countries, and that this variation will likely grow over the next decade as mortality declines. Generalized health intervention packages, while easier to implement on an international level, are likely to be increasingly less cost-effective in this changing environment.

Second, many observers of the experience of the 1980s have concluded that governments, donors, and international agencies are going to have to face the issue of institution building (i.e., strengthening or building a primary health care system) head-on during the 1990s if gains in children's health are to continue. The route to building a primary health care system may be through institutionalization of SPHC-type interventions, but the experience of the 1980s shows that simply having SPHC programs in place does not automatically guarantee institutional strengthening (Gadomski et al., 1989; Unger, 1991). The need to face the issue of institution building does not arise either because EPI and other SPHC have been ineffective (in fact, many SPHC programs have been quite effective) or because of the problem of "replacement mortality" (which for many diseases is probably much less of a concern that many previously thought). Rather, efforts to build an effective primary health care system are important because of the difficulty of sustaining effective SPHC interventions and of dealing with important health conditions such as ARI, pregnancy, and diarrhea, in the absence of such a system.

REFERENCES

Aaby, P., J. Bukh, I.M. Lisse, and A.J. Smits
1981 Measles vaccination and child mortality. *Lancet* 2:93.

Caldwell, J.
1986 The role of mortality decline in theories of social and demographic transition. *Consequences of Mortality Trends and Differentials*. Population Studies No. 95,ST/ESA/SER.A/95. New York: United Nations, Department of International Economic and Social Affairs.

Ewbank, D., and S. Zimicki
1990 The interim is over: Implications of the changing cause-structure of mortality for the design of health interventions. In K. Hill, ed., *Child Survival Programs: Issues for the 1990s*. Baltimore, Md.: Institute for International Programs, School of Hygiene and Public Health, Johns Hopkins University.

Foster, S.
1984 Immunizable and respiratory diseases and child mortality. In W.H. Mosley and L. Chen, eds., *Child Survival: Strategies for Research*. Supplement to *Population and Development Review* 10:119-140.

Gadomski, A., and R.E. Black
1990 Impact of direct interventions. In K. Hill, ed., *Child Survival Programs: Issues for the 1990s*. Baltimore, Md.: Institute for International Programs, School of Hygiene and Public Health, Johns Hopkins University.

Gadomski, A., R. Black, and W.H. Mosley
1989 Constraints to the potential impact of the direct intervention for child survival in developing countries. *Health Transition* 2.

Gareaballah, E.-T., and B.P. Loevinsohn
1989 The accuracy of mothers' reports about their children's vaccination status. *Bulletin of the World Health Organization* 67(6):669-674.

Garenne, M., and O. Fontaine
1988 Enquete sur les causes probables de deces en milieu rural au Senegal. In J. Vallin, S. D'Souza, and A. Palloni, eds., *Mesure et Analyse de la Mortalite: Nouvelles Approches*. Paris: Presses Universitaires de France.

Gerein, N.M., and D.A. Ross
1991 Is growth monitoring worthwhile? An evaluation of its use in three child health programs in Zaire. *Social Science and Medicine* 32(6):667-675.

Goldman, N., and A.R. Pebley
1992 Health cards, maternal recall, and immunization coverage in Guatemala. Mimeo.

Grodos, D., and X. de Bethune
1988 Les interventions sanitaires selectives: Un piege pour les politiques de sante du tiers monde. *Social Science and Medicine* 26(9):879-889.

Habicht, J.-P., and P.A. Berman
1980 Planning primary health services from a body count? *Social Science and Medicine* 14C:129-136.

Hill, K., and A.R. Pebley
1989 Child mortality in the developing world. *Population and Development Review* 15(4):657-687.

Holt, E.A., R. Boulos, N.A. Halsey, L.M. Boulos, and C. Boulos
1990 Childhood survival in Haiti: The protective effect of measles vaccination. *Pediatrics* 85(2):188-194.

Hull, H.F., P. Williams, and F. Oldfield
1983 Measles mortality and vaccine efficacy in rural West Africa. *Lancet* 1:972-975.

Kalish, S.
1992 Child survival and the demographic "trap." *Population Today* 20(2):8-9.
Kasongo Project Team
1981 Influence of measles vaccination in developing countries. *Lancet* 4 (April):764-767.
Knodel, J.
1982 Child mortality and reporductive behavior in german villages in the past: A micro-level analysis of the replacement effect. *Population Studies* 36(2):177-200.
Manshande, J.P., and P. De Caluwe
1981 Measles vaccination and survival. *Lancet* 6 (June):1271.
Martorell, R., and T.J. Ho
1984 Malnutrition, morbidity, and mortality. In W.H. Mosley and L. Chen, eds., *Child Survival: Strategies for Research.* Supplement to *Population and Development Review* 10:119-140.
Mata, L.J.
1978 *The Children of Santa Maria Cauque: A Prospective Field Study of Health and Growth.* Cambridge, Mass.: MIT Press.
Mensch, B.S.
1985 The effects of child mortality on contraceptive use and fertility in Colombia, Costa Rica, and Korea. *Population Studies* 39(2):309-328.
Molineaux, L.
1985 The impact of parasitic diseases and their control with an emphasis on malaria and Africa. Pp. 103-137 in J. Vallin and A.D. Lopez, eds., *Health Policy, Social Policy and Mortality Prospects.* Liège: Ordina Editions.
Morgan, L.M.
1990 International politics and primary health care in Costa Rica. *Social Science and Medicine* 30(2):211-219.
Mosley, W.H.
1985 Will primary health care reduce infant and child mortality? In J. Vallin and A.D. Lopez, eds., *Health Policy, Social Policy and Mortality Prospects.* Liège: Ordina Editions.
1988 Is there a middle way? Categorical programs for PHC. *Social Science and Medicine* 26(9):907-908.
Mosley, W.H., and S. Becker
1990 Demographic models for child survival: Implications for program strategy. *Health Policy and Planning* 6(3):218-233.
Newell, K.W.
1988 Selective primary health care: The counter revolution. *Social Science and Medicine* 26(9):903-906.
Notestein, F.
1945 Population: The long view. In T.W. Schultz, ed., *Food for the World.* Chicago: University of Chicago Press.
Rifkin, S., and G. Walt
1986 Why health improves: Defining issues concerning "Comprehensive Primary Health Care" and "Selective Primary Health Care." *Social Science and Medicine* 23:559-566.
Ruel, M.
(in press) Growth monitoring as an educational tool, an integrating strategy and a source of information: A review of experience. In P. Pinstrup-Anderson, D. Pelletier, and H. Alderman, eds., *Beyond Child Survival.* Ithaca, N.Y.: Cornell University Press.

Stephens, P.W.
1984 Morbidity and mortality from measles in Ngayokheme: A case study of risks and their associated factors. University Microfilms: Ph.D. dissertation, University of Pennsylvania.

Sullivan, J.M.
1991 The pace of decline in under-five mortality: Evidence from the DHS surveys. Paper presented at the DHS World Conference, Washington, D.C., August 5-7.

Taylor, C., and R. Jolly
1988 The straw men of primary health care. *Social Science and Medicine* 26(9):971-977.

Unger, J.-P.
1991 Can intensive campaigns dynamize front line health services? The evaluation of an immunization campaign in the Thies health district, Senegal. *Social Science and Medicine* 32(3):249-259.

Unger, J.-P., and J. Killingsworth
1986 Selective primary health care: A critical view of methods and results. *Social Science and Medicine* 20:1001-1012.

UNICEF
1990a *First Call for Children: World Declaration and Plan of Action from the World Summit for Children.* New York: UNICEF.
1990b *The World Summit for Children: A UNICEF Contribution to the World Summit for Children.* New York: UNICEF.

Van Lerberghe, W., and K. Pangu
1988 Comprehensive can be effective: The influence of coverage with a health centre network on the hospitalisation patterns in the rural area of Kasongo, Zaire. *Social Science and Medicine* 26(9):949-955.

Walsh, J.A., and K.S. Warren
1979 Selective primary health care: An interim strategy for disease control in developing countries. *New England Journal of Medicine* 301:18.

Warren, K.S.
1988 The evolution of selective primary health care. *Social Science and Medicine* 26(9):891-898.

World Health Organization
1987 *Key Issues in Measles Research: A Review of the Literature.* Expanded Programme on Immunization Global Advisory Group Meeting. November. EPI/GAG/87/Wp.10.

Zimicki, S.
1988 L'enregistrement des causes de deces par des non-medecins: Deux experiences au Bangladesh. In J. Vallin, S. D'Souza, and A. Palloni, eds., *Mesure et Analyse de la Mortalite: Nouvelles Approches.* Paris: Presses Universitaires de France.

APPENDIX

Goals for Children and Development in the 1990s
(From UNICEF, 1990a:31-35)

I. Major goals for child survival, development and protection

(a) Between 1990 and the year 2000, reduction of infant and under-5 mortality rate by one-third or to 50 and 70 percent per 1,000 live births, respectively, whichever is less
(b) Between 1990 and the year 2000, reduction of maternal mortality rate by half
(c) Between 1990 and the year 2000, reduction of severe and moderate malnutrition among under-5 children by half
(d) Universal access to safe drinking water and to sanitary means of excreta disposal
(e) By the year 2000, universal access to basic education and completion of primary education by at least 80 percent of primary school-age children
(f) Reduction of the adult literacy rate (the appropriate age group to be determined in each country) to at least half its 1990 level with emphasis on female literacy
(g) Improved protection of children in especially difficult circumstances

II. Supporting/sectoral goals

A. Women's health and education
(i) Special attention to the health and nutrition of the female child and to pregnant and lactating women
(ii) Access by all couples to information and services to prevent pregnancies that are too early, too closely spaced, too late, or too many
(iii) Access by all pregnant women to prenatal care, trained attendants during childbirth, and referral facilities for high-risk pregnancies and obstetric emergencies
(iv) Universal access to primary education with special emphasis for girls and accelerated literacy programs for women

B. Nutrition
(i) Reduction in severe, as well as moderate, malnutrition among children under 5 by half of 1990 levels
(ii) Reduction of the rate of low birthweight (2.5 kilograms or less) to less than 10 percent
(iii) Reduction of iron deficiency anemia in women by one-third of the 1990 levels

(iv) Virtual elimination of iodine deficiency disorders
(v) Virtual elimination of vitamin A deficiency and its consequences, including blindness
(vi) Empowerment of all women to breastfeed their children exclusively for four to six months and to continue breastfeeding, with complementary foods, well into the second year
(vii) Growth promotion and its regular monitoring to be institutionalized in all countries by the end of the 1990s
(viii) Dissemination of knowledge and supporting services to increase food production to ensure household food security

C. Child health
(i) Global eradication of poliomyelitis by the year 2000
(ii) Elimination of neonatal tetanus by 1995
(iii) Reduction by 95 percent in measles deaths and reduction by 90 percent of measles cases compared to preimmunization levels by 1995, as a major step toward the global eradication of measles in the longer run
(iv) Maintenance of a high level of immunization coverage (at least 90 percent of children under 1 year of age by the year 2000) against diphtheria, pertussis, tetanus, measles, poliomyelitis, and tuberculosis and against tetanus for women of childbearing age
(v) Reduction by 50 percent in the deaths due to diarrhea in children under the age of 5 years and 25 percent reduction in the diarrhea incidence rate
(vi) Reduction by one-third in the deaths due to acute respiratory infections in children under 5 years

D. Water and sanitation
(i) Universal access to safe drinking water
(ii) Universal access to sanitary means of excreta disposal
(iii) Elimination of guinea-worm disease (dracunculiasis) by the year 2000

E. Basic education
(i) Expansion of early childhood development activities, including appropriate low-cost family- and community-based interventions
(ii) Universal access to basic education, and achievement of primary education by at least 80 percent of primary school-age children through formal schooling or nonformal education of comparable learning standard, with emphasis on reducing the current disparities between boys and girls
(iii) Reduction of the adult literacy rate (the appropriate age group to be

determined in each country) to at least half its 1990 level, with emphasis on female literacy

(iv) Increased acquisition by individuals and families of knowledge, skills, and values required for better living, made available through all educational channels, including mass media, other forms of modern and traditional communication and social action, with effectiveness measured in terms of behavioral change

F. Children in difficult circumstances

Provide improved protection of children in especially difficult circumstances and tackle the root causes leading to such situations

Distributional Implications of Alternative Strategic Responses to the Demographic-Epidemiological Transition—An Initial Inquiry

Davidson R. Gwatkin

INTRODUCTION

Over the past decade, transitions in the developing world's demographic and epidemiological situations have become increasingly obvious. Mortality and fertility have been declining, and disease patterns have been shifting. Illness and death among the young caused by the diarrhea-malnutrition-pneumonia triad have been progressively giving way to newer configurations dominated by chronic and degenerative diseases among adults and the elderly.

These changes raise the possibility that the time has come for a corresponding shift in developing countries health strategies. No longer can one simply assume that it remains adequate to continue stressing oral rehydration, immunization, and related approaches. As the epidemiological and demographic transitions proceed, it would seem reasonable to anticipate a need to become increasingly concerned with preventing strokes and heart attacks as well.

Were societies epidemiologically and demographically homogeneous, the case for such a shift would be straightforward. But societies are not homogeneous. Different groups in them suffer from different kinds of diseases at different ages. A change in focus from one set of diseases and age groups to another could benefit some groups at the expense of others.

This question of who gains and who loses from a change in priorities is

---

Davidson R. Gwatkin is director of the International Health Policy Program. The author wishes to thank Jun Zhu for his effective research assistance and the many readers of earlier drafts for their valuable suggestions.

of particular interest in health because of the egalitarian tendencies that have typified professional thinking in the field during recent years.[1] From an egalitarian perspective, any change is to be welcomed to the extent that its benefits accrue to the poor, and to be resisted to the degree that the gains go instead to the better-off and leave the poor at an even greater disadvantage than before.

For those adhering to this viewpoint, is a shift in priorities from communicable diseases among infants and children toward chronic diseases at older ages to be welcomed or resisted? To the extent it is to be resisted, what alternative responses to the demographic and epidemiological transitions might be considered? Such are the questions toward which this exploration into the distributional consequences of different approaches to the Third World's changing health conditions is directed.

THE OVERALL SITUATION

Although most of this exploration focuses on the country level that is of particular interest, it can best begin with a brief look at the situation of the Third World as a whole and of the major regions within it. Such a look can provide both a sense of how central a place the demographic and epidemiological transitions deserve in designing health improvement strategies and an initial hint about the possible distributional consequences of these strategies. The inquiry is facilitated by the availability of recent figures produced at the World Bank on cause- and age-specific mortality in the Third World as a whole and in its major regions. A summary of these figures appears in Tables 1A and 1B (Bulatao and Stephens, 1989).

The most immediately obvious feature of these tables is the shift in overall age- and disease-specific mortality patterns that they were developed to document. This shift is very large. If mortality trends in the developing world proceed according to the Bulatao-Stephens projections for example, the percentage of total deaths occurring among children less than

[1] This thinking is typified by the widely used expression "health for all" and the accompanying belief that an emphasis on the poor and disadvantaged is required to achieve this objective. To many, the greater intergroup equality in health status implied by health for all would also be a more equitable situation than that which currently prevails. For those adhering to such a belief, this is a paper not simply about distribution and equality, but also about equity and justice. However, the equation of equity with equality of health status involves a value judgment that some have felt requires further justification than is possible in the limited space available here. For this reason, the paper focuses on such empirically measurable features of a society's situation as the intergroup distribution and equality of health status, which are notably less value laden than is the concept of equity. This focus, however, cannot be said to remove all value considerations since the paper's underlying assumption continues to be that, for whatever reason, reduced intergroup disparities in health status are desirable.

TABLE 1A Deaths by Age (percent)

Region and Age Group	Year 1970	1985	2000	2015
Less Developed Countries				
0-14	50.0	42.9	26.7	18.5
15-64	27.8	28.9	33.2	34.3
65 +	22.2	28.2	40.0	47.2
Total	100.0	100.0	99.9	100.0
Life expectancy at birth (years)	(57.5)	(62.0)	(66.0)	(68.5)
Latin America and the Caribbean				
0-14	38.3	33.3	19.2	10.4
15-64	28.7	27.6	30.4	31.1
65 +	33.1	39.0	50.3	58.6
Total	100.1	99.9	99.9	100.1
Life expectancy at birth (years)	(62.5)	(66.5)	(70.5)	(72.5)
Asia				
0-14	48.5	37.1	18.5	10.7
15-64	27.9	30.6	34.2	34.2
65+	23.5	32.3	47.4	55.1
Total	99.9	100.0	100.1	100.0
Life expectancy at birth (years)	(59.0)	(64.0)	(68.0)	(70.0)
Middle East and North Africa				
0-14	51.6	54.5	34.7	25.8
15-64	28.2	23.9	33.9	37.2
65+	20.3	21.6	31.4	36.9
Total	100.1	100.0	100.0	99.9
Life expectancy at birth (years)	(53.0)	(60.0)	(64.5)	(66.5)
Sub-Saharan Africa				
0-14	60.3	58.8	50.2	41.9
15-64	26.5	27.0	31.4	34.6
65+	13.2	14.2	18.4	23.5
Total	100.0	100.0	100.0	100.0
Life expectancy at birth (years)	(45.0)	(51.5)	(57.0)	(61.0)

SOURCE: Bulatao and Stephens (1989:44, 61-62).

TABLE 1B Death by Cause (percent)

	Year			
Region and Cause of Death	1970	1985	2000	2015
Less Developed Countries				
Infectious and parasitic diseases	42.1	36.2	25.9	19.4
Neoplasms and circulatory disorders	21.6	26.0	39.6	48.9
Other	36.4	37.7	34.6	31.8
Total	100.1	99.9	100.1	100.1
Life expectancy at birth (years)	(57.5)	(62.0)	(66.0)	(68.5
Latin America and the Caribbean				
Infectious and parasitic diseases	33.3	24.4	15.1	9.3
Neoplasms and circulatory disorders	30.3	35.9	51.6	61.2
Other	36.4	39.7	33.3	29.5
Total	100.0	100.0	100.0	100.1
Life expectancy at birth (years)	(62.5)	(66.5)	(70.5)	(72.5
Asia				
Infectious and parasitic diseases	41.2	33.6	21.3	14.6
Neoplasms and circulatory disorders	22.8	28.5	45.5	55.7
Other	36.0	37.9	33.2	29.7
Total	100.0	100.0	100.0	100.0
Life expectancy at birth (years)	(59.0)	(64.0)	(68.0)	(70.0
Middle East and North Africa				
Infectious and parasitic diseases	41.4	40.4	29.5	23.2
Neoplasms and circulatory disorders	19.1	22.0	32.7	40.8
Other	39.5	37.6	37.8	36.0
Total	100.0	100.0	100.0	100.0
Life expectancy at birth (years)	(53.0)	(60.0)	(64.5)	(66.5)
Sub-Saharan Africa				
Infectious and parasitic diseases	48.2	47.2	41.8	36.5
Neoplasms and circulatory disorders	13.9	16.0	20.7	26.7
Other	37.9	36.8	37.5	36.8
Total	100.0	100.0	100.0	100.0
Life expectancy at birth (years)	(45.0)	(51.5)	(57.0)	(61.0)

SOURCE: Bulatao and Stephens (1989:44, 15-16).

15 years of age would decline from 50 to 18 between 1970 and 2015, while that attributable to people more than 65 years old would rise from 22 to 47. Similarly, the percentage of deaths caused by infectious and parasitic diseases would fall from 42 to 19, and the percentage resulting from neoplasms and circulatory disorders would climb from 22 to 49.

These overall shifts represent only part of the story, however. Of greater interest from a distributional perspective are the interregional differences in the numbers presented, especially differences between high- and low-mortality regions. When these differences are examined, a clear pattern emerges: The poorer a region's health status, the greater is the importance of deaths at earlier relative to older ages, and from communicable relative to chronic diseases. This pattern is clearly visible in each of the time periods shown in Tables 1A and 1B. In general, when the life expectancy of a region is 50 years, about 60 percent of deaths occur among children under 15 years, about 20 percent at age 65 or above. When a region's life expectancy is 70 years, the percentage of deaths occurring at less than 15 years is only 10-12, compared to almost 50 percent at age 65 or above. The interregional differences in the cause of death are equally sharp: when a region's life expectancy is 50 years, approximately 50 percent of deaths are caused by infectious/parasitic diseases and 10-15 percent by neoplasms/circulatory disorders. When a region's life expectancy is 70 years, the proportions are about 20 percent and 45-50 percent, respectively.[2]

This pattern suggests that a health strategy focusing on chronic diseases among adults and the elderly might be considerably more relevant for regions with low mortality levels than for high-mortality regions. For example, an emphasis on adult mortality would seem quite sensible for a region in which overall life expectancy is 70 years or so, in which almost 90 percent of deaths take place among people over 15. But its likely efficacy would appear questionable when life expectancy is only 50 and the distinct majority of deaths occurs among infants and children younger than 15.

This point appears to have been at least implicitly accepted within the international health profession in that calls for a review of health priorities seem to arise much more frequently with reference to the more advanced Latin American and Asian countries than with respect to high-mortality sub-Saharan African nations. What seems much less well recognized is the possibility that differences analogous to those just noted with respect to

[2]The figures presented are estimated from linear regression equations in which the percentage of deaths at a specific age or from a specific cause serves as the dependent variable, and a group's life expectancy at birth is the independent variable. Each equation is based on 16 observations, one for each of the four regions of the developing world and for each of the four dates covered by the Bulatao and Stephens figures.

regions might also exist within regions and within the individual countries of which regions are composed.

Should analogous intracountry differences exist, a health strategy oriented toward communicable diseases among infants and children would seem much more relevant for a society's disadvantaged groups than a strategy focusing on chronic diseases of older ages. This raises the possibility that shifting from the former to the latter could benefit the better-off more than the poor, thereby increasing the degree of inequality between them.

How great is such a possibility? To find out, it is necessary to turn to the information available about individual countries and about differences in health conditions among population groups within them.

RANGE OF INTRACOUNTRY MORTALITY DIFFERENCES

The best way to begin the examination is with a look at intergroup differences in overall mortality levels—that is, at differences in mortality at all ages and from all causes together. These differences are of interest both in themselves and, as will be seen later, because of the use to which they can be put in assessing age- and cause-specific patterns. Also, the data that exist about differences in overall levels are considerably better than those available for differences in the distribution of deaths by age and cause; these data make it possible to begin by drawing upon observations taken directly from the countries concerned before proceeding to the necessarily more synthetic data featured in later stages of the discussion.

Data based on such direct observations are presented in the appendix to this paper. They represent 14 countries that are broadly representative of the widely diverse conditions found in the Third World, for which relatively recent information is available. For each of the countries there is information on one of four attributes commonly used in discussions of mortality differentials: income, place of residence, women's educational status, and race. To facilitate comprehension, the figures presented in the appendix focus on one particularly important dimension of intergroup mortality differences: the range between a society's healthiest and least healthy groups. To the extent feasible, the figures seek to compare the situation of the top 10-20 percent with that of the bottom 10-20 percent of the population in the country concerned.[3]

The many limitations of the data significantly restrict the uses to which

[3]Such a comparison can be meaningfully attempted only with respect to income and place of residence. For women's educational status and race, the number of groups is too small and the proportion of the population in each is too large and/or too different to permit identification of comparably sized groups at the two ends of the mortality spectrum.

the figures may legitimately be put.[4] The figures can, however, serve to substantiate the ubiquitous presence of significant intrasocietal differences in mortality and to give an initial sense of the general orders of magnitude typically involved. For example, the figures show that in all but one of the fourteen societies covered, infant mortality in the most disadvantaged group is more than twice as high as that of the most advantaged. In four of the fourteen, the difference is three times or more; in two, it is more than fourfold. Similarly, life expectancy of the most privileged groups is 25 percent or more than that of the most disadvantaged in all but three of the societies. In at least one case, the difference is greater 50 percent.[5]

Beyond this are suggestions with respect to differences in mortality status according to place of residence and education, the two attributes for which the most information is available:

- The information with respect to place of residence gives rise to a "10-20" rule of thumb. That is, in most settings the life expectancy of the top 10-20 percent of the population as measured by place of residence appears to be somewhere on the order of 10-20 years higher than that of the lowest 10-20 percent of the population defined in a similar manner.[6] This rule of thumb, which is broad enough to cover all of the six situations based

---

[4]In addition to the wide variations in intergroup size referred to in the preceding note, these limitations include the multiplicity of attributes used in differentiating among population groups and the reliance on only one statistical measure (i.e., the range) of intergroup disparities.

[5]The cross-sectional figures available cannot address the question of whether the differences cited have been widening or narrowing as countries' epidemiological transitions have proceeded: whether, in other words, the least healthy groups have benefited less or more from the transitions than the groups that were healthiest to begin with. In light of the connection between income and health status, one would expect trends in the distribution of health status to follow at least approximately those of income distribution. If so, the voluminous literature on income distribution trends suggests two possibilities concerning the evolution of disparities in health status. One, derived from the well-known "Kuznets hypothesis" on income distribution, is that disparities would normally widen in the initial stages of development, narrow in the later. The second, based on empirical research into the Kuznets hypothesis, would be that no generalization is possible: that disparities widen in some countries and narrow in others, depending on the particular development and health service strategies adopted. (The findings of the only known examination of this issue, for Mexico, suggest that interregional disparities have been widening, with mortality in areas where it was initially low declining much more rapidly than in regions where it was initially high. This finding, which is giving rise to what the authors call a "health polarization," is in line with the initial part of the first hypothesis presented above while leaving open the question of whether or when the second part might occur (Bobadilla et al., 1993).

[6]The country concerned is divided into 10-20 or so geographical units. The magnitude of the difference between upper and lower groups can normally be expected to vary directly with the number of geographical units being observed, rising as the number increases and declining as the number falls.

on place of residence in section B of the appendix, implies a two- to fourfold difference in infant mortality between the uppermost and lowest 10-20 percent of the population.

- The children of the relatively few women with secondary or college education, which qualifies them for consideration as members of their countries' social and economic elite, can expect to live 10-20 years longer than the children of women with no education, who belong to the core of the most disadvantaged groups in those societies. Here, too, the implied difference in infant mortality is roughly two- to fourfold. This variation of the 10-20 hypothesis suggested above would cover five of the six groups for which figures by education are presented in section C of the appendix.

FRAMEWORK

Placed in an appropriate framework, this knowledge about differences in overall conditions between a society's healthiest and least healthy groups can play a central role in the examination of intergroup differences in age- and cause-specific patterns of mortality. The most appropriate framework, of course, is that of the developing country population within which the observed differences exist; however, fully satisfying studies can be undertaken only at a national (or subnational) level. However, an initial look at illustrative country situations based on composite data can be instructive both in introducing an approach of potential relevance for those national studies and in providing findings to guide policies in the interim prior to the studies' completion.

For this purpose, two illustrative populations can serve as the basis for an examination of age- and cause-specific mortality patterns: one population with mortality and fertility levels characteristically found in societies of sub-Saharan Africa, the area of the Third World where overall mortality is highest; the other broadly representative of Latin America, the developing world's lowest-mortality region. Within each, the age- and cause-specific mortality patterns of the healthiest and least healthy 10-20 percent of the population can be compared.

The overall mortality levels of the two societies can be established through reference to the World Bank's figures cited in Tables 1A and 1B, which showed 1985-1990 life expectancy to be 51.5 years in sub-Saharan Africa, 66.5 years in Latin America and the Caribbean. An upward rounding to allow for increases that have presumably taken place since 1985-1990 leads to the selection of 55.0 years as the average life expectancy of the high-mortality society, 67.5 years as that of the low-mortality society.

Based on the 10-20 hypothesis established through the figures for developing countries presented in the appendix, the difference between the most-advantaged 10-20 percent and least-privileged 10-20 percent of the population is set at 15.0 years[7], assumed to be centered at the mean. These assumptions yield population groups with life expectancies of 47.5 and 62.5 years in the high-mortality society and life expectancies of 60.0 and 75.0 years in the low-mortality society.

The fertility levels are determined through reference to World Bank data. An examination of these data suggests that on average, a woman in an African population group with a life expectancy of 47.5 years will bear about 6.7 children. When life expectancy is 62.5 years, the average number of children will be around 5.1. In Latin America, the corresponding figures for children born are 4.9 (when life expectancy is 60.0 years) and 2.3 (when life expectancy is 75.0 years), respectively (Bulatao et al., 1989, 1990).

The same World Bank data are also used to establish the age distribution of each population group. This estimation is done with reference to the three or four national populations whose life expectancies are closest to that of the group concerned: two below, two above. Thus, for example, the age structure for the least healthy group in the high-mortality society is the unweighted average of those of the four African countries whose 1985-1990 life expectancies are closest to the 47.5 years of that group: Mali and Burkina Faso, whose life expectancies of 47.2 and 47.3 years, respectively, are just below 47.5 years; and Senegal and Mozambique, whose life expectancies of 47.6 and 48.1 years are just above. The population distributions of the other groups are determined in an analogous manner, by using data from Africa for the other group in the high-mortality society, and from Latin America and the Caribbean for the two groups in the low-mortality society.[8]

The resulting population distribution figures appear in Table 2, which also presents the mortality and fertility levels referred to earlier. The higher fertility and mortality of the least healthy groups combine to produce populations that are younger than those of the most healthy groups, particularly in the low-mortality society, with only around 25 percent of the healthiest population being under 15 years of age, compared with more than 40 percent of the least healthy population. At the upper end of the age spectrum, the situation is reversed: more than 9 percent of the healthiest population is

---

[7]This difference is approximately the same as the mean difference of 14.7 years between the highest and lowest groups in the fourteen country examples presented in the appendix, and the mean difference of 15.2 years in the seven examples in which the groups compared represent approximately the uppermost and lowest 10-20 percent of the country's population.

[8]Thanks to Ansley Coale for suggesting this approach based on country data, rather than on stable populations derived from the fertility and mortality rates. The age distributions appearing in stable population tables are based on the assumption that fertility and mortality have remained constant over an extended period prior to the observation date, and as Coale noted, this assumption is not valid for most developing countries, in which mortality and fertility have been declining.

TABLE 2 Demographic Characteristics of Population Groups With Differing Life Expectancies and Fertility Levels

	High-Mortality Country		Low-Mortality Country	
Characteristic	Least Healthy 10-20% of Population	Healthiest 10-20% of Population	Least Healthy 10-20% of Population	Healthiest 10-20% of Population
Life expectancy (years)	47.5	62.5	60.0	75.0
Total fertility rate	6.7	5.1	4.9	2.3
Distribution by age group				
0-14	45.3	42.0	42.6	25.5
15-44	40.9	42.9	42.7	49.0
45-64	10.7	11.3	11.3	16.4
65 +	3.1	3.8	3.4	9.2
Total	100.0	100.0	100.0	100.1

65 years of age or older, compared with much less than 4 percent of the least healthy population.

AGE-SPECIFIC MORTALITY

Within societies such as those just described, how different are the age- and cause-specific patterns of mortality? What are the implications of these differences for the distributional consequences of alternative health improvement strategies?

These questions may be more easily addressed with respect to age, because age at death has been the subject of intense study by demographers over the past several decades. The results of this study cannot be considered fully definitive because it has not yet proceeded to the point at which it can provide reliable direct information about the Third World's higher-mortality countries. There are, however, model life tables or standardized compilations of age-specific mortality data from developed and advanced developing countries that are generally considered trustworthy. These have long been routinely used by the United Nations, the World Bank, and national statistical offices to assist demographic analyses in a wide range of developing countries with insufficient data of their own. Although obviously less suitable than reliable direct observations, they have withstood the test of time well enough to justify at least a modest degree of confidence in their applicability for the development of broad illustrations such as those pictured here.

The figures in Table 3 show what one of the most frequently used sets of model life tables has to say about age-specific mortality in populations with life expectancies corresponding to those of the four groups presently under consideration. Age-specific mortality displays the well-known "U-shaped" pattern featuring high death rates at the youngest and oldest ages, separated by a period of much lower mortality during the intervening years. In each case, death rates for the least healthy are higher at every age. Of particular interest in the present context is the magnitude of the difference between the two groups, which is not constant.

In the high-mortality society, for example, the death rate of the high-mortality group's children aged 1-5 is about 3.6 times that of children in the low-mortality group. This difference declines sharply with age: it is only

TABLE 3 Age-Specific Mortality Rates (per 1,000 population) of Population Groups With Differing Life Expectancies

	High-Mortality Country			Low-Mortality Country		
Age (1)	Least Healthy 10-20% of Population (2)	Healthiest 10-20% of Population (3)	Ratio (2)/(3) (4)	Least Healthy 10-20% of Population (5)	Healthiest 10-20% of Population (6)	Ratio (5)/(6) (7)
0	148.80	62.49	2.38	74.45	13.31	5.59
1	20.15	5.58	3.61	7.37	0.44	16.79
5	4.50	1.61	2.80	2.00	0.23	8.54
10	3.37	1.24	2.72	1.53	0.20	7.58
15	4.73	1.96	2.42	2.35	0.39	6.04
20	6.39	2.71	2.36	3.24	0.55	5.95
25	7.13	3.00	2.38	3.60	0.58	6.18
30	8.15	3.44	2.37	4.12	0.70	5.92
35	9.43	4.19	2.25	4.96	0.97	5.13
40	11.16	5.42	2.06	6.27	1.55	4.04
45	13.42	7.43	1.81	8.34	2.77	3.01
50	17.97	10.75	1.67	11.87	4.70	2.53
55	24.00	15.76	1.52	17.05	8.10	2.11
60	35.09	24.06	1.46	25.80	13.42	1.92
65	50.31	37.03	1.36	39.16	23.19	1.69
70	75.49	58.64	1.29	61.35	40.08	1.53
75	115.04	93.60	1.23	97.06	69.09	1.40
80	175.81	146.80	1.20	151.54	112.60	1.35
85	270.64	231.02	1.17	237.54	183.27	1.30
90	413.43	360.62	1.15	369.37	295.78	1.25
95	626.93	557.93	1.12	569.41	472.27	1.21
100	949.35	860.99	1.10	875.70	751.40	1.17

SOURCE: Average figures for males and females from West model life tables in Coale and Demeny (1983:46, 50, 53).

one-half as large among people 45 years of age in the two groups, and the mortality prospects of the few people in each group who attain 100 years are almost identical.

The differences in the low-mortality society follow the same general trend, reaching a maximum in the same 1- to 5-year age group and then falling. However, the magnitude of the differences is notably greater at each age. Between 1 and 5 years of age, for example, the death rate in the least healthy group is more than 16 times that of the most healthy group in the low-mortality society, compared with a difference of three-plus times in the high-mortality society.

The implications of this pattern can be seen by weighting the age-specific mortality rates that lie behind these curves by the proportion of the population in each age group shown in Table 2, to provide an estimate of the percentage of total deaths occurring at each age. These results appear in Table 4.

The results show that infant and child deaths occupy a far more prominent place in society's least healthy groups than in its most healthy ones. In the least healthy group of the high-mortality society, for instance, there are nearly four times as many deaths in the age group 0-14 as in the age group 65+; in the healthiest group of that society, the number of deaths in each age category is approximately equal. The situation in the low-mortality society is similar: there are 50 percent more deaths at ages 0-14 than at ages 65 and over, less than one-tenth as many in the healthiest group.

The potential consequences of these differences from a distributional perspective may be illustrated through a simple example. Suppose it were possible to reduce mortality equally in all of a society's population groups by a given amount—one-third, for example—in any specified age category

TABLE 4 Total Deaths by Age (percent)

	High-Mortality Country		Low-Mortality Country	
Age Group	Least Healthy 10-20% of Population	Healthiest 10-20% of Population	Least Healthy 10-20% of Population	Healthiest 10-20% of Population
0-14	56.5	35.0	40.4	4.2
15-44	16.5	15.5	16.5	6.2
45-64	12.2	17.0	16.7	15.2
65+	14.8	32.5	26.4	74.4
Total	100.0	100.0	100.0	100.0
Ratio of deaths at ages 0-14 to deaths at age 65+	3.8	1.1	1.5	0.1

through the introduction of additional resources.[9] What would be the distributional consequences of such a mortality reduction in any one of the four broad age categories presented in Table 4, relative to those of reducing it in another age category?

The answer to this question appears in Table 5. If mortality among infants and children under 15 years were to decline by one-third in all groups, the result would be distinctly progressive in that the least healthy would benefit more than the healthiest, and the gap between the two groups would narrow. The number of deaths in the least healthy group of the high-mortality society would fall by 18.8 percent, a reduction 1.6 times as large as the 11.7 percent decline of the healthiest group. In the low-mortality society, the differences would be greater: deaths would fall by 13.4 percent in the least healthy group, nearly 10 times as much as the 1.4 percent reduction in the healthiest one.

The result would become steadily less progressive and more regressive as the age of those affected by the mortality decline increases. An emphasis on ages 65+ would be clearly regressive in each society, benefiting the healthiest twice or more as much as the least healthy.[10]

---

[9]This formulation produces what might be called an "equal-output" (or, more precisely, an "equiproportionate-output") scenario, where output is defined in terms of mortality reduction. Such a scenario needs to be distinguished carefully from an "equal-input" scenario, in which the *per capita* allocation of resources to each health status or age group is equal. The equal-output and equal-input scenarios will produce the same results only if the output-input ratios (i.e., the amount of mortality reduction produced per unit of resource invested) are the same for all groups. The equal-output scenario has been selected for presentation here partly to permit ready comprehension, and partly out of concern for the reliability of the available information about input-output relationships that an input-based scenario requires. A next step in the line of inquiry initiated by this paper is to be an input-based approach, allowing variation in both the level and the effectiveness of inputs by group. In the meantime, brief references to the results that can be expected from use of this approach appear in footnotes 10 and 11.

[10]The distinctions would be even sharper if the resources needed to reduce mortality in any particular age category were to be drawn from activities benefiting people in some other age category, instead of being introduced exogenously as assumed in the calculations underlying the figures in Table 5. (For instance, diverting resources from children's programs to serve people in older ages under the conditions specified in the example would reduce the progressive influence of those programs in addition to introducing the more regressive effect of the new ones.) The distinctions would also become sharper under an input-based approach such as that alluded to in footnote 9 incorporating the view, held by many, that infant and child deaths can be prevented less expensively than deaths among adults and the elderly under present technology. Use of an input-based approach incorporating the assumption that deaths at all ages are less expensive to prevent among the least healthy than among the healthiest would increase the progressive effect of funds allocated to the least healthy at each age. This would raise the age above which there would be a regressive effect in absolute terms. In the absence of variations in the age-specific cost-effectiveness differential between groups, however, there would be no change in relative terms because the progressive effect of dealing with unhealthy infants and children would be increased by an amount comparable to that of the increase at older ages.

TABLE 5 Change in Number of Deaths Attributable to One-Third Reduction of Mortality in a Particular Age Group (percent)

Age Group	High-Mortality Country			Low-Mortality Country		
	Least Healthy 10-20% of Population (1)	Healthiest 10-20% of Population (2)	Ratio (1)/(2) (3)	Least Healthy 10-20% of Population (4)	Healthiest 10-20% of Population (5)	Ratio (4)/(5) (6)
One-third reduction in deaths from all causes						
0-14	–18.8	–11.7	1.6	–13.4	–1.4	9.6
15-44	–5.5	–5.2	1.1	–5.5	–2.1	2.6
45-64	–4.1	–5.7	0.7	–5.6	–5.1	1.1
65 +	–4.9	–10.8	0.5	–8.8	–24.8	0.4

This result holds even though, as noted earlier, mortality rates among the least healthy are higher than among the healthiest at every age level— including age 65 and older— because of a situation somewhat analogous to that of the famous international trade example that David Ricardo presented nearly 200 years ago. That is, what matters is not so much the absolute difference in mortality levels between two groups at a given age level, but rather the comparative difference (i.e., the magnitude of the difference at that age level relative to the magnitude of the difference at another age level) considered in conjunction with differences in the age structure of the groups concerned resulting (primarily) from differing fertility levels.

The example also shows that the regressive effects of shifting attention toward older ages would by no means be limited to high-mortality societies. The low-mortality societies in which the case for a shift in emphasis seems particularly strong would also be affected, and under some circumstances and by some measures, the effect would be considerably more significant than in high-mortality populations. As indicated above, for example, a focus on infants and children in the illustrative low-mortality society would benefit the least healthy groups almost 10 times as much as the healthiest group, compared with less than twice as much in the high-mortality one. An upward movement in the age-specific focus would bring a far greater fall in this ratio in the high- than in the low-mortality society because of the age structure effects of the larger fertility differences between groups in the low-mortality society and from the much greater intergroup differences in child mortality.

As such an outcome indicates, what matters in determining the distributional impact of a policy change is not a society's overall health status, but rather the pattern of intergroup differences in demographic and health conditions within the society. The distributional consequences of changing priorities may be considerably more severe in a low-mortality society marked by large intergroup differences than in a high-mortality society where intergroup differences are relatively small.

None of the quantitative findings reported here can be considered definitive, of course. The example from which they emerged has been consciously oversimplified to facilitate communication about a general point, and as a result, the numbers presented cannot be legitimately applied to any particular situation without far more careful analysis than is possible here. This being said, however, the logic that underlies the figures suggests that the concern raised in the earlier investigation of regional data is well founded. That is, the health problems of infants and children appear likely to loom much larger among the less healthy than among the healthier groups of a national population, suggesting that shifting priorities away from them toward the health problems of older people would divert attention toward issues of primary relevance for the better-off and away from those of greatest concern to the least healthy.

CAUSE-SPECIFIC MORTALITY

The approach just used to look at age-specific mortality can also be employed to examine the distributional implications of alternative disease-oriented program foci, although the results that it produces must be viewed with considerably greater caution for several reasons. One is the inherent complexity of disease patterns, which defy easy categorization. A second is the smaller amount and less certain reliability of the information about cause of death. A third is the more limited experience in inferring cause-specific mortality patterns in the Third World from developed country data.

Even so, reliance on developed country data when assessing the Third World's evolution appears to be becoming an increasingly accepted practice in leading professional institutions, as demonstrated by the central role it has played in such major works as the two World Bank studies that represent the most careful extant examination of developing country trends (Feachem et al., 1992; Jamison and Mosley, 1993). This reliance and the importance of the topic suffice to justify at least a passing look at what the figures in current use have to say about the distributional consequences of alternate disease-specific foci.

Table 6 presents estimates of cause-specific mortality rates for our four populations that are based on estimates from Bulatao and Stephens (1992). As can be seen from columns 4 and 7 of the table, mortality from most causes is higher in the least healthy groups than in the healthiest ones. However, there is one exception: neoplasm, a noncommunicable disease particularly important at older ages. For the single most important set of noncommunicable diseases in adults and the elderly—circulatory and certain degenerative diseases—death rates are only modestly (15-20 percent) higher among the least healthy than among the healthiest. In contrast, people in the least healthy groups are 2.2 to 3.6 times as likely to die as are those in the healthiest from infections and parasitic diseases, the largest category of communicable ailments.

The implications of these patterns, when viewed in conjunction with the inter-group differences in age structure, can be seen in from Tables 7 and 8. These two tables, developed in a manner analogous to that used to produce Tables 5 and 6, show the cause-specific distribution of deaths and the effect on each group of a society-wide one-third reduction of mortality in a particular disease category.

As can be seen from Table 7, the principal communicable diseases are of far greater importance than the principal noncommunicable diseases for the least healthy than for the healthiest segments of society. In the high-mortality society, communicable diseases kill three times as many of the least healthy as do noncommunicable diseases; among the healthiest, about the same number of people die from each type of disease. When overall mortality is low, the least healthy die around 40 percent more often from

TABLE 6 Cause-Specific Mortality Rates (per 1,000 population) of Groups With Differing Life Expectancies

	High-Mortality Country			Low-Mortality Country		
Cause of Death (1)	Least Healthy 10-20% of Population (2)	Healthiest 10-20% of Population (3)	Ratio (2)/(3) (4)	Least Healthy 10-20% of Population (5)	Healthiest 10-20% of Population (6)	Ratio (5)/(6) (7)
Circulatory system and certain degenerative diseases	5.70	4.91	1.16	6.13	5.25	1.17
Infectious and parasitic diseases	7.99	3.65	2.19	4.64	1.30	3.57
Neoplasms	1.33	1.44	0.92	1.68	1.83	0.92
Injury and/or poisoning	0.84	0.69	1.22	0.76	0.64	1.19
Perinatal conditions	0.70	0.37	1.89	0.35	0.16	2.19
Complications of pregnancy	0.14	0.06	2.33	0.07	0.01	7.00
Other causes	5.51	3.50	1.57	4.47	2.43	1.84

SOURCE: Calculated by using functional relationships between overall life expectancy and age-cause-specific mortality rates prepared by Bulatao and Stephens (1989:Supplementary Tables). (Figures for both groups in high-mortality countries are based on stationary age structures at country mean life expectancy (55.0 years) in order to neutralize intergroup fertility differences. For the same reason, figures for both groups in low-mortality countries are calculated for stationary population age structures at country mean life expectancy of 62.5 years.)

TABLE 7 Total Deaths by Cause (percent)

	High-Mortality Country		Low-Mortality Country	
Cause of Death	Least Healthy 10-20% of Population	Healthiest 10-20% of Population	Least Healthy 10-20% of Population	Healthiest 10-20% of Population
Infectious and parasitic diseases	47.2	32.8	36.6	10.7
Circulatory system diseases and neoplasms	15.5	30.0	26.0	59.4
Other causes	37.3	37.2	37.4	30.0
Deaths from infectious and parasitic diseases relative to deaths from circulatory system diseases and neoplasms	3.0	1.1	1.4	0.2

communicable than from noncommunicable diseases; the healthiest die only about 20 percent as frequently.

Accordingly, it should come as no surprise to find that the least healthy would be the principal beneficiaries of a reduction of mortality from communicable diseases produced in a manner comparable to that described earlier in the section on age-specific mortality. As indicated by the figures in columns 3 and 6 of Table 8, a society-wide decline in mortality from communicable diseases would benefit the least healthy around 1.4 times as much as the healthiest in the high-mortality society, and more than three time as much in the low-mortality society. A decline in mortality from noncommunicable diseases would produce the opposite effect: the least healthy would gain only about one-half as much as the healthiest in each society, and the gap between the two groups would widen. According to the figures in Table 8, in other words, an emphasis on communicable diseases is progressive; a focus on the noncommunicable diseases is regressive.[11]

Although figures like these can be considered no more than suggestive,

[11]As indicated in footnote 9, these figures have been produced through the equal-outcome approach described there and would not necessarily be the same as figures resulting from an input-based approach. The principal sources of possible differences between results yielded by the two approaches are analogous to those for different age groups, as discussed in footnote 10. As is the case with respect to age, use of an input-based approach seems more likely to strengthen than to weaken the overall conclusion produced through the equal-outcome approach employed here.

TABLE 8 Change in Number of Deaths Attributable to One-Third Reduction of Mortality from Particular Causes (percent)

	High-Mortality Country			Low-Mortality Country		
	Least Healthy 10-20% of Population (1)	Healthiest 10-20% of Population (2)	Ratio (1)/(2) (3)	Least Healthy 10-20% of Population (4)	Healthiest 10-20% of Population (5)	Ratio (4)/(5) (6)
One-third reduction in deaths from infectious and parisitic diseases	–15.7	–10.9	1.4	–12.2	–3.6	3.4
One-third reduction in deaths from circulatory system diseases and neoplasms	–5.2	–10.0	0.5	–8.6	–19.8	0.4

they are nonetheless of interest both in themselves and for the reinforcement they give to and derive from the age-specific mortality figures presented earlier. The fact that an emphasis on reducing mortality from leading communicable diseases produces the same distributional effect as a focus on reducing deaths at early ages is what one would expect in light of what is known about the generally direct relationships that exist between the two, as is the fact that emphasizing noncommunicable diseases has the same distributional consequences as stressing mortality reduction among adults and the elderly.

OTHER CONSIDERATIONS

In moving from the suggestions emerging from the simple arithmetic exercises presented here toward the definitive conclusions needed for effective policy formulation, many other considerations will have to be taken into account. An adequate treatment of any of them would require far more space than presently available and will thus have to await another time. It is, however, both possible and valuable to note some of the most important.

Among the most significant considerations is one that has already been mentioned: the wide variations among countries that could limit the relevance of generalizations such as those developed here in any particular setting. However, the generalizations' illustrative value should not be denigrated. The demographic and epidemiological parameters developed for the high- and low-mortality societies presented in the preceding sections are far from hypothetical. Rather, they are based on information about sub-Saharan Africa and Latin America drawn from standard sources and used routinely for a wide range of analytical purposes. The results presented can thus be reasonably considered at least broadly representative of each of those regions as a whole. There are, however, wide differences within each region; and many important developing countries lie in neither one. The strengths of the effects of a shift in age- and disease-specific focus in particular settings could thus well vary from those presented above in a manner that can be determined only through the fuller country-level investigations that this initial exploration hopes to inspire.

A second consideration is the limited nature of the indicator of health status used in the illustrations (see Preston in this volume for a fuller discussion). The number of deaths suffered or prevented in a group is obviously important, but it is by no means a complete representation of the group's health status or of changes in it. Compared to a more appealing indicator such as the number of quality-adjusted years lost or added, a focus on the number of deaths prevented is deficient in two respects. First, it ignores differences in the number of years of life added per death prevented at different ages or from different causes. A death prevented in childhood obviously adds many more years of life than does a death averted at an advanced age. To overlook this difference is to bias the arguments advanced against infant and child health programs and against many communicable disease initiatives. Second, it overlooks morbidity. If the morbidity/mortality ratio differs across age and/or disease groups, and if people in the groups concerned place a high value on morbidity relative to mortality reduction, a failure to take morbidity into account could lead to distorted results. Whether any such distortion actually exists is difficult to determine. Little is known about the morbidity/mortality ratios of diseases suffered at different ages and caused by different agents.[12] Even less knowledge exists about the relative importance that different population groups in developing countries attach to morbidity relative to mortality.

The third consideration is the question of the interrelationships among deaths (and illnesses) at different ages and from different causes. The examples presented here assume that no such relationships exist. But in fact, they clearly do. The two-way relationship between death and poor health at different ages has been a topic of particular attention. Deaths among adults are thought to produce a significant decrease in the survival probabilities of their children. Conversely, deaths among infants and children have well-known effects on fertility and thus on maternal health; more generally, unhealthy children are believed to become less healthy adults who are more prone to early death (see Mosley and Gray in this volume). The effects work in both directions, and it is possible that they are of adequately similar magnitudes to cancel each other. Should this be the case, the failure to account for the effects in the illustrations would not bias the illustrations' results, but one cannot be certain without a careful investigation.

The fourth consideration is the previously noted possibility of differences in the cost-effectiveness of interventions available to prevent deaths at different ages and from different causes. The conclusions reached in the illustrations are valid only if the cost of preventing a death in the most

---

[12]At first glance, chronic diseases at older ages might seem to be particularly "morbidity intense" because of the extended period of disability and suffering that often precedes death. Yet such morbidity, while perhaps more visible than that caused by communicable diseases early in life, is not necessarily more prevalent. Communicable diseases among infants and children also produce a great deal of illness for every death attributable to them. For each childhood death from diarrhea, for example, some 100 children are thought to fall ill and remain so for two to three days each, implying 200-300 days—roughly six to ten months—of morbidity per death. This estimate is clearly shorter than the period of morbidity suffered by some older victims of the strokes or heart attacks that represent the most frequent causes of death among them. But it is also considerably longer than the duration of illness among the many others whose strokes and heart attacks lead to almost immediate death. What counts are the averages, and these remain to be determined.

prevalent category is equal to or less than the cost of preventing a death in the less prevalent categories.[13] In view of what is currently known about the cost-effectiveness of dealing with different age- and disease-specific groups (Jamison and Mosley, 1993), the inclusion of cost-effectiveness considerations would seem unlikely to upset many of the conclusions reached in situations where communicable diseases and deaths at an early age appear to deserve highest priority. However, the costs of the traditional approaches to averting deaths among older people from chronic diseases are notoriously high, which raises the possibility that the illustrations in which such diseases emerge dominant overstate the case for according priority to them.[14]

A fifth consideration concerns the existence of wide differences in the distributional implications of dealing with specific problems within each of the broad age and disease categories covered. Even if a general focus on adults and the elderly or on noncommunicable diseases is less progressive or more regressive than an overall emphasis on communicable diseases or on infants and children, such will not necessarily be the case with respect to each and every noncommunicable condition that occurs primarily at older ages. The figures in Table 6 on deaths resulting from complications of pregnancy illustrate the point. Deaths from this cause, a condition of young adults that is not communicable in the standard sense of the term, represent too small a proportion of total deaths at older ages to justify their use as the basis of any generalization (Bulatao and Stephens, 1989). Unlike other, more frequent causes of death from noncommunicable diseases, however, they clearly affect the least healthy groups far more severely than the healthiest groups: more than twice as severely in the high-mortality population and seven times as severely in the low-mortality one. If comparable figures available were for malnutrition, the results would probably be similar. Such examples serve as important reminders that, although a primary overall focus on communicable diseases and an overall emphasis on infants and children might well be justified, the careful examinations necessary for the formulation of intelligent policies are likely to find at least some activities

[13]Otherwise, in a situation of limited resources, a greater number of deaths would be prevented by first directing those resources against that minority of deaths that can be averted at relatively low cost and only then paying attention to the more difficult majority.

[14]Unless one assumes that any general shift in priorities toward chronic diseases at older ages is accompanied by a major change in the way in which these diseases are approached. A shift away from high-technology curative approaches that are currently predominant in the treatment of noncommunicable diseases among adults and the elderly, toward the simpler treatment and behavioral measures advocated by reformers, would lead to cost-effectiveness ratios apparently comparable to those of the approaches currently in use for dealing with communicable diseases at younger ages. This shift would reduce or eliminate any overstatement that might exist.

outside those rubrics that deserve inclusion in a program oriented toward disparity reduction.

The sixth consideration is the possibility of modifying the distributional effects of efforts to reduce mortality by targeting specific population groups to benefit from them. By careful targeting, a program with any age- or disease-specific focus can be shaped to benefit the least healthy more than the healthiest. For example, even a tertiary-care facility specializing in rare cardiovascular conditions will benefit the least healthy more than the healthiest and thereby reduce inequalities if it is located in a poor neighborhood and its services are made available only to the poorest residents of that neighborhood. However, the magnitude of the distributional improvement thereby achieved would obviously be far smaller than that which brought about by applying the same resources to an approach more closely aligned with the epidemiological conditions prevailing in the poor community being served. As the example demonstrates, targeting has an extremely important role to play in the development of programs to help the disadvantaged, but it cannot by itself lead to the efficient reduction of disparities that represents the logical objective of such efforts. To reduce disparities, targeting must be used in conjunction with a clear appreciation of the target population's demographic-epidemiological situation and with cost-effectiveness considerations.

CONCLUSION

The importance of the considerations presented in the preceding section point to a clear need for further research in many areas to assist in the development of effective approaches to the reduction of differences in health status. One can only urge and hope that such research will proceed as rapidly as possible.

In the meantime, thousands of health policymakers will be making hundreds of thousands of decisions concerning health policies that will benefit different groups in different manners. Can guidance, however preliminary and provisional, be drawn from what is now known and presented here in order to help them decide how to respond to the demographic and epidemiological transitions?

At the heart of any such guidance would have to be a warning against responding to overall trends such as those portrayed by the data presented in tables 1A and 1B by a general shift in health priorities toward a greater emphasis on problems caused by noncommunicable diseases among adults and the elderly. These data are societal averages. To rely on them is to overlook the differences that exist among groups within society and, in the process, to give as much weight to problems concentrated in society's most privileged groups as to those of greatest relevance for the least healthy. The information presented here suggests that the least healthy can be much better served by a strategy based on a careful study of their particular needs and that such a strategy is likely to give highest priority to communicable diseases among the young.

REFERENCES

Bobadilla, J.L., J. Frenk, T. Frejka, R. Lozano, and C. Stern

1993 The epidemiological transition and health priorities. In D.T. Jamison and W.H. Mosley, eds., *Disease Control Priorities in Developing Countries.* New York: Oxford University Press for the World Bank.

Bulatao, R.A., and P.W. Stephens

1989 Estimates and projections of mortality by cause: A global overview, 1990-2015. Unpublished manuscript, World Bank, Washington, D.C.

1992 Estimates and projections of mortality by cause: A global overview, 1970-2015. *Policy Research Working Papers.* Washington, D.C.: World Bank.

Bulatao, R.A., E. Bos, P.W. Stephens, and M.T. Vu

1989 Africa regional population projections (1989-1990 edition). Policy Planning and Research Working Paper. No. WPS 330 (November). Population and Human Resources Department of the World Bank, Washington, D.C.

Bulatao, R.A., E. Bos, P.W. Stephens, and M.T. Vu

1990 Latin America and the Caribbean region population projections, 1989-1990 edition. Policy Planning and Research Working Paper. No. WPS 329 (November). Population and Human Resources Department of the World Bank, Washington, D.C.

Coale, A.J., and P. Demeny, with B. Vaughan

1983 *Regional Model Life Tables and Stable Populations*, 2nd ed. New York: Academic Press.

Feachem, R., T. Kjellstrom, C.J.L. Murray, M. Over, and M.A. Phillips, eds.

1992 *The Health of Adults in the Developing World.* New York: Oxford University Press for the World Bank.

Jamison, D.T., and W.H. Mosley.

1993 Disease control priorities in developing countries. In D.T. Jamison and W.H. Mosley, eds., *Disease Control Priorities in Developing Countries.* New York: Oxford University Press for the World Bank.

APPENDIX

Intergroup Differences in Mortality Within Developing Countries

A. Populations differentiated by income status

Brazil:

The highest mortality group for 1970 is based on households with monthly incomes below Cr$100, representing 21.0 percent of the total population. Infant mortality rate (IMR) was 127.4 per 1,000 live births and life expectancy at birth (e_0) was 48.9 years. The lowest mortality group is based on households with monthly incomes above Cr$1,000, representing 22.0 percent of the total population. IMR was 60.8 per 1,000 live births and e_0 was 62.2 years.
IMR relative difference: 2.10 times; IMR absolute difference: 66.6 deaths per 1,000 live births.
e_0 relative difference: 1.27 times; e_0 absolute difference: 13.3 years.

Charles H. Wood and José Alberto Magno de Carvalho, *The Demography of Inequality in Brazil*, (Cambridge, New York, New Rochelle, Melbourne, Sydney: Cambridge University Press, 1988), p. 190. (Infant mortality derived through application of model life tables to life expectancy figures provided in text.)

B. Populations differentiated by place or residence

Kenya:

The highest mortality group for 1974 is based on residents of Coast and Nyanza Provinces, representing 26.1 percent of the total population. IMR was 140.3 per 1,000 live births and e_0 was 46.7 years. The lowest mortality group is based on residents of the Central Province, representing 15.3 percent of the total population. IMR was 58.0 per 1,000 live births and e_0 was 62.9 years.
IMR relative difference: 2.42 times; IMR absolute difference: 82.3 deaths per 1,000 live births.
e_0 relative difference: 1.36 times; e_0 absolute difference: 16.2 years.

W. Henry Mosley, "Will Primary Care Reduce Infant and Child Mortality? A Critique of Some Current Strategies, with Special Reference to Africa and Asia," in Jacques Vallin and Alan D. Lopez, eds. *Health Policy, Social Policy, and Mortality Prospects: Proceedings of a Seminar at Paris, France, February 28-March 4, 1983*, (Place of publication not indicated: Ordina Publications for the Institut National d'Etudes Démographiques and the International Union for the Scientific Study of Population, 1985), p. 109. (Infant mortality and life expectancy derived through application of model life tables to figures for child deaths by age 2 per 1000 live births presented in text.)

Sudan:

The highest mortality group for 1973 is based on residents of Bahr El Ghazal Province, representing 9.4 percent of the total population. IMR was 227.5 per 1,000 live births and e_0 was 34.2 years. The lowest mortality group is based on residents of the Khartoum Province, representing 7.8 percent of the total population. IMR was 107.6 per 1,000 live births and e_0 was 52.5 years.
IMR relative difference: 2.11 times; IMR absolute difference: 119.9 deaths per 1,000 live births.
e_0 relative difference: 1.54 times; e_0 absolute difference: 18.3 years.

Abdul-Aziz Farah and Samuel H. Preston, "Child Mortality Differentials in Sudan," *Population and Development Review*, vol. 8, no. 2 (June 1982). (Infant mortality derived through application of model life tables to life expectancy figures presented in text. Figures for percentage of total population calculated from 1973 census.)

India:

The highest mortality group for 1986 is based on residents of Uttar Pradesh State, representing 16.2 percent of the total population. IMR was 132.0 per 1,000 live births and e_0 was 48.0 years. The lowest mortality group is based on residents of Kerala, Maharashtra, and Punjab States, representing 15.3 percent of the total population. IMR was 54.9 per 1,000 live births and e_0 was 63.5 years.
IMR relative difference: 2.40 times; IMR absolute difference: 77.1 deaths per 1,000 live births.
e_0 relative difference: 1.32 times; e_0 absolute difference: 15.6 years.

Office of the Registrar General, Ministry of Home Affairs, Government of India, *Registrar General's Newsletter*, vol. XIX, no. 1 (January 1988), p. 16. (Life expectancy derived through application of model life tables to infant mortality figures provided in text. Figures for percentage of total population calculated from 1981 census.)

Philippines: The highest mortality group for 1986 is based on residents of Western and Central Mindanao Regions, representing 10.0 percent of the total population. IMR was 101.4 per 1,000 live births and e_0 was 53.2 years. The lowest mortality group is based on residents of the National Capital Region, representing 12.9 percent of the total population. IMR was 36.3 per 1,000 live births and e_0 as 67.5 years.
IMR relative difference: 2.79 times; IMR absolute difference: 65.1 deaths per 1,000 live births.
e_0 relative difference: 1.27 times; e_0 absolute difference: 14.3 years.

Panfila Ching, "Factors Affecting the Demand for Health Services in the Philippines," (unpublished manuscript, 1989), pp. 10-21, 29.

Mexico: The highest mortality group for the period 1982-1988 is based on residents of eight southern states, representing 16.6 percent of the total population. IMR was 92.0 per 1,000 live births and e_0 was 55.5 years. The lowest mortality group is based on residents of the seven northern states, representing 14.8 percent of the total population. IMR was 28.0 per 1,000 live births and e_0 was 70.2 years.
IMR relative difference: 3.29 times; IMR absolute difference: 64.0 deaths per 1,000 live births.
e_0 relative difference: 1.26 times; e_0 absolute difference: 14.7 years.

José-Luis Bobadilla et al., "The Epidemiological Transition and Health Priorities," draft manuscript prepared for the World Bank Disease Control Priorities Review, December 1989, p. 14a. (Life expectancy derived through application of model life tables to infant mortality figures presented in text. Figures for percentage of total population calculated from 1980 census.)

Peru: The highest mortality group for 1967-1968 is based on residents of the Southern Region, representing 18.6 percent of the total population. IMR was 173.0 per 1,000 live births and e_0 was 42.0 years. The lowest mortality group is based on residents of the Metropolitan Region, representing 24.4 percent of the total population. IMR was 78.0 per 1,000 live births and e_0 was 58.2 years.
IMR relative difference: 2.22 times; IMR absolute difference: 96.0 deaths per 1,000 live births.
e_0 relative difference: 1.39 times; e_0 absolute difference: 16.2 years.

Hugo Behm and Alfredo Ledesma, *La Mortalidad en Los Primeros Años de Vida en Paises de La America Latina: Peru, 1967-1968*, (Serie A. No. 1029) (San José: Centro Latinoamericano de Demografia, Mayo de 1977), pp. 11, 38.

C. Populations differentiated by women's educational status

Burundi: The highest mortality group for the period 1981-1987 is based on children of women with no education, representing 80.2 percent of the total population. IMR was 90.0 per 1,000 live births and e_0 was 55.8 years. The lowest mortality group is based on children of women with secondary or higher education, representing 2.2 percent of the total population. IMR was 32.0 per 1,000 live births and e_0 was 69.2 years.
IMR relative difference: 2.81 times; IMR absolute difference: 58.0 deaths per 1,000 live births.
e_0 relative difference: 1.24 times; e_0 absolute difference: 13.4 years.

"Burundi 1987: Results from the Demographic and Health Survey," *Studies in Family Planning*, Vol. 20, No. 3 (May/June 1989). (Life expectancy derived through application of model life tables to infant mortality figures provided in text.)

Dominican Republic The highest mortality group for the period 1982-1985 is based on children of women with no education, representing 4.8 percent of the total population. IMR was

102.0 per 1,000 live births and e_0 was 53.5 years. The lowest mortality group is based on children of women with higher education, representing 8.4 percent of the total population. IMR was 34.0 per 1,000 live births and e_0 was 68.5 years.
IMR relative difference: 3.00 times; IMR absolute difference: 68.0 deaths per 1,000 live births.
e_0 relative difference: 1.26 times; e_0 absolute difference: 15.0 years.

"Dominican Republic 1986: Results from the Demographic and Health Survey," *Studies in Family Planning*, Vol. 19, No. 2 (March/April 1988). (Life expectancy derived through application of model life tables to infant mortality figures provided in text.)

Ecuador: The highest mortality group for the period 1982-1987 is based on children of women with no education, representing 7.8 percent of the total population. IMR was 106.0 per 1,000 live births and e_0 was 52.8 years. The lowest mortality group is based on children of women with higher education, representing 9.2 percent of the total population. IMR was 22.0 per 1,000 live births and e_0 was 71.9 years.
IMR relative difference: 4.82 times; IMR absolute difference: 84.0 deaths per 1,000 live births.
e_0 relative difference: 1.36 times; e_0 absolute difference: 19.1 years.

"Ecuador 1987: Results from the Demographic and Health Survey," *Studies in Family Planning*, Vol. 20, No. 2 (March/April 1989). (Life expectancy derived through application of model life tables to infant mortality figures provided in text.)

Indonesia: The highest mortality group for the period 1984-1987 is based on children of women with no education, representing 23.2 percent of the total population. IMR was 99.0 per 1,000 live births and e_0 was 54.1 years. The lowest mortality group is based on children of women with secondary or higher education, representing 13.1 percent of the total population. IMR was 34.0 per 1,000 live births and e_0 was 65.6 years.

IMR relative difference: 2.91 times; IMR absolute difference: 65.0 deaths per 1,000 live births.
e_0 relative difference: 1.27 times; e_0 absolute difference: 14.4 years.

"Indonesia 1987: Results from the Demographic and Health Survey," *Studies in Family Planning*, Vol. 20, No. 5 (September/October 1989). (Life expectancy derived through application of model life tables to infant mortality figures provided in text.)

Senegal:

The highest mortality group for the period 1981-1986 is based on children of women with no education, representing 77.2 percent of the total population. IMR was 96.0 per 1,000 live births and e_0 was 54.7 years. The lowest mortality group is based on children of women with higher education, representing 9.3 percent of the total population. IMR was 50.0 per 1,000 live births and e_0 was 64.7 years.
IMR relative difference: 1.92 times; IMR absolute difference: 46.0 deaths per 1,000 live births.
e_0 relative difference: 1.16 times; e_0 absolute difference: 10.0 years.

"Senegal 1986: Results from the Demographic and Health Survey," *Studies in Family Planning*, Vol. 19, No. 6 (November/December 1988). (Life expectancy derived through application of model life tables to infant mortality figures provided in text.)

Thailand:

The highest mortality group for the period 1982-1987 is based on children of women with no education, representing 9.7 percent of the total population. IMR was 54.03 per 1,000 live births and e_0 was 63.7 years. The lowest mortality group is based on children of women with secondary or higher education, representing 7.7 percent of the total population. IMR was 19.0 per 1,000 live births and e_0 was 72.9 years.
IMR relative difference: 2.84 times; IMR absolute difference: 35.0 deaths per 1,000 live births.
e_0 relative difference: 1.14 times; e_0 absolute difference: 9.2 years.

"Thailand 1987: Results from the Demographic and Health Survey," *Studies in Family Planning*, Vol. 20, No. 1 (January/February 1989). (Life expectancy derived through application of model life tables to infant mortality figures provided in text.)

D. Populations differentiated by race

South Africa: The highest mortality group for the period 1981-1985 is based on the black population, representing 68.0 percent of the total population. IMR was ranged from 94.0 to 124.0 per 1,000 live births and e_0 ranged from was 49.4 to 55.1 years. The lowest mortality group is based on the white popuation, representing 18.2 percent of the total population. IMR was 12.3 per 1,000 live births and e_0 was 75.3 years.
IMR relative difference: 7.64-10.08 times; IMR absolute difference: 81.7-111.7 deaths per 1,000 live births. e_0 relative difference: 1.37-1.52 times; e_0 absolute difference: 20.2-25.9 years.

D. Yach, "Infant Mortality Rates in Urban Areas of South Africa, 1981-1985," *South African Medical Journal*, vol. 73 (1988), p. 234. (Life expectancy derived through application of model life tables to infant mortality figures presented in text. Figures for percentage of total population calculated from 1980 census.)

NOTES

The data here are drawn from the 14 studies referred to in the text. These studies employed a wide range of approaches that required conversion into a standardized format. Three aspects of this conversion process are worthy of note:

1. None of the studies presented information divided precisely into the population groups desired: that is, the top 10 or 20 percent and the bottom 10 or 20 percent of the total population. To provide workable approximations, an effort was made to identify groups of roughly the same size equaling as closely as possible the highest and lowest 15 percent of each population under study. For this purpose, smaller groups were combined, and weighted averages of the relevant parameters were prepared when necessary. As can be seen and as noted in the text, it was possible to come reasonably close to the desired objective for studies categorizing health status by income and place of residence, but not possible to approach it when the basis of categorization was educational status or race, because of the limited number of categories and uneven distribution of population among them. (A follow-up inquiry is planned to gather information from more countries at different points in time and to organize it in terms of

a common distributional index—such as the Gini coefficient—in order to permit intercountry and intertemporal comparisons.)

2. Only two of the fourteen studies (Peru and the Philippines) included both life expectancy and infant mortality figures. One (Kenya, in which mortality was expressed in terms of survival probabilities from birth through age 2) provided neither. The remaining eleven presented either life expectancy or infant mortality, but not both. The missing life expectancy and/or infant mortality figures were estimated using the average of female and male figures taken from the Coale-Demeny West model life tables. An indication of which figures were calculated in this manner is provided in a parenthetical note accompanying each data source.

3. Four of the studies (India, Mexico, South Africa, and Sudan) lacked the information about group-specific population sizes needed to estimate the proportion of the population. In these cases, the information provided in the studies has been supplemented by census data. Information about the years of the censuses used appears in the parenthetical notes accompanying each relevant data source.

Health, Government, and the Poor: The Case for the Private Sector

Nancy Birdsall and Estelle James

INTRODUCTION

An important current issue in the health sector in developing countries concerns the appropriate degree of reliance on the private sector and on private spending for the provision of health care. Proponents of user charges and greater privatization claim that such reliance will conserve scarce public funds and promote efficiency in the sense of cost-effectiveness and responsiveness to consumer preferences (Akin et al., 1987; Jimenez, 1987). Opponents retort with two arguments. The first is an efficiency and effectiveness argument: that in the past in developing countries, the public sector has been successful in providing health care. The second is an equity argument: that because of their reliance on ability to pay as a rationing criterion, user charges for public services and privatization will have negative distributional effects that are likely to outweigh any efficiency gains (e.g., see Gertler et al., 1987, and Gertler and van der Gaag, 1990, on user charges for health care in Peru and Côte d'Ivoire).

In this paper, we argue that neither argument is correct, given current and likely future trends—and that there is a case for limited and selective employment of user charges and privatization of health in most developing countries. In the first section we set forth a brief statement of public choice theory, which predicts that, in general, government actions may be neither efficient nor equitable. Instead, they may be directed toward increasing the

Nancy Birdsall and Estelle James are with the World Bank. This draft draws heavily on ideas developed in and excerpts from two papers by Birdsall (1989), and by Birdsall and James (1990). The views expressed are not necessarily those of the World Bank.

real income of influential middle- and upper-income groups, often in inefficient ways. The next section draws, as a central point of this paper, an important corollary of public choice theory for the health field: that the past successes of the public sector are not likely to be repeated in the future. The reason is an increasing tension between the health needs of the rich versus the poor, with the greatest potential mortality gains coming from attention to the latter but political forces often dictating a flow of resources to the former. The third section provides numerous examples of this misallocation and suggests ways that selective use of fees and privatization may improve equity, efficiency, and returns to future public health spending.

In the conclusion, we summarize the crux of the political economy problem raised in the earlier sections. If the inefficiency and inequity of government health programs are endogenous and politically determined, how can they be fixed? How do we break into the chain of causation and bring about a new equilibrium, more efficient and more redistributive, that is apparently not in the interest of the main actors or it would have happened already?

WHY IS GOVERNMENT HEALTH SPENDING BOTH INEFFICIENT AND INEQUITABLE?

Why are governments often inefficient and inequitable? This section contrasts a normative (welfare theory) and positive (public choice theory) approach to government behavior, and argues that the pessimistic conclusions of the latter are most applicable to developing countries. The following section extends public choice theory to the health sector in developing countries and shows how it implies a deteriorating effectiveness of government spending and a need to place greater reliance on private spending, in order to improve both efficiency and equity.

Welfare Theory Versus Public Choice Theory

Classical welfare theory gives us a *normative* view of what government *should* do. The main economic role of government is to correct market failure by funding public goods, by subsidizing (or taxing) goods that generate (positive or negative) externalities, and by compensating for capital market or insurance market failure, in addition to simply setting the framework within which private enterprise will function.[1]

[1]When efforts of government to correct for market failure in themselves introduce some efficiency losses—because of transaction costs or the distortionary effects of taxes—we are operating in a second-best world in which the benefits of intervention must be weighed against the costs. But much of classical welfare theory can nevertheless be depicted as a pursuit of the first best.

With respect to distribution, the "maximum" point of social welfare is acknowledged by most economists to depend on equity as well as efficiency. Opinions vary widely on whether a "social welfare function" exists, what an "equitable" distribution would be, and whether it is possible to aggregate diverse preferences to arrive at a consensus on this matter.[2] However, despite this ambivalence about the redistributive role of government, most economists agree that if there is to be any redistribution, it should be from rich to poor and not vice versa—the "Robin Hood" function of government (Birdsall, 1992). We use the term "equity" as a shortened form of Robin Hood redistribution in this paper.

A second, more recent, and less benevolent view of government activities stems from public choice theory, which gives us a *positive* model of what the government *will* do, under the presumption that the chief agents act to maximize individual utility rather than social welfare. According to this theory, politicians do not seek to maximize efficiency but rather to maximize their own chances of staying in power; bureaucrats seek to maximize their budgets; and individuals use governments to augment their real income via the creation of protected market positions and the direct provision of services and transfers (Mueller, 1979; Borcherding, 1985).

Politicians and political parties have some discretionary power because of barriers to entry and because they are in a position to shape as well as respond to people's tastes. At the same time, threats from actual or potential competitors limit the scope of their monopoly power. Thus, natural selection operates in political life as well as in economic or biological life. In terms of the entire spectrum of issues, among which different groups of voters have different trade-offs, the politicians who survive to make policy are those who assess these trade-offs correctly and give influential groups what they want on issues that are most salient to them. Where democracy does not exist, a similar process often occurs, but with greater discretionary monopoly powers for government officials who control the political market.

---

[2]A vast literature has developed on the question of whether actual compensation or simply the potential for compensation should be used to compare the relative desirability of two alternative allocations. In the latter case, distribution is essentially deemed irrelevant, whereas in the former, the nature of compensatory mechanisms is crucial. Opinions vary on how much the government should intervene to alter the market distribution (see Rawls, 1971, and Nozick, 1974, for strongly contrasting views). The strongest advocates of redistribution argue that it is justified on efficiency as well as equity grounds—if people care about the utility of others or if there exists a set of "merit goods" (health, education) about which society does not trust consumers to make the "right" consumption decisions (Meade, 1964; Musgrave, 1959; Hochman and Rogers, 1969). Skeptics point to the lack of consensus on the desired distribution and to the disincentive effects of redistribution. Bourgignon (1989), for example, sets out a model in which the pursuit of equity, through education and health programs that build human capital or through transfer programs such as food subsidies for the poor, requires that governments generate tax revenues, which reduce overall efficiency.

Public policies designed to maximize private interests will not necessarily be inefficient. Indeed, politically influential groups would have a potentially larger pie to capture if the Pareto frontier were reached; compensatory mechanisms could then make everyone better off. Taxes could be imposed on some (less influential groups) and transferred to others.

However, the allocation of resources resulting from public choice politics is often inefficient, for the following reasons:

Veil of Ignorance

In a context of imperfect information, people may not know the degree and direction of redistribution going on. If well-defined groups know they are "losers" they are more likely to mobilize and foment opposition to existing policies; therefore, the "gainers" benefit from perpetuating a "veil of ignorance." Suppose that the most efficient form of transfers is also more obvious (e.g., transfers in cash are more transparent than those in kind). In that case, efficiency imposes cost to the "gainers" by reducing the amount they will be potentially able to extract; they are therefore likely to choose inefficient transfer mechanisms. Most commonly, some private goods may be publicly provided and oversupplied because they benefit a politically influential group of people in a nonobvious way (see Becker, 1983; Borcherding et al., 1983).

Fiscal Illusion

Our second point is closely related: Imperfect information and uncertainty also surround the relationship between the tax structure and the bundle of public services provided. Although these may be interdependent components of a long-run political equilibrium (e.g., if the benefits of a group rise, its tax burden may also rise), taxes and services may appear to be independent of each other in the short run—a kind of "fiscal illusion." In that case, some public or quasi-public goods may be undersupplied because their benefits accrue to dispersed, less influential individuals, and it is not clear (to the influential "loser") that the tax share of the gainers can be adjusted upward commensurately with their benefits. Similarly, some goods may be oversupplied because their chief beneficiaries are politically powerful and expect to avoid much of the tax burden (Buchanan, 1967; Pommerehne and Schneider, 1978).

High Costs of Public Sector Provision

The real costs of publicly produced private goods may be above minimal levels because government imposes bureaucratic rules and red tape (in part as a substitute for the profit motive) and often lacks competitive pressures for internal efficiency (perhaps because politicians reap a surplus from monopolistic provision). Heads of bureaucratic agencies who wish to maximize their prestige and perks, and have greater information than the politicians and citizens they supposedly serve, are often able to argue successfully for larger budgets than are needed for least-cost production. In addition, distortionary tax financing also raises the nonprogram costs of publicly produced private goods (Niscanen, 1971; Romer and Rosenthal, 1978; Borcherding et al., 1983).[3]

Rent Seeking

The diversion of entrepreneurial energies toward extracting a surplus from public agencies rather than toward productivity-enhancing market activities also impedes private sector efficiency and growth. Rent-seeking activities thus misallocate private as well as public resources (Krueger, 1974; Buchanan et al., 1980).

The resulting distribution of real income is likely to depend upon political power as well as market power. Political power, of course, will vary across societies and through time, depending on the size of different producer and consumer groups, the coalitions among them, and the long-run "rules of the game" that have been set up (e.g., through constitutions) for allocating voting rights. Given that the distribution of voting rights is ordinarily more equal than the distribution of income, one might expect political decision making to be relatively egalitarian.[4] However, low-income people often do not vote, and economic power can also buy political power, for example, through campaign contributions and purchases of media influence that shape other people's votes. Because producer groups are likely to be more concentrated and better organized than consumer groups, because upper- and middle-income groups are generally more articulate and politically active than poorer groups, and because lines of communications and mobility often are strong among government agencies, their bureaucratic chiefs, and the private industries or professions they supposedly regulate, public choice theory predicts that producer and upper-income groups

[3]Program costs may exceed minimal levels even when politicians and bureaucrats wish to choose an efficient product and factor mix. The non-price rationing that often exists for distributional reasons under public funding, and the civil service procedures governing wages, hiring, and firing—procedures that substitute for managerial discretion under public production—mean that prices do not serve as a measure of the real benefits and costs of a program, as they do in the private market.

[4]Thus, Meltzer and Richard (1978, 1981) have argued that redistribution is likely to flow to the median voter whose income is generally less than average, and Demsetz (1982) ties this tendency to the extension of the franchise.

will benefit disproportionately from implemented government policies (see Stigler, 1970, 1971; Peltzman, 1976, 1980; Fiorina and Noll, 1978).

Public Choice in Developing Countries

How could we expect these divergent forces to sort themselves out in the developing country context? On the one hand, the gulf between rich and poor and the relative number of poor people are much greater there, so under "one man, one vote" we would expect to find the poor gaining from politically induced redistributions. Indeed, in a few countries (e.g., Malaysia) an economically disadvantaged group has used its political advantage effectively to increase its share of the national income. However, differences in education (hence, in organizational and communication skills) are also much greater in developing countries, and democratic institutions are often primitive, limiting the power of the poor. We would expect the latter tendency to dominate in most cases.

This is not to say that there will be no redistribution to the poorer classes. In fact, even when the rich are in control, we would expect to find some such redistribution of income. For example, people voluntarily donate to beggars and use the government as an efficient mechanism for donating to disadvantaged groups, in part because the extremes of poverty and socioeconomic immobility raise fears of crime or revolution that will ultimately hurt the rich. In developed countries, historically, the provision of certain merit goods to the poor (e.g., basic health and education services, social insurance) has been viewed as an effective way to combat these problems.

In addition, in developing countries, where there are many more poor people than rich, the desire to constrain the popularity of opposition parties encourages some distribution to lower-income groups on grounds of expediency. Out-of-power groups must be appeased by giving them "just enough" to prevent opposition parties from gaining strong support (a "contestable market" view of political equilibrium), but just enough may not be very much. For example, it may imply that the poor are given low-cost services or very limited access to high-cost services from which the rich are the main beneficiaries. Governmental expenditures on high-quantity, low-quality primary-level school systems and on selective high-cost universities are common illustrations of these two phenomena. In short, in many situations, perverse distributional rather than efficiency or equity criteria determine the allocation of government funds, and these criteria imply large benefits to powerful upper-income groups, combined with small redistributions to the poor (Behrman and Birdsall, 1988). We believe that these pessimistic predictions of public choice theory are consistent with the observed actions of developing countries in health today.

FUTURE EFFECTIVENESS OF GOVERNMENT SPENDING ON HEALTH

There is little doubt that governments have played a major role in bringing about extraordinary postwar mortality decline and the accompanying improvements in health in developing countries (see Table 1)—most obviously through direct interventions such as immunizations and malaria control, but also through more general public investments in education, sanitation, and improved communications and transportation, which have reduced the mortality toll once taken by limited information and periodic famine (Birdsall, 1989).

Can the past success of governments in reducing mortality and improving health be maintained? In this section we argue that, on grounds of public choice theory, there are strong reasons for doubt about the future contribution of government. Past gains have come from expenditures that benefited a wide spectrum of the population. However, future gains will require additional expenditures targeted toward the poor, behavioral changes among the poor, and indeed, the elimination of some aspects of poverty. But, for the reasons given above, governments are unlikely to spend dispro-

TABLE 1 Crude Death Rate and Life Expectancy at Birth, by Region, 1950-1985

	Crude Death Rate (deaths per 1,000 persons per year)				Life Expectancy at Birth (years)	
Region	1950	1965	1980	1985-1990	1950-1955	1985-1990
Sub-Saharan Africa	29.3	22.8	17.7	15.3		51.5
Middle East/ North Africa	24.0	18.1	12.6	10.9		59.0
South Asia	28.8	20.6	14.5	12.2	38.9	55.8
East Asia (except China)	27.1	16.3	10.5	7.3		67.9
China	27.3	16.0	7.9	6.7	40.8	69.0
Latin America/ Caribbean	16.6	11.7	8.5	7.2		66.6
Developing countries					41.1	59.1
Industrialized countries	10.5	9.6	9.1	9.3	65.8	73.1

SOURCES: Reproduced from Birdsall (1989); World Bank (1984:5); World Bank projections, 1985-1990 (for death rates); and United Nations (1986, for life expectancies).

portionately on the poor, and the behavior of the poor is unlikely to change rapidly; hence, the gains of the past are unlikely to continue into the future.

This tension between rich and poor is exacerbated by the tension between old and young. As the population ages, its disease profile changes; the prevalence of cancer, heart disease, and other diseases of adulthood and old age increases (Feachem et al., 1992). These are expensive diseases to treat, requiring hospitalization and modern technology, in comparison to the relatively low cost of inoculating children against measles and polio.[5] This fact alone would tend to reduce the rate of return to public health expenditures, unless these continue to be spent on preventing diseases of the young and are not heavily siphoned off for treating diseases of the old.

Yet public choice theory again tells us that this is unlikely to be the case: Children do not vote or make political contributions, as older people do. Moreover, their parents come disproportionately from lower-income groups (where birth rates are higher), whereas people who live to adulthood and old age come disproportionately from middle- and upper-income groups (where life expectancy is longer, in part because they have enjoyed better health care).[6] Thus, the latter are likely to win in the competitive struggle for public health resources against the children and their parents, giving us another powerful reason for predicting that the past successes of the government in reducing mortality will not be maintained in the future.

These arguments are developed in further detail below.

Correlation Between Mortality and Poverty

The most obvious success of the state in reducing mortality in developing countries has come via programs based on new technologies, programs

---

[5]This is not to say that the cost-effectiveness of treating all childhood diseases is higher than the cost-effectiveness of treating all adult diseases. Jamison and Mosley (1991:18) point out that among the most cost-effective interventions in developing countries are such adult health interventions as antismoking campaigns plus tobacco taxes, passive case finding and short-course chemotherapy for tuberculosis, and the use of condoms to prevent AIDS transmission. However, because many other adult health interventions are so costly and the burden of chronic diseases increases as populations age, the authors also note that this increasing burden is "initially likely to affect the relatively more affluent and politically vocal older groups who are growing in numbers. This being the case, governments will need to take great care to assure that the infectious diseases which predominantly affect children and the poor are not neglected in the face of resource demands placed in large measure by the more affluent."

[6]Preston (1984) makes this point in explaining the shift in public spending from the young to the old in the United States. This description of low- and high-income groups is based on lifetime income. In terms of current income, parents of young children and older age groups are both at relatively low points on their age-earnings profiles, while middle-age adults are at relatively high points. However, the current income and asset situation of the parents is probably worst of all since older people with high lifetime incomes have at least had the opportunity to save.

to immunize people and to control malaria and other endemic diseases. In some cases (e.g., malaria control), these programs provided "public goods" that were automatically available to all. In other cases (e.g., immunizations), they provided "quasi-public goods" that were ostensibly available to all but, in fact, had a large private component that was rationed to the people (typically middle and upper class) who were most likely to perceive and capture these benefits. This group was the easiest clientele to reach and serve; hence, such expenditures bore a high rate of return, as well as strong political support.

Further mortality declines will be much harder to achieve; they will depend much more than in the past on behavioral changes, particularly among people who have been most resistant to such change, (i.e., the poor and uneducated), and on public expenditures specifically targeted toward these groups.[7] Moreover, these are the politically disenfranchised groups in many societies. Thus, such policies will be costlier, will bear a lower rate of return, and, for political economy reasons, are unlikely to be adopted.

What is the evidence that further mortality declines will be harder to achieve—because they will have to reach the poor? First, within developing countries, the differentials in mortality associated with income and other measures of socioeconomic status have persisted, even when overall mortality has fallen substantially. In Brazil, deaths from infectious and parasitic diseases have declined drastically. These accounted for 45 percent of all deaths in 1930 but only 11 percent in 1980 (Briscoe, 1990). Other causes of death, however, are highly concentrated among the poor. Infant mortality rates among the rural poor in the northeast of Brazil are two to three times higher than rates in the wealthier, more urbanized south. For eight developing countries in which households were surveyed in the mid-1980s, infant mortality among mothers with no education was two to three times higher than among mothers with secondary education and three to six times higher than among mothers with more than secondary education (Mosley et al., 1990). The poverty rate works better than average income as a predictor of infant mortality and life expectancy in a sample of 86 developing countries (Anand and Ravallion, 1993). These continuing differences suggest that progress in reducing mortality among the very poor and uneducated requires new, and probably more expensive, initiatives (including the reduc-

---

[7]Hill and Pebley (1988) report that over the past 25 years, there has not been stagnation in the pace of mortality decline. However, the pace of mortality decline has been markedly slower in Africa than in other regions; this was true even before the economic crisis of the 1980s. Mosley et al. (1990:350) note the difficulty in Africa of reducing mortality, where reduction of mortality "from diarrhea and acute respiratory infections will require increased food production, environmental improvements, and behavioral changes, along with improvements in the efficiency and effectiveness of the health system."

tion in poverty) than those that succeeded in reducing aggregate mortality in the past.

Second, there is a difference in the nature of diseases that kill people in developing countries today and those that predominated in developed countries when they had similar overall mortality levels. For example, the proportion of deaths due to diarrhea is much higher in the developing world than it was in the West when overall mortality levels were similar, in large part because the prevalence of other diseases has been reduced by technological interventions (Preston et al., 1972; World Health Organization, 1989; J.L. Bobadilla, personal correspondence, 1991). Diarrhea is a disease of the poor; it is found along with, and contributes to, malnutrition, and it is caused by lack of access to clean water, simple health services, and basic education. To date, diarrhea has been relatively impervious to the programs and technologies that have reduced other causes of mortality. It has been hoped that the "new technology" of oral rehydration therapy (ORT) can reduce mortality due to diarrhea, but use of ORT itself requires change in the behavior of mothers and other caretakers. Moreover, it is not clear that repeated handling of diarrhea through ORT actually reduces mortality in environments in which infants are likely to die from other diseases of poverty (Mosley and Chen, 1984).

Third, there is evidence across countries of continuing huge disparities in disease risks, including risk of chronic disease, that are also clearly associated with overall differences in income, education, and the effectiveness of the public health infrastructure. For example, the annual risk of infection from tuberculosis is 50 to 200 times greater in developing than in developed countries (Mosley et al., 1990).

Reductions in mortality will continue in developing countries at a moderate rate, if further increases in educational opportunities, especially for women, and in family income are assumed. But the dramatic declines in mortality of the past are unlikely—unless public expenditures are concentrated much more heavily on the poor, to ensure delivery of good- quality personal health services. Of critical importance are family planning, nutritional supplementation for children, prenatal and obstetrical care, clean water, and the correct use of effective drugs (against respiratory infections, tuberculosis, and malaria). However, for such services to be effective, not only must they be readily available, they must be sought, understood, and used voluntarily by their clientele. Such behavioral change will occur only if the time and money costs of health services to the poor decline and/or if the poor receive information that changes their underlying tastes and choices.

The time and money costs will decline only if government targets its health spending to the poor, making basic health services easily accessible in the rural areas and urban neighborhoods where the poor are concentrated. For the reasons of political economy given above, such targeting appears unlikely. Similarly, it will be difficult to inform the poor and change their health habits (e.g., concerning nutrition, sanitation, and drug regimes to handle tuberculosis) unless their educational levels increase, which also requires a heavy and unlikely targeting of public (educational) expenditures toward the poor. Indeed, if the poor had access to substantially improved and heavily subsidized health, education, water, and sanitation facilities, there would be drastic improvements in their mortality rates and therefore the overall mortality rates of their countries, but a drastic redistribution of real income and utility would be implied. In this sense, continued high rates of health improvement and income redistribution go hand in hand, and both will be opposed by powerful groups intent on maintaining the distributional status quo.

Population Aging and Disease Patterns

The aging of the population in developing countries, a result of fertility declines over the last two decades and falling death rates, means that the prevalence of such chronic "adult" diseases as cancer, hypertension, and heart disease (in comparison to parasitic diseases and childhood infectious and diarrheal diseases) is increasing. The number of people over age 65 in developing countries will more than double between 1985 and 2015. By the year 2025, this elderly group will exceed 10 percent of the population in many developing countries, a proportion close to that in the United States today (Mosley et al., 1990; World Bank, 1991).

Brazil provides a telling example of the effects of past improvements in health technology and future changes in demographic structure on the pattern of disease. In 1950, heart disease, stroke, cancer, and accidents accounted for 20 percent of deaths there; in 1980, they accounted for approximately 50 percent. The increase in their relative contribution over the period was due largely to a decline in the proportion of deaths caused by infectious and parasitic diseases. However, the changing age structure means that from now on their prevalence is likely to rise as the proportion of the elderly in the population increases. Age structure changes alone imply a 60 percent increase in deaths due to these diseases from 1980 to 2020 (Briscoe, 1990).

Increases in age-specific death rates from some of these chronic diseases will further change epidemiological patterns. Age-specific death rates are likely to rise because of increasing exposure to such risks as smoking, poor diet, and urban pollution. For example, increases in tobacco consumption in the developing world over the last 40 years are likely to cause increases in the incidence of lung cancer comparable to the large increases experienced in Great Britain in the 1960s and 1970s, and in the United States more recently (in both places the peak has already been passed; Jamison and Mosley, 1991).

These changing demographic and epidemiological patterns will put new financial pressure on health systems in developing countries. By 1980 in Brazil, the allocation of public health resources for curative care had increased to 85 percent of all spending (from 36 percent in 1965), and the treatment of patients with heart disease accounted for an estimated 25 percent of all inpatient costs. Per capita health expenditures on persons over 60 were 3.5 times greater than the average for the population.[8]

Unfortunately, continuing increases in spending on hospital services for the care of chronic disease, although very expensive, will have little effect on the high death rates in developing countries among the poor.[9] The estimated cost (per discounted healthy life years gained) for such services as maternal and child health care, immunization, vitamin A supplementation, antismoking campaigns, and short-course therapy for tuberculosis is $50 to $150; the estimated cost per life saved through curative treatment (e.g., at the extreme for coronary bypass surgery and hospital management of lung and stomach cancers) is more than $1,000 (Jamison and Mosley, 1991; Akin et al., 1987). The latter costs are likely to rise still further because of continuing pressure to use high-cost technologies, such as open-heart surgery, organ transplants, and kidney dialysis.

Thus, the marginal cost of reducing mortality would appear to be much lower if societies concentrated on diseases of the young (and the poor), and the marginal benefit, in terms of years of life expectancy added, would be much higher; hence such an allocation would seem to be efficient by these criteria. However, political pressures from influential groups have led most societies to spend disproportionately on diseases of adults, particularly curative hospital care, as described in detail later. The problem is exacerbated because the young come disproportionately from lower-income groups and the old from middle- and upper-income groups; the problem is currently being experienced in developed countries as well. However, its consequences are (and will be) even more marked in developing countries, where income and health disparities are greater. The argument of the previous section sug-

[8]The cost burden could also rise because of the spread of AIDS, especially in Africa. The cost of treating AIDS patients in a typical African country could be as high as 10 percent of its current spending on health, even if modest estimates of current spending per patient on care (compared, for example, with spending in the United States); see Over (1988).

[9]It is worth clarifying at this point that hospital care need not be costly and, even when costly, is not necessarily cost-ineffective. Small hospitals (of 50 or fewer beds) can be a critical part of an effective overall health system in which consumers can count on referral to higher levels of the system. In general in this text, however, the term hospital care refers to hospitals at the tertiary level (i.e., facilities offering specialized and relatively high-cost services). Even these may be a necessary part of an overall system that is cost-effective, in the sense of providing the full range of services society desires at minimum costs.

gests that unless funding mechanisms change, the battle will be won by the wealthier, older groups whose rapidly accelerating health care costs will use up public resources that could more productively, and equitably, be spent on the younger and poorer members of society.

Endogeneity of Medical Research

This argument is strengthened if we ask: Why are expensive high-technology procedures aimed disproportionately at curing diseases of the old? We believe that the allocation of research and developmental resources in this direction is not accidental. Instead, we believe that the allocation process within the medical research arena is itself endogenous, governed by the same political economy forces described above with regard to service delivery. (For a much fuller discussion of the endogeneity of medical research, particularly its response to alternative insurance systems, see Weisbrod, 1991.)

A large share of medical research is carried on by pharmaceutical and other private companies in industrial countries, with the object of patenting and selling the life-prolonging drugs and equipment that they develop. The generous health insurance coverage received by the old, in part because of their political power, combined with the rapidly aging population profile in these countries, assures these companies of a ready market for their new products. On the other hand, the proportion of children in the population is declining, and they come disproportionately from low-income families who are less likely to have health insurance or to use it if they have it. Along similar lines, insurance often covers curative treatment rather than preventive. Therefore, companies in developed countries have less incentive to direct their research efforts toward children and preventive treatment than toward old people and cures. As a result, the developing countries, which utilize the new products and methods that emerge from this process, are faced with expensive medical technologies aimed at prolonging the life of the old rather than preventing illness among the young, and also with political pressures from the influential older groups in society for public spending to make these technologies accessible to them.

Other Reasons for Pessimism

Other reasons for pessimism include increased fiscal pressures on the government, leading it to divert expenditures from health care; political pressures from workers that often cause these cuts to be made in inefficient ways; and cost escalations in health care that diminish the productivity of the remaining expenditures, ceteris paribus.

The expenditure of central governments in developing countries rose dramatically from 5 percent of the gross national product (GNP) in 1945 to almost 20 percent in the early 1970s. It has continued to rise since then, though more slowly, and in 1985 was about 22 percent of GNP (World Bank, 1988b). Excluding expenditures on social security (which are higher in industrial countries) the share of the public sector in GNP in developing countries now exceeds that in industrial countries. In general, public expenditures have risen faster than revenues, so that annual deficits in developing countries have increased from less than 3 percent to more than 4 percent of GNP since the early 1970s (World Bank, 1988b).

The growing deficits do not bode well for spending on health or on education, which has potentially positive effects on health in addition to its other benefits. Between the early 1970s and 1985 in developing countries, the share of central government budgets directed toward health fell from 7 to 4 percent; the share for education fell from 14 to 10 percent (World Bank, 1988b). In some countries, particularly in Africa, the falling shares translated into real overall declines and even larger declines on a per capita basis. Though state and local governments may have taken up some of the slack, the dominance of the central government in most of the developing world means that expenditures of other governmental levels are not likely to have compensated.

Fiscal pressures in the 1980s also contributed to a reduction in the efficiency of government spending on health. Although in the long run the public sector may react to reduced resources for health by altering its mix of services, the short-run reaction has been to maintain the product mix and protect spending on personnel while cutting expenditures on nonpersonnel operating costs, including drugs, fuel for vehicles, and maintenance of physical plant and equipment (Akin et al., 1987). People are not easily laid off from public service jobs. Moreover, scarce foreign exchange is critical to the purchase of drugs, fuel, and equipment but not to the payment of wages. Because the nonpersonnel inputs are usually a small portion of total costs (less than 20 percent), they must be cut drastically to reduce total spending by a relatively modest amount. The price of a small financial saving is a large drop in the effectiveness of the system as a whole.

Finally, these problems have been exacerbated by the extension of health insurance without adequate cost containment measures in some developing countries. For example, in Latin America, the system of automatic reimbursement by the public sector insurer to charges of private providers has fueled the rapid growth of prices and spending on curative care, leaving fewer resources to be spent on more productive basic health services that are not covered by insurance.

All of these forces lead us to conclude that governments will simply not perform as effectively in the future as they have in the past; that this is due in part to growing tensions between the health needs of the rich and poor, old and young, in the face of increasingly constricted state resources; and that a radical restructuring of public-private roles may simultaneously improve equity, efficiency, and health outcomes.

EXAMPLES AND THE PRIVATIZATION SOLUTION

This section provides examples of our assertion that allocations within the health sector often disregard the benevolent prescriptions of welfare theory and instead fulfill the more pessimistic predictions of public choice theory. The frequent designation of health services as "externality-generating goods" or merit goods for lower-income groups has provided justification for government intervention along classic welfare theory lines. Our examples suggest that once this intervention begins, ostensibly to correct for market imperfections, improve health outcomes, and benefit poor consumers, more influential consumer and producer groups are often able to divert resources to the costly overprovision of services that predominantly benefit upper-income groups and have a much lower social rate of return. The influential groups are typically urban and older and require costly, curative treatments. Thus, these allocations are both inefficient and inequitable.

Second, we show how a shift of financing, particularly hospital financing, from public to private sources could alleviate this pressure on public resources, thereby permitting reallocations that increase equity and efficiency. Finally, potential pitfalls of these "privatization" policies are considered, as well as ways of guarding against the pitfalls.

The efficiency and equity criteria discussed in the first section and used here deal mainly with the question of who *finances* quasi-public services. Another set of efficiency considerations deals with the question of who *produces* these services, and how much private choice and public controls are involved. (For the distinction and connections between these issues, see Birdsall, 1992; James, 1990.) Below, the focus is on the benefits of shifting some of the financing of quasi-public services to the private sector, irrespective of whether the private or the public sector manages and provides the service.[10]

Examples of Inefficient and Inequitable Public Health Spending

As discussed earlier, efficiency criteria would dictate government ex-

[10]This focus also abstracts from the possible links between financing and provision that can arise in the real world for institutional or political economy reasons (e.g., the amount raised via user charges may be greater if the provider retains control over the resources; private provision with partial public subsidy may be more sustainable politically than public provision with partial user charges; and public regulations may accompany public subsidies).

penditures for such programs as immunization (generating externalities), improved water supply (a public good), monitoring minimum standards for pharmaceuticals and pesticides, and generating publicity about lifestyles that promote good health (such as antismoking and pronutrition campaigns) to help consumers make better-informed utility-maximizing decisions (Birdsall, 1989). The provision of basic medical services to low-income groups and to rural regions that cannot support a private competitive market in medical services is also warranted if people care about the health of others and wish to reduce the overall incidence of illness and mortality. Maternal and child health programs are particularly important examples of the latter since these affect the health of entire generations, in which there may be a large societal interest. Because they have public good characteristics, all the above programs are not likely to be provided by the private market; hence they are logical candidates for public funding.

We have argued that these basic services and informational programs would raise health standards and reduce mortality in the most cost-effective way (Birdsall, 1989; Akin et al., 1987). They would most help the poor, where mortality loss is currently highest. They would also help the young, where potential gain in life expectancy is the greatest. On both efficiency and equity grounds, these are the programs that merit public spending.

However, in many countries we observe relatively little public health money going to these cost-effective programs. Instead, a large proportion of public health budgets is spent on hospitals, usually located in urban areas, even in countries where the vast majority of the population lives in rural areas and suffers from high mortality rates caused by diseases that need not be treated in hospitals. In virtually all developing countries, the total health expenditure for curative care is between 70 and 85 percent, leaving only 15 to 30 percent for spending on preventive care and community services.

More specifically, in Bangladesh in 1986 hospitals consumed more than 80 percent of recurrent public health spending. In Brazil in 1982, 70 percent of public health funds was spent on reimbursement for physician and hospital care, including expensive high-technology procedures (kidney dialysis, coronary bypass, caesarean section). In Zimbabwe, which has tried to make its health sector more egalitarian, two-thirds of Ministry of Health expenditures are for hospital services, and 60 percent of these expenditures was absorbed by four hospitals in Harare. In Tanzania, which has made a special effort to improve rural clinics, 60 percent of the recurrent health budget was nevertheless spent on hospitals in 1983-1984 (Griffin, 1989; World Bank, 1988b).

Typically, these hospitals are located in urban centers of population and they serve the middle and upper classes; the superior public hospitals (e.g., armed forces or social security hospitals) serve the elite. Most of their patients are middle aged or older. Because hospital services are parceled out to their patients, they have a large private benefit component and could therefore be financed privately. But once government undertakes the task of financing hospitals, resources are crowded out and financing absorbs a large share of the public budget, because of the high cost of modern medical technology.

How Shifting to Private Spending Could Help

Suppose instead that many urban hospitals were turned over to private bodies, with fees to be covered by mandated health insurance (which might be administered by government but financed by premiums paid by the beneficiaries or their employers). Along similar lines, user charges could be instituted at the remaining public facilities, and the use of competitive, privately managed services might improve their effectiveness. Public funds would then be freed up to provide the externality-generating health programs listed above and also to subsidize health insurance for the poor. We contend that these changes would bring about a net improvement in health indicators, far beyond that which would be experienced under current funding mechanisms.

Examples of countries with such experiments are Zambia, where the university hospital at Lusaka is being turned into a parastatal that charges clients for services, with public funds thereby released to finance new maternal, child health, and family-planning services; Zimbabwe, where a fee has been introduced for patients who bypass lower levels of the health system and those who want a private hospital room; and The Gambia, where fees charged for drugs are turned over to village development councils for further health improvement (Akin et al., 1987). In Jamaica, costs declined when housekeeping and food services at public hospitals were contracted to private firms (Griffin, 1989). In Chile, increased reliance on private hospitals during the past decade was accompanied by a shift toward less expensive medical personnel (more nurses and midwives, fewer doctors), by structural changes to improve incentives, and by the targeting of government services toward primary health care and other services for the poor (Griffin, 1989).

Moreover, to the extent that reliance on government funds has limited hospital expansion, access to private funds (including insurance reimbursement) may increase the supply of hospital services and thereby improve overall access to health services. In the Philippines in the 1970s, after a policy change that allowed private expenditures, the greatest expansion of hospitals occurred in the poorest regions served (Griffin, 1989).

Pitfalls and Problems

In any privatization program, considerable thought and research must be given to potential pitfalls and methods of guarding against these pitfalls. For example, private hospitals are sometimes accused of taking actions designed to maximize their profits at the expense of ill-informed clients; they may downgrade quality, refuse to carry out important but costly services, recommend an excessive number of lucrative surgical and laboratory procedures, and deny admission to indigent patients. Possible remedies to these problems include regulations that require hospitals to provide crucial services and admit poor patients (but monitoring may be difficult); self-regulation and peer review to safeguard quality and reduce excessive surgery (but self-dealing, logrolling, and conflict of interest are pitfalls here); reliance on nonprofit rather than for-profit hospitals (but there is little evidence to prove that nonprofits are more trustworthy than for-profits, although some economic theories of nonprofits argue that this is the case); and mandatory insurance, subsidized for the poor, so that no one is left out of the system (but this introduces moral hazards, discussed below).

Another pitfall to avoid is the possibility that public funds will not be reallocated in an efficient, equitable way, even after private financing and service delivery are introduced. For example, in Brazil about half of health care expenditures are private, many private hospitals exist (70 percent of the total), and health maintenance organizations privately funded by workers and their employers are a rapidly growing urban phenomenon, demonstrating the viability of the market in health. Nevertheless, most of the public health funds are spent on hospital procedures with a large private benefit component (including public reimbursement of private hospitals) for upper-income groups (World Bank, 1988a).

In general, the availability of medical insurance plays a key role in all these scenarios that shift responsibility for hospital care to the private sector. Insurance, of course, raises the problem of moral hazard, hence overspending, which must be addressed or the efficiency gains just described will be reduced and perhaps eliminated. Indeed, uncontrolled private hospitals together with mandatory medical insurance may be the worst combination of all from this point of view (Birdsall, 1989). Procedures for dealing with this problem are requiring coinsurance (e.g., an annual deductible and/or a copayment for each treatment), exempting small costs from coverage, paying hospitals on the basis of diagnosis rather than procedures, reviewing recommendations for surgery and unusually high surgical rates, and building in competition among insurance carriers—in general, greater reliance on market incentives to contain costs. At the same time, it must be recognized that cost escalation in the health field is a problem whose first-best solution has not yet been found in any country. Perhaps all that is possible is a second-best solution, in which the burden does not fall disproportionately on the public treasury or on the lowest-income groups in society.

CONCLUSION AND POLITICAL STRATEGIES

Our policy recommendation is thus for a reallocation of public funds to public goods and to quasi-public goods targeted to lower-income groups, together with a shift of responsibility for "private" services to the private sector. The shift involves expanded financial and producing responsibilities for the private sector, combined with a reallocation of government funds within the public sector. For the reasons given above, this shift holds out the promise of increasing both efficiency (i.e., greater improvement in health indicators at lower cost) and equity (i.e., greater health gains for the poor). The central premise of this paper is that in the contemporary health context, equity is a necessary precondition for efficiency, and a reassignment of public and private roles is one of the few economically and politically feasible ways to accomplish both goals and to continue into the future the rapid mortality decline and health improvement that developing countries have experienced in the past.

In the absence of political change, however, this shift will not be easy to accomplish, since the current "misbehavior" of government (inefficiently producing private health and other services that benefit influential groups) has come about precisely because people with political power gain therefrom and will resist relinquishing this source of real income. The current situation is the outcome of a political process, and possibly a political equilibrium, in which each group has tried to maximize the utility it can extract from the system: the payoffs for the rich are superior hospitals, whereas the poor receive low-quality and limited rural health services. If we now disturb or constrain one element of this equilibrium, other elements will change as a reaction, so that the end result may be quite different from what was sought with the initial step.

For example, suppose the upper classes feel their benefits have declined when a shift is made from funding private to public goods by government (e.g., from financing medical operations to financing malaria control and immunization campaigns); they may then lobby successfully for a corresponding tax cut, so that government has less to spend, or for a shift in the structure of taxes, so that relatively more is collected from the lower classes. (Tax cuts in the Reagan years in the United States could thus be viewed, in part, as a reaction to the buildup of poverty programs in the 1960s and early 1970s.) The elite may try to recapture their higher real income in other ways (e.g., by increasing the level of bribery and corruption elsewhere in the economy). Ultimately, large changes in the distribution of benefits from government spending will occur only if there is a corresponding change in the distribution of political power.[11]

Although the above comments sound pessimistic, there are a few sources of hope. First, as discussed initially, many inefficient and inequitable policies are stimulated and perpetuated by imperfect information. The "losers" do not always know how much they are losing and the "winners" incur costs to hide information from them. Spreading more accurate information may thus in itself alter the feasible political equilibrium. Along similar lines, politicians do not know people's preferences or the intensity of these preferences with certainty, and if their perceptions of preferences are changed, the policies they deem politically optimal may also change.

Second, the current fiscal crisis in many countries may make politicians more willing to consider cost-effective reallocations, even if these hurt some of their supporters. The fiscal crisis may also indirectly reduce subsidies to the rich by leading them to abandon the public systems as they deteriorate in quality.[12]

Third, if service delivery becomes more efficient, as a consequence of the privatization policies discussed in this paper, this will free up some resources that could be used (at least theoretically) to make everyone better off. If the surplus is distributed in such a way that there are more winners than losers, including some influential winners, then political pressure to once again expand the public sector inefficiently might be offset.

Finally, the power structure may be changed through the intervention of external actors such as local and international nonprofit nongovernmental organizations, the World Bank, and other aid agencies—although the scope for action here is obviously limited. External actors are probably most effective over the long run when they provide new information and new ways of looking at old problems.

[11]For example, as the urban working class grew in size and became enfranchised in nineteenth and twentieth century Europe, it also acquired greater power to influence government-policies. Enfranchisement of black voters in the U.S. South, which accelerated with the Civil Rights Act of 1964, has increased the access of blacks to the benefits of state-sponsored social programs. Obviously, changes in the internal power structure are very slow and difficult to achieve. On the other hand, a temporary change in power can sometimes be multiplied and become permanent if it is used to alter the long-run rules of the game via constitutional change, precedent-setting judicial interpretations, irreversible extensions of voting rights, reapportionment, etc.

[12]For example, the fiscal crisis in Mexico appears to have contributed to the deterioration of the public university system and the evolution of financially autonomous elite private institutions; these now cater to the rich and reduce public spending on high-income university students.

REFERENCES

Akin, J., N. Birdsall, and D. de Ferranti
1987 *Financing Health in Developing Countries: An Agenda for Reform.* Washington, D.C.: World Bank.

Anand, S., and M. Ravallion
1993 Human development in poor countries: On the role of private income and public services. *Journal of Economic Perspectives* (7) (forthcoming).

Becker, G.S.
1983 A theory of competition among pressure groups for political influence. *Quarterly Journal of Economics* (98):371-400.

Behrman, J., and N. Birdsall
1988 The equity-productivity tradeoff: Public school resources in Brazil. *European Economic Review* 32(8):1585-1602.

Birdsall, N.
1989 Thoughts on good health and good government. *Daedalus* 118 (1)(Winter):89-124.
1992 Pragmatism, Robin Hood and other themes: Good government and social well-being in developing countries. In L.S. Chen, A.M. Kleinman, and N.C. Ware, eds., *Social Dimensions of Health Transitions: An International Perspective.* New York: Oxford University Press.

Birdsall, N., and E. James
1990 Efficiency and equity in social spending: How and why governments misbehave. World Bank Working Paper Series No. 294. World Bank, Washington, D.C.

Borcherding, T.
1985 The causes of government expenditure growth: A survey of the U.S. evidence. *Journal of Public Economics* 28:359-382.

Borcherding, T.E., W.W. Pommerehne, and F. Schneider
1983 Comparing the efficiency of private and public production: The evidence from five countries. *Zeitschrift fur National o Ekonomie/Journal of Economics* sup. 2:127-156.

Bourgignon, F.
1989 Optimal poverty reduction, adjustment and growth: An applied framework. World Bank draft report, Washington, D.C.

Briscoe, J.
1990 *Brazil: The new challenge of adult health.* World Bank Country Study, 1990. Washington, D.C.: World Bank.

Buchanan, J.M.
1967 *Fiscal Institutions and Individual Choice.* Chapel Hill: University of North Carolina Press.

Buchanan, J.M., R.D. Tollinson, and G. Tullock
1980 *Toward a Theory of a Rent-Seeking Society.* College Station, Texas: Texas A&M University Press.

Demsetz, H.
1982 The growth of government. *Economic, Legal and Political Dimensions of Competition.* de Vries lectures, no. 4. Amsterdam: North Holland Press.

Feachem, R.G.A., T. Kjellstrom, C.J.L. Murray, M. Over, and M.A. Phillips, eds.
1992 *The Health of Adults in the Developing World.* New York: Oxford University Press.

Fiorina, M., and R.G. Noll
1978 Voters, bureaucrats and government growth: A rational choice perspective on the growth of bureaucracy. *Journal of Public Economics* 9:239-254.

Gertler, P. and J. van der Gaag
1990 *The Willingness-to-Pay for Medical Care: Evidence from Two Developing Countries.* Baltimore, Md.: The Johns Hopkins University Press.
Gertler, P., L. Loray, and W. Sanderson
1987 Are user fees regressive? The welfare implications of health care financing proposals in Peru. *Journal of Econometrics* 36:67-88.
Griffin, C.
1989 Strengthening health services in developing countries through the private sector. World Bank draft report, Washington, D.C.
Hill, K., and A. Pebley
1988 Levels, trends, and patterns of child mortality in the developing world. Paper presented at seminar on Child Survival Programs: Issues for the 1990s, November 21-22, Johns Hopkins University School of Hygiene and Public Health.
Hochman, H.M., and J.D. Rogers
1969 Pareto optimal redistribution. *American Economic Review* 59:542-557.
James, E.
1990 Public policies toward private education. *International Journal of Educational Research* 15(5):359-376.
Jamison, D.T., and W.H. Mosley
1991 Disease control priorities in developing countries: Health policy responses to epidemiological change. *American Journal of Public Health* 81(1):15-22.
Jimenez, E.
1987 *Pricing Policy in the Social Sectors: Cost Recovery for Health and Education in Developing Countries.* Baltimore, Md.: Johns Hopkins University Press.
Krueger, A.
1974 The political economy of the rent-seeking society. *American Economic Review* 64(3):291-303.
Meade, J.E.
1964 *Efficiency, Equality and Ownership of Property.* London: Allen and Unwin.
Meltzer, A.H., and S.F. Richard
1978 Why government grows (and grows) in a democracy. *Public Interest* 52:111-118.
1981 Tests of rational theory of the size of government. *Journal of Political Economy* 89:914-927.
Mosley, W.H., and L.C. Chen
1984 Child survival: Strategies for research. *Population and Development Review* (supplement to volume 10).

Mosley, W.H., D.T. Jamison, and D.A. Henderson
1990 The health sector in developing countries: Problems for the 1990s and beyond. *Annual Review of Public Health* 11:335-358.
Mueller, D.C.
1979 *Public Choice.* New York: Cambridge University Press.
Musgrave, R.A.
1959 *The Theory of Public Finance: A Study in Political Economy.* New York: McGraw-Hill.
Niscanen, W.A.
1971 *Bureaucracy and Representative Government.* Chicago: Aldine-Atherton.
Nozick, R.
1974 *Anarchy, State and Utopia.* Oxford: Basil Blackwell.
Over, M.
1988 Testimony to the United States Presidential Commission on the human imunodeficiency virus epidemic. World Bank, Washington, D.C.

Peltzman, S.
1976 Toward a more general theory of regulation. *Journal of Law and Economics* 19:211-240.
1980 The growth of government. *Journal of Law and Economics* 23:209-287.
Pommerehne, W.W., and F. Schneider
1978 Fiscal illusions, political institutions, and local public spending. *Kyklos* 31:381-408.
Preston, S.H.
1984 Children and the elderly in the U.S. *Scientific American* 251:44-49.
Preston, S.H., N. Keyfitz, and R. Schoen
1972 *Causes of Death: Life Tables for National Populations.* New York: Seminar Press.
Rawls, V.
1971 *A Theory of Justice.* Cambridge, Mass: Harvard University Press.
Romer T., and H. Rosenthal
1978 Political resource allocation, controlled agendas and the status quo. *Public Choice* 33:27-43.
Stigler, G.
1970 Director's law of public income distribution. *Journal of Law and Economics* 13:1-10.
1971 The theory of economic regulation. *Bell Journal of Economics and Management Science* 2:3-21.
United Nations
1986 *World Population Prospects: Estimates and Projections as Assessed in 1984.* New York: United Nations.
Weisbrod, B.
1991 The health care quadrilemma: An essay on technological change, insurance, quality of care and cost containment. *Journal of Economic Literature* XXIX:523-552.
World Bank
1984 *World Development Report.* New York: Oxford University Press.
1988a *Policies for Reform of Health Care, Nutrition and Social Security in Brazil.* World Bank Report No. 6741-BR, Washington, D.C.
1988b *World Development Report.* New York: Oxford University Press.
1991 *World Development Report.* New York: Oxford University Press.
World Health Organization
1989 *World Health Statistics.* Geneva: World Health Organization.

Roles of Women, Families, and Communities in Preventing Illness and Providing Health Services in Developing Countries

John C. Caldwell and Pat Caldwell

INTRODUCTION

The informal sector plays a vital role in the provision of health services. Families, individuals, and societies all have rules that govern the type of treatment an individual receives for a given illness. As societies modernize, health usually improves owing to greater availability of health services and to changes in attitudes and norms pertaining to women's behavior and the value of life. In this paper we examine aspects of society and of behavior that encourage or discourage health, concentrating on the areas we know best, South Asia, sub-Saharan Africa, and to a lesser extent, the Middle East. Inevitably, the main measurement of ill-health is mortality because perceptions of illness vary across cultures and limited access to health services impedes gathering data on morbidity. Much of this paper focuses on child deaths, partly because they still form the majority of mortality in the poorer Third World societies and partly because we can locate the living carers for most dead children in contrast to the situation in the more difficult area of self-care that characterizes much of adult mortality.

The central argument of this paper is that the persons with the greatest interest in children's health and survival, and with the greatest willingness to devote time to their protection and to care for them in sickness, are children's mothers. Children may receive less than optimal attention both in health and in sickness because their mothers are prevented from giving

John C. Caldwell and Pat Caldwell are at the Health Transition Centre, National Centre for Epidemiology and Population Health, Australian National University, Canberra.

them the needed attention, lack sufficient resources from the larger family or their husbands, or lack self-confidence about their ability to care and make health decisions. Many of these elements still exist and restrict the rate of health improvement not only for the children but for their mothers as well. Moreover, these restrictions on women probably also jeopardize their husbands' health and survival chances.

This restriction on women limits the resources available to children and younger women so that men and the elderly receive what is regarded as their rightful share. However, the main reason for controlling women is to ensure the operation of the male-dominated, ancestor-oriented, patriarchal, larger family (not necessarily defined by a common residence). Only men or the elderly should confidently make decisions. A young woman should not divert her husband's primary obligations, duties, and affections away from his parents and brothers toward herself and her children. It is often the task of the mothers-in-law to see that this diversion does not occur. Such a structure once facilitated largely subsistence agricultural production but has retained a justification of its own as economies change.

In much of the Third World the most rapid gains against mortality can be made by giving women, especially young wives and mothers, greater confidence, more decision-making power, and greater access to resources for care and treatment. Women can be empowered as caregivers by education and by female home health visitors. They can also be empowered by social scientific "health transition" research which, as the findings become part of public knowledge, convinces men that women's powerlessness is endangering their children, even their sons. The same end is achieved through gains made by the women's movement in claiming greater gender equality as a question of social justice.

Women are helped in their caring mission by access to resources of such types as free advice and assistance from health visitors, and easy access to free or inexpensive health services. If these services are not free or of minimal cost, then there must be some way of ensuring that women can obtain immediate treatment for themselves or their children without having to wait for family budgetary decisions. In a fee-for-service system, women may have no way of obtaining quick access to the money necessary to pay those fees and may feel unable to take actions that would have to be covered by payment.

Women are often so immobile that the services must be close at hand. Because the traditional medical system has the loyalty of many people and is more often seen as offering complementary rather than adversarial services, the aim should usually be not confrontation with that system but rather an ever greater attempt to steer patients toward the modern system when it has the best treatment to offer, especially if the illnesses are life-threatening.

Populations of less developed countries need to consider more seriously the change, occurring in adult and old-age mortality. Males' health is threatened by the structure of the patriarchy and by the emphasis on masculine virtues, and in this area too, gains are to be made from the feminization of care, treatment decisions, and resource control. Here, too, the findings of health transition research need to become part of the public consciousness.

TRADITIONAL SOCIETY AND HEALTH BELIEFS

All traditional societies existing before the massive imports of culture and technology that have increasingly characterized the present century have very different beliefs about the nature of illness and its causes than those espoused by modern biomedical science. At their simplest, they merely put forward an alternative explanation for each individual type of sickness. In the absence of any access to modern health services these explanations were not necessarily harmful, although in both India and Nigeria (Cantrelle and Locoh, 1990) the cure involved contacting more persons than the sufferers tended normally to do. The real danger of traditional beliefs about disease causation is that when modern health services do become available, the sick or their parents may fail to use the services or may delay using them.

These dangers are not always as great as they seem, but they do have policy implications. In both Asia and Africa, most people regard the alternative systems not as being in conflict but rather as two different but valid roads to recovery. They are willing to alternate between the two systems, and frequently employ modern health services for life-threatening complaints and traditional services for those endemic conditions for which modern medicine has little to offer. In Asia, traditional healers take a rather similar view and most Indian *Ayurvedic* practitioners dispense modern medicine as well as prescribing ancient herbal cures. However, they may store medicines incorrectly, prescribe inappropriate dosage levels, and misdiagnose the condition for which medicines should be given. They go along with modern practice only as far as providing medicines, but not in other behavioral advice. In Africa, traditional doctors have rarely moved into this "halfway house," and their patients rarely receive whatever benefits modern medicine may confer. In the 1973 Changing African Family Project study of Ibadan, Nigeria, the children of traditional practitioners had higher mortality than almost any other occupational group (Caldwell, 1977).

Perhaps the greatest problem about traditional health beliefs is that they readily divert behavior into incautious patterns. In Africa there is a strong belief that the person of physical and psychological vigor cannot easily succumb to serious illness. This belief has resulted in continued high-risk behavior in such areas as sexuality, contributing to the spread of sexually transmitted diseases and AIDS (Caldwell et al., 1991). In both Africa and

Asia, people still believe that the future—or at least the timing of death—is predetermined, which may encourage incautious health behavior and weaken the belief in personal responsibility. Much sickness is regarded as a punishment for sins in this world or beyond. In sub-Saharan Africa, for example, there is often little attempt to obtain assistance during difficult childbirths because it is believed that the women can overcome the problem by admitting the adultery that caused it.

Another serious problem with regard to traditional medicine is the belief that the healer identifies the sickness at sight and prescribes the best treatment. If it does not work, then nothing will. In rural south India this practice means that illiterate women bringing sick children even to a modern physician do not overly exert themselves to explain the history of the sickness and, if the child fails to recover, frequently do not return for further treatment because they believe that the best available treatment has already been given.

On the other hand, not all traditional health precepts are in conflict with modern medicine. The historic Sri Lankan sensitivity to illness and the belief that doing nothing about it was inexcusable have fitted in well with the modern health system (Caldwell et al., 1989).

The policy implication in all but the most modern Third World societies is to avoid confrontation between traditional and modern providers. The public should be educated that the modern health system is the place of first resort for serious, sudden, or life-threatening sickness, without scorning the solace that the traditional system can provide for sufferers of rheumatism or even inoperable cancer. Where there is a well-established practice of traditional healers dispensing modern medicine, as in India, it is probably best to attempt to guide rather than prohibit this activity, given the paucity of modern doctors. The lack of confrontation is foremost a public reaction to the kind of health that is wanted and can be afforded. Politicians have moved slowly, and the modern medical profession more slowly still, in working out some kind of arrangement, but a nonconfrontational compromise is probably in the best interests of public health.

TRADITIONAL FAMILY AND COMMUNITY STRUCTURE—IMPLICATIONS FOR CARE AND HEALTH DECISIONS

In rural south India (Caldwell et al., 1988) and much of South Asia, the mother of young children is usually still a young woman and is likely to be living with her husband's family. She has been chosen by his parents primarily as a female member of the younger generation of the household rather than as his wife. In south India she may be living far away from her own family, and in north India this is almost inevitable. Her work and her life are controlled by her mother-in-law. The marriage must not undermine the structure and solidarity of the larger family, and the young wife must not seem to be emotionally too close to her husband, to influence him too much, or to seek his advice too frequently. She must not try to crystallize her nuclear family from the larger family. Her children are the children of the household, and her parents-in-law have direct control over them as their grandchildren.

This family structure influences health behavior decisions. The young mother keeps the closest watch over her babies and young children because they improve her status in the family. She is usually the first to notice that her child is ill, but in few cases does she take physical action and rarely does she even tell others; rather, she waits for her mother-in-law or her husband to notice (Caldwell et al., 1988). Her position is weakened further in the lower castes by working for long hours in the fields as an agricultural laborer while her mother-in-law cares for the child and regards herself as the child's main caregiver. The older woman would be insulted if the younger woman claimed that the child was sick and would regard it as a slur on her child-caring abilities. Consequently, taking action about sickness is delayed and the health decisions that are made are often strongly influenced by an older, uneducated woman. In parts of north India the patriarchy is so strong that most women, even the older ones, and especially the illiterates, feel little confidence in their abilities to make decisions and often take no action (Khan et al., 1989).

Education or the presence of educated women may modify these traditional structures. In south India, the older women usually regards an educated daughter-in-law as not only having rights to make health decisions, but as being more likely to make correct ones. Indeed, rural families now state that the second greatest advantage of an educated daughter-in-law is being more likely to ensure the safety and survival of the grandchildren. The young mother's independence is reinforced by the presence of government-sponsored family-planning workers who have caused the older women to retreat. In Sri Lanka, a system of female health visitors, who develop a relationship with the young women, has strengthened the decision-making ability of young mothers. Research in Sri Lanka indicates that half of the health decisions are made by the mother without consultation; most health decisions have been made this way in Kerala since at least the last century (Sushama, 1990, citing Mateer, 1883).

African women experience situations ranging from those not very different from India—among the Luo of East Africa—to those of West Africa where women have great independence but also great responsibilities that are not provided for by a joint family budget. Whyte and Kariuki (1991) indicate that among the Luo, although the mother is the most immediate caretaker of children and is usually held responsible when the children have accidents or suffer from sickness, she is constrained by the attitudes and traditional practices of men and family members. What is eaten, for example, and even the order in which people eat, are in many ways the most central aspects of culture. Women alone change what and how the family eats or even what they and their children eat. Yet nutritional education programs often direct themselves only at the women and avoid coming into conflict with the men and older women who make the actual decisions.

On the other hand, in West and Middle Africa, women are more independent, partly because of the prime social role of descent lineage and partly because of the existence of very high levels of polygyny, which renders each wife and her children a separate economic unit. In many settings, if a woman can find the resources, she can usually treat herself and her children as she sees fit, but the treatment may be more costly than she can afford from her farming or marketing income. In this case, she may have to seek money from her husband or the child's father. Involving others in the decision-making results in delays and in yielding power about treatment to the person who pays. Bledsoe (1990) indicates that the West African position to be more complex when a mother has to find the resources to pay for her child's treatment if her husband is not the father; she is also unlikely to try as hard if she is not the child's biological mother.

In South Asia, as in much of the Middle East, North Africa, and East Asia, society constrains a mother by placing more emphasis on the survival of sons than daughters. This emphasis is most dangerous among children ages 1-9, who are no longer receiving the equal nourishment and antibody protection provided by breastfeeding and are not yet old enough to look after themselves. Muhuri and Preston (1991) have demonstrated lower mortality in Bangladesh among the first two sons and the first daughter, showing that a care component exists that causes differential mortality. However, it is not clear to what degree attention or neglect affects mortality, or whether the mechanisms occur through feeding, maintaining good health in other ways, or securing timely curative treatment. In sub-Saharan Africa, where there is no excess female child mortality, girls are probably more protected by a bridewealth system than would be the case under a dowry system, although it is still in many ways a man's society. Perhaps the main factor protecting little girls in Africa is that children are very largely brought up by their mothers, who both take the responsibility and make the decisions.

What kind of care can be provided in a traditional society by a mother, and what is its likely effect? The kinds of effective care that can be offered by a mother in a traditional society include protection from accidents, protection from infectious disease, and treating a sick child in a way that will maximize the chance of recovery by allowing the child rest. They can also include elements of foresight about providing warm clothes or bedding and protection from the weather in other ways (cf. LeVine and Dixon, 1990). The provision of adequate feeding can often be achieved by the transfer of an almost insignificant amount of food from adults to the very young. The All India Nutrition Institute decided that the prime reason for the relatively high levels of malnutrition in traditional households where neither parent was literate was that they really did not think that such tiny persons needed very much food. They were also more likely to regard breast milk as a free gift not needing supplementing even when the baby was a year old.

There is another important dimension to child care in traditional society related to absolute and relative commitment to child survival, which has been well captured in a paper by Simons (1989). In most traditional societies, mothers are not as careful about their child's survival as they might be. They do not take as much responsibility as they might, partly because the family system does not dictate that the final responsibility is theirs and partly because they feel powerless to change the inevitable course of events. Child minding is usually very far from being the exclusive province of mothers, and in many small villages, children tend to run around together, with the community as a whole keeping an eye on them. Galel el Din (1977a; 1977b; personal communication, 1977) has described how mothers in Sudan who took such a system for granted subsequently changed as they were educated or migrated to towns and began to protect their children by intervening in the crowd and often withdrawing them into the home.

Community factors can also reduce the care a woman gives a child. In many Muslim societies, seclusion means that a woman cannot act easily to obtain treatment for herself or her children. Seclusion may be why educated women in the Middle East and North Africa do not have as low child mortality as their incomes and education would suggest; their problem is usually compounded because they do not have the education that such income levels in other parts of the world would ensure. In Bangladesh a young mother cannot take a sick child a few hundred yards across an open field to a dispensary until her husband or mother-in-law is available to accompany her. She cannot go herself to a hospital unless a curtained bicycle rickshaw can be obtained. Seclusion may explain why even in Matlab, with a hospital and four additional health centers, only 11 percent of women who die in childbirth are seen by a physician before death (Fauveau et al., 1989).

TRANSITIONAL SOCIETY

Traditional societies begin a phase of transition when they become more closely linked with the global economy and society; this phase is characterized by the growing importance of education and market economies. The traditional society passes when schools and health centers appear. Urbanization, too, and even the potential ability to migrate to a town also weaken the old system. Although family and social structure changes during these transitions, the changes are often not sufficiently fast to make full use of the new health services.

The aim of this analysis has been to show how social and behavioral change can be directed to improving health. The optimum path in most Third World societies is dominated by the need to modify the nature of the traditional family and the position of women in it, which is not to imply that health is improved by excision from the family. Such would be least likely to be true precisely in those societies where the family is all-embracing, and the solitary widow without surviving sons in India is subject to an appallingly high-mortality risk. Nevertheless, the traditional family does provide support and even health care, although these are subject to its own priorities toward the old and those of working age, and usually toward boys. Family priorities in South Asia seem to favor most the main contributors to its survival, especially working adult males, but in sub-Saharan Africa, priority is often given to old men, who will soon become powerful ancestors. To secure its physical and competitive survival, as well as give men what they feel they deserve, the traditional family is, in most societies, strongly masculine in attitudes and priorities. The evidence from transitional societies seems to show that the faster it is feminized (usually to only a modest extent), the more rapidly does mortality fall, even in the case of males. The process has often been most rapid where women's status has been highest in traditional or early transitional society, as in matrilineal Kerala or in Sri Lanka after the Buddhist Revival Movement of the late nineteenth century.

The role of the community is even more ambiguous. The community also can be patriarchal and oligarchic, reinforcing masculine and assertive values that are essentially anticare and, in transitional societies, monopolizing the new health care systems for the use of the powerful. In some transitional societies such as Kerala, community pressure can make the new health systems work efficiently, but these new community pressure groups appear to be an outgrowth of grass-roots, radical, and democratic tendencies that have flourished because of the weakness of older structures. They have been reinforced by modern political organization, which they have brought into existence, rather than being based on older community structures.

In recent years, research has demonstrated that child mortality declines steeply as the mother's education increases and that perhaps half of this effect remains when economic and other factors are controlled. This finding has elucidated the role of care in both transitional and traditional societies. We believe that it works partly through strengthening the individual internal locus of control and the commitment to child survival, making mothers feel personally responsible for what happens to their children and less likely to believe that it is inevitable (Caldwell et al., 1990). Girls who go to school identify themselves with other aspects of modernization ranging from nationalism to health centers, and modern medicine. They believe that they are the kinds of persons who can and should go to see doctors. Lindenbaum et al. (1989) examined mortality in rural Bangladesh and concluded that much of the lower-risk behavior of girls who had been to school arose not so much from the ideas they had absorbed but from the fact that they had learned to behave as the educated should—to dress themselves and their children cleanly, to wash their hands, and so on. As schooling continues, however, it probably has additional influences. Lessons are taught about health and hygiene—the need to boil water and to wash one's hands—as well as about modes of infection. Although most of this knowledge is probably lost, especially in nonreceptive family circumstances, some still remains. Probably the more important reason is the assault on nonscientific and nonrational thinking (Goody, 1971; Caldwell, 1982). Although students do not necessarily disown all traditional beliefs, they are taught to believe in the efficacy of modern science and may have two parallel interpretations of the world. They are much more likely to have some faith in modern medicine and to resort to it than are illiterate women. Although education and sensitivity to ill-health are not enough to produce very low levels of mortality, they tend to intensify effective maternal care, as Orubuloye and Caldwell (1975) showed. The big advance in reducing child mortality in Sri Lanka occurred when free modern health services became accessible. Cleland and van Ginneken (1989) found that much of the effect of maternal education on child survival depended on interaction with health services. They also established that there was a very considerable unexplained residual, which must largely be a measure of domestic care or health maintenance, that leads children not to become sick or have accidents in the first place.

A difficult challenge found more commonly in transitional rather than traditional societies is the rise of faith-healing Christian churches. In Nigeria, it is estimated that their membership may be as large as 25 million—one half of the Christian population and one-fourth of the national total. The growth of these churches may be related to charges for modern drugs, but they also affect behavior where there is no cost (e.g., the substitution of praying over water for boiling it). A recent study of a large town showed that modern maternity facilities were almost unused while babies were delivered in faith-healing church clinics without the benefit of sterilized instruments, boiled water, or any medicines (Adetunji, 1992). Here again, the best policy may be to avoid conflict and attempt to convince the churches that demarcation of services needs to exist.

There appears to be little doubt that when comprehensive health services are spread through a society over a period too short for social change or substantial alteration of educational levels, major mortality decline has occurred (Halstead et al., 1985; Caldwell, 1989). Two provisos should be made: (1) the successful health programs were essentially democratic and

(2) the successful services were often established in countries that were poor but had high levels of female education.

The community and its political structure affect not only a woman's capacity to visit the health service but also the way that service works. The extent to which doctors listen to less educated or poorer women is very much the product of social attitudes. If the doctors are also drawn from a group that is economically better-off or more powerful, they may give less attention to the poor and may work neither long hours nor conscientiously. Mosley (1989) has provided examples of studies of Asian societies, where social stratification and patriarchal attitudes rendered health services ineffective for most people. Even in more egalitarian West Africa, Okediji (1975) revealed the extent to which Nigeria's middle class monopolized the free government hospital services in the city of Ibadan.

The other side of the picture is the extent to which community attitudes and pressures make the health system work in Kerala. Popular emotions can run high and politicians quickly enter the fray. The pressures on health staff can be unfair, but they are compelled to work long and efficiently and to give due consideration to the poor. They see that drugs are ordered on time and make themselves available for emergencies outside normal hours, maximizing the access of women and children. But difficulties may arise in implementing these factors elsewhere because having adequate local control is really an agenda for political and social change extending far beyond the health service.

Democracy at the national level can ensure greater expenditure on high-quality, less expensive, and more accessible educational and health services, and greater equality for women. For this to happen, the government must have a radical and egalitarian element; otherwise, the chief thrust may be for lower taxes and the least governmental intervention. Left-wing revolutionary governments, especially in their early populist phase, can do the same. There are some interesting anomalies. Infant and child mortality decline appeared to falter under the early Pinochet regime in Chile but subsequently fell faster than ever. The explanation may have been partly the improvement of an economy that had found itself in severe difficulties, and partly the fact that external assistance and advice by donor governments determined that the experiment under way should succeed socially as well as economically. There is little doubt that in Indonesia popular pressures appear to be generated at the community level, which make health and other services work, yet in ultimate origin are autocratic rather than democratic.

Communities can influence health services in a number of ways. They can demand modern health service provision, usually more successfully in a representational democratic system. The new health system can be identified with their community, encouraging people to use it. This identification may be most successful if the community plays some role in the health center's administration and in the selection and employment of its staff. Perhaps more important is community pressure and spontaneous anger to ensure that the staff serve the people efficiently and without discrimination by wealth, gender, or education. Communities normally do not interfere in household care, although programs for weighing children and periodically examining their health can result in the community taking an interest in individual families and indirectly—or directly—exerting pressure.

There is evidence of education catalyzing a range of caring behavior in developing countries. We shall start with the interaction with the health system, if only because it is easier to measure, and outline our findings in rural South India (Caldwell et al., 1988), which are probably broadly similar to the situation in many countries. The young mother who had been to school probably crystallized in her own mind that her baby was sick somewhat earlier than did the illiterate mother and demanded that something be done. She was more likely to be allowed to do something herself because illiterate mothers-in-law concede that educated daughters-in-law understand what is of value in the new world. If the young mother was a Muslim this concession was more likely to be made over the doubts of local religious leaders about the necessity for her taking such public action. She was less likely to accept traditional explanations for the sickness but might rely on them if the doctor's treatment failed. The time she spent explaining the problem to the doctor was proportional to her education. The illiterate woman may fail to communicate for three reasons: (1) she thought that the doctor already understood what was wrong; (2) she lacked the words and concepts to make an easy explanation; and (3) the doctor shortened the time with the mother because he did not expect to understand her. This can be disastrous in view of Christakis and Kleinman's (1989) estimate that at least 80 percent of the correctness of diagnoses in rural developing areas can be attributed to the histories of the complaints as presented by the parents or patients. The more educated mother is also told at greater length by the doctor what should be done. She is more likely to buy the drugs, because she may be better-off and has the determination to secure the prescribed drugs, and she is more likely to use them properly. Also, the more education a mother had, the sooner she was likely to report back that the treatment was not working. The failure of illiterates to do so arose partly from the belief, based on the traditional medical system (which contained no probabilistic element with regard to diagnosis), that the disease had certainly been identified and the best treatment already given, and partly because they did not believe that they belonged to the same world as the doctor and, in their own words, could not tell him that he had been wrong. A number of policy interventions that might improve the situation are, clearly, encouraging the original determination that something should be done, attendance at a modern health facility, interaction with the doctor, obtaining the prescribed drugs, and reporting to the system that recovery has not taken place.

The maternal care that does not involve attendance at a health facility is much harder to measure. It has most often been assessed through specific behaviors. Bhuiya and colleagues (1990) showed that in rural Bangladesh, educated mothers were more likely to know that boiled water was safer to drink and were more likely to wash their hands after they had defecated or their children had done so. Owing to cultural proscriptions and practical difficulties, however, they were no more likely to confine the family source of water to the tube well. Chen and colleagues (1989) showed that for the Matlab area of Bangladesh, daughters received less food than sons and suffer from greater malnutrition based on standardized tests. They were also less likely to be taken to free clinics when suffering from diarrhea, which may have had a greater effect on mortality than differential feeding. In rural South India we found that educated mothers restricted other expenditures when food was in short supply, concentrating on adequate nutrition for the whole family. Our observations showed them making less distinction than uneducated mothers between old and young, or male and female, although, as Cleland and van Ginneken (1989) point out, the latter is not the usual finding in South Asia.

IDENTIFYING POLICY PATHS

What follows from the above discussion with regard to policy interventions that may help women as carers both in health maintenance and in curative interaction with modern health services?

The diffusion of social science research almost certainly has a central role to play. Public debate, fueled by social science research, contributed to world fertility decline by impinging on both governments and individuals (Caldwell and Caldwell, 1986). It is similarly inevitable that sufficient debate about the cultural, social, and behavioral determinants of health will influence governments at every level. The most patriarchal government or father is disturbed to find that some boys are dying unnecessarily because their mothers have too little education or too little autonomy, both in general and specifically with regard to health decisions and behavior. Clearly, the women's movement also has an important role to play in this area, both in securing women sufficient autonomy to make them more effective carers and in showing that some daughters are dying unnecessarily.

Lower fertility has a role to play in a sense that can be demonstrated by history rather than by comparing the fate of children in large and small families. Dramatic declines occurred in Western infant and child mortality in the first decades of the present century, following rather than preceding the movement toward the small family. Undoubtedly, a substantial component of this decline was behavioral, although to a considerable extent this was probably also due to new biomedical knowledge and techniques. As the family became smaller, more care and resources were diverted to children and there was greater determination that all should survive. This change occurred not only in the family but also at the level of governments and national organizations. In Australia and New Zealand, and presumably elsewhere, the emotional driving force of the infant welfare movement was the national responsibility for ensuring that all the children of these unexpectedly smaller cohorts should survive to support national growth and security. The responsibility for this care was laid even more firmly on the mother. Although this shift saddled her with more responsibility, it also backed her decision-making powers by a social consensus. It might be noted that the first deliberately contrived small families in Ibadan, Nigeria, experienced extraordinarily low mortality (Caldwell and Caldwell, 1978), and it appears that this differential has also held true in China's one-child families (Caldwell and Srinivasan, 1984). The children of sterilized mothers in rural South India have abnormally low mortality, partly because of family planning workers' concerns for child survival (Caldwell et al., 1988).

Perhaps the most promising policy interventions on the social and behavioral side for reducing infant and child mortality are to provide mothers, especially young mothers, with more self-confidence and more decision-making power. These two matters are not identical but are usually interrelated. Part of the answer is continuing public debate and media attention to these issues and their consequences for child health. In circumstances where fees for services or transport costs are involved, women need automatic access to the family budget or some sort of funds. The trend toward charging for health services jeopardizes children's health not only because it squeezes the family budget but also because it dramatically reduces the capacity of mothers to take quick action because they have the least access to family budgets.

One way to strengthen the position of wives and young women in the family relative to old women is the establishment of women's groups. These can be specifically related to child health and linked with health services. They can help ensure that all women and children receive a fair deal from both their families and the health system. Such groups existed in Australia earlier in this century, but their sole purpose seems to have been putting pressure on inadequate mothers.

An effective intervention in Sri Lanka and Botswana has been female health visitors. The visitors are usually educated young women from the specific area in which they are going to work. This experience and similar experiments elsewhere have shown that the visitors should be trained adequately by some kind of health authority and infused with some expertise, self-confidence, and realization of what their role is going to be. If possible, they should be given the backing and moral support of both the local community organizations and the local health facility. They should concentrate on identifying pregnant women and giving them support through pregnancy, birth, and the infancy of the child. The system succeeds not merely by providing advice but by being active within the family. The visitor suggests decisions and offers the young mother moral support in carrying them out. The health worker may also suggest when prenatal checkups are due, may make appointments for them, and may help not only with the logistics of transport but with seeing that the woman can get away from the home. She may also do all these things with regard to the birth itself and subsequent treatment of infant sickness or securing immunization. One of the advantages of institutional birth-delivery is that for a critically short period an even stronger organization takes the decision-making power out of family hands. The health visitor may even serve as a role model for the girls and young women of the area.

The health visitor will find it hardest to be effective in matters concerning family or culture. Such areas may include the family allocation of food, the work allocation of children, and the ability to rest when sick. At their most difficult, these decisions may involve the allocation of resources between the old and the young, the extent to which access to medical treatment is permitted, or whether continuation of girls' schooling beyond menarche should have priority over female modesty or seclusion. Community leadership and community meetings may be the mechanism for inducing such changes. In Indonesia this approach has been effective, although the emphasis is on securing community consensus on an issue rather than encouraging initiatives originating from the meetings themselves.

A different range of interventions is available to make the health system work better for mothers and children. The most important issues are the provision of adequate services for the poor, illiterate, or inarticulate; the ensuring of alternative treatments if the initial treatment is unsuccessful; and a devotion to duty that encompasses the constant availability of providers and medicines. Better training in medical and nursing schools, a better atmosphere in the health bureaucracy, an adequate surveillance system, and routine checks on patients who have not reported back—all can improve health status and conditions. Although the Kerala experience cannot be reproduced, it is clear that many of these objectives will be fully achieved at the local level, and even at the governmental and medical school levels, only if community pressures can be exerted. Local representative bodies need a voice in controlling health services.

If cost recovery is going to become a significant element in Third World health systems, there will have to be ways for ensuring that service is immediately available for sick children even if the cost is later recouped from their fathers. This difficult matter, involving both the collection of money and the guarantee that neither the mother nor the children will suffer because of incurring such debts, is probably something that community organizations do best.

OTHER STAGES OF THE EPIDEMIOLOGIC TRANSITION AND QUESTIONS OF ADULT MORTALITY

For much of the Third World we know far less about the structure of adult mortality, especially deaths outside hospitals, than we know about child mortality. Cardiovascular disease and illnesses linked to diabetes may be far more important than we thought; so may accidents and other violent deaths. There are regions such as mainland South Asia where mortality in late middle age or older, especially among men, appears to be almost inexplicably high, given the changes that have been achieved in younger mortality levels. Low levels of education and relatively low abilities for self-protection may be part of the explanation. The failure of adults to look after themselves may have causes very similar to those of the failure to care adequately for the young.

Among younger women, one obvious area for intervention is childbirth. Research at Matlab suggests that the entire excess female mortality in the reproductive-age range, which is observed throughout South Asia, can be explained by causes of death related to reproduction (Chen et al., 1974). The solution seems to be institutionalized childbirth, which overcomes the problem both of traditional birth attendants and of family unwillingness to allow modern care when difficulties with delivery arise. The fact that this female excess mortality is explained by maternal mortality does not mean that no gender discrimination is involved, for if men were subject to such risks, the resources for creating the necessary institutions would probably have been found long ago. The Matlab research shows that such mortality can also be reduced by more family planning so as to limit the number of births per woman and possibly prevent the premarital or extramarital conceptions that so often lead to fatal illegal abortions or domestic violence.

Little attention has been given to the fact that although the patriarchy diverts resources toward older men, it probably also places them in considerable danger. The emphasis on masculinity can mean a *macho* disregard for illness and its treatment. Our research in South India, an area characterized by a high excess of male mortality at older ages, showed only half as many adult men coming to the health center for treatment as adult women. It is probable, too, that in harsh, poor rural conditions, women, who are past reproductive age, provided they do not become widows without surviving sons, are subject to less physical adversity than old men. Farming, at this age, can be both strenuous and involve exposure to the rigors of the climate.

Finally, little attention has been given to self-inflicted damage from deleterious behavior in the Third World, partly because it is felt that there should be some solace for a harsh life and, in any case, death will probably come early. This attitude may lead to an underestimation of the level of deaths attributable to drinking (often impure and dangerous forms of alcohol), smoking, betel chewing, addictive drugs, and violence. The issue of high-risk behavior, however, now has to be faced in sub-Saharan Africa and elsewhere because of the occurrence of AIDS.

Many Third World countries are now entering an era in which health will no longer be dominated by infectious disease and early mortality. Indeed, much of Latin America, East Asia, and Southeast Asia are far along this path. It is a common experience for researchers in the poorer regions of the world, especially in rural areas of mainland South Asia and sub-Saharan Africa, to find that most people believe that mortality has risen over the past few generations. This belief is not prevalent in the more developed and better educated societies furthest along in the epidemiologic transition, if only because their educational levels and the better national data collection systems make their populations "developed" in depending on the media and on statistical services to determine their viewpoints.

There is little problem with the recognition that a need exists in these epidemiologically advanced societies to move from a health system dominated by protecting the young from infectious disease to treating the old for degenerative disease. Third World countries have been so dominated by models from the West, by the demands of their own urban elite, and by the views of the medical establishment in their capital cities that there has always been enormous pressure to accelerate such shifts. It has been expert reports, often written by teams with external membership, and the advice of such international bodies as World Health Organization (WHO), UNICEF, and the World Bank that have kept this tendency partly in check. The real challenges go behond this shift in the provision of services.

The first is to persuade the more epidemiologically advanced countries that a broader approach is needed to combat the degenerative diseases. Lifestyle changes, as well as medical provision, are necessary. This message may not be difficult to impart, given the extent to which these populations now read material originating with the Western media. The more difficult task will be to persuade market-oriented, development-focused governments and international organizations that the whole burden of the new old-age sickness should not fall on the women in Third World families and that the Western model of community assistance with the provision of subsidized hospitals, nursing homes, and old-age accommodations should, in forms suitably modified for the culture, be followed.

The second is to persuade the international health community that even in countries with life expectancies still in the range of 55-60 years of age, much of the battle against infectious disease has now been won and a growing proportion of deaths in the population over 40 years of age are now avoidable or deferable. This change has come about for two reasons. One is that the onslaught of infectious disease is being defeated for a range of reasons including the UNICEF insistence on worldwide immunization. The other is the change in age structure as fertility continues to fall in most of Asia and Latin America and begins to fall in Africa. Our ignorance of this mortality change in countries with incomplete death registration is partly the product of deficient demographic techniques for measuring adult mortality, let alone trends and rates of change, and partly a woeful lack of cause-of-death data except from the minority who die in hospitals.

The best health agenda for the Third World is reasonably clear: more investment in education, especially for females; more female empowerment, by direct intervention and through "health transition" research, which brings the social causes of unnecessarily high mortality into the public domain; more accessible and democratic health services identified with themselves by the local community; and a gradual reorientation toward attempting to reduce middle- and old-age mortality.

REFERENCES

Adetunji, J.

1992 Health behaviour among the Yoruba of Nigeria. Ph.D. thesis, Demography Program, Australian National University, Canberra, to be submitted.

Bhuiya, A., K. Streatfield, and P. Meyer

1990 Mothers' hygienic awareness, behaviour and knowledge of major childhood diseases in Matlab, Bangladesh. Pp. 462-477 in J.C. Caldwell, S. Findley, P. Caldwell, J. Braid, and D. Broers-Freeman, eds., *What We Know About Health Transition: The Cultural, Social and Behavioural Determinants of Health.* Proceedings of an International Workshop, May 1989, Health Transition Centre, Australian National University, Canberra, 2 vols.

Bledsoe, C.

1990 Differential care of children of previous unions within Mende households in Sierra Leone. Pp. 561-583 in J.C. Caldwell, S. Findley, P. Caldwell, J. Braid, and D. Broers-Freeman, eds., *What We Know About Health Transition: The Cultural, Social and Behavioural Determinants of Health.* Proceedings of an International Workshop, May 1989, Health Transition Centre, Australian National University, Canberra, 2 vols.

Caldwell, J.C., ed.

1977 *The Persistence of High Fertility: Population Prospects in the Third World.* Changing African Family Monograph. Canberra: Australian National University, 2 vols.

Caldwell, J.C.

1982 Mass education as a determinant of the timing of fertility decline. Pp. 301-330 in J.C. Caldwell, *Theory of Fertility Decline.* New York: Academic Press.

1989 Routes to low mortality in poor countries. Pp. 1-46 in J.C. Caldwell and G. Santow, eds., *Selected Readings in the Cultural, Social and Behavioural Determinants of Health.* Canberra: Australian National University.

Caldwell, J.C., and P. Caldwell

1978 The achieved small family: Early fertility transition in an African city. *Studies in Family Planning* 9(1):2-18.

1986 *Limiting Population Growth and the Ford Foundation Contribution.* Dover, N.H.: Frances Pinter.

Caldwell, J.C., and K. Srinivasan

1984 New data on nuptiality and fertility in China. *Population and Development Review* 10(1):71-79.

Caldwell, J.C., P.H. Reddy, and P. Caldwell

1988 *The Causes of Demographic Change: Experimental Research in South India.* Madison, Wis.: University of Wisconsin Press.

Caldwell, J.C., I. Gajanayake, P. Caldwell, and I. Peiris

1989 Sensitization to illness and the risk of death: An explanation for Sri Lanka's approach to good health for all. Pp. 222-248 in J.C. Caldwell, and G. Santow, eds., *Selected Readings in the Cultural, Social and Behavioural Determinants of Health.* Canberra: Australian National University.

Caldwell, J.C., S. Findley, P. Caldwell, J. Braid, and D. Broers-Freeman, eds.

1990 *What We Know About Health Transition: The Cultural, Social and Behavioural Determinants of Health.* Proceedings of an International Workshop, May 1989, Health Transition Centre, Australian National University, Canberra, 2 vols.

Caldwell, J.C., I. Orubuloye, and P. Caldwell

1991 Underreaction to AIDS in sub-Saharan Africa. *Health Transition Working Paper* No 9. Canberra: Australian National University.

Cantrelle, P., and T. Locoh

1990 Cultural and social factors related to health in West Africa. Pp. 251-274 in J.C. Caldwell, S. Findley, P. Caldwell, J. Braid, and D. Broers-Freeman, eds., *What We Know About Health Transition: The Cultural, Social and Behavioural Determinants of Health.* Proceedings of an International Workshop, May 1989, Health Transition Centre, Australian National University, Canberra, 2 vols.

Chen L.C., M.C. Gesche, S. Ahmed, A.I. Chowdhury, and W.H. Mosley

1974 Maternal mortality in rural Bangladesh. *Studies in Family Planning* 5(11):334-341.

Chen, L.C., E. Huq, and S. D'Souza

1989 Sex bias in family allocation of food and health care in rural Bangladesh. Pp. 247-263 in J.C. Caldwell, and G. Santow, eds., *Selected Readings in the Cultural, Social and Behavioural Determinants of Health.* Canberra: Australian National University.

Christakis, N.A., and A.M. Kleinman

1989 Illness behavior and the health transition in the developing world. Unpublished mimeograph, Harvard University.

Cleland, J.G., and J. van Ginneken

1989 Maternal education and child survival in developing countries: The search for pathways of influence. Pp. 79-100 in J.C. Caldwell, and G. Santow, eds., *Selected Readings in the Cultural, Social and Behavioural Determinants of Health.* Canberra: Australian National University.

El Din, M.

1977a The economic value of children in rural Sudan. Pp. 617-632 in J.C. Caldwell, ed., *The Persistence of High Fertility: Population Prospects in the Third World.* Changing African Family Monograph. Canberra: Australian National University, 2 vols.

1977b The rationality of high fertility in urban Sudan. Pp. 633-658 in J.C. Caldwell, ed.,

The Persistence of High Fertility: Population Prospects in the Third World. Changing African Family Monograph. Canberra: Australian National University, 2 vols.

Fauveau, V., B. Wojtyiniak, M.A. Koenig, J. Chakraborty, and A.I. Chowdhury, eds.
1989 Epidemiology and cause of deaths among women in rural Bangladesh. *International Journal of Epidemiology* 18(1):139-145.

Goody, J.
1971 *Technology, Tradition and the State in Africa.* London: Oxford University Press.

Halstead, S.B., J.A. Walsh, and S. Warren, eds.
1985 *Good Health at Low Cost.* Proceedings of a Conference held at Bellagio Conference Center, Bellagio, Italy, April 29-May 2. New York: Rockefeller Foundation.

Khan, M.E., R. Anker, S.K. Ghosh Dastidar, and S. Bairati
1989 Inequalities between men and women in nutrition and family welfare services: An in-depth enquiry in an Indian village. Pp. 175-199 in J.C. Caldwell, and G. Santow, eds., *Selected Readings in the Cultural, Social and Behavioural Determinants of Health.* Canberra: Australian National University.

LeVine, R.A., and S. Dixon
1990 Child survival in a Kenyan community: Changing risks over thirty years. Pp. 420-424 in J.C. Caldwell, S. Findley, P. Caldwell, J. Braid, and D. Broers-Freeman, eds., *What We Know About Health Transition: The Cultural, Social and Behavioural Determinants of Health.* Proceedings of an International Workshop, May 1989, Health Transition Centre, Australian National University, Canberra, 2 vols.

Lindenbaum, S., M. Chakraboorty, and M. Elias
1989 The influence of maternal education on infant and child mortality in Bangladesh. Pp. 112-131 in J.C. Caldwell, and G. Santow, eds., *Selected Readings in the Cultural, Social and Behavioural Determinants of Health.* Canberra: Australian National University.

Mateer, S.
1883 *Native Life in Travancore.* London: W.H. Allen.

Mosley, W.H.
1989 Will primary health care reduce infant and child mortality? Pp. 261-294 in J.C. Caldwell and G. Santow, eds., *Selected Readings in the Cultural, Social and Behavioural Determinants of Health.* Canberra: Australian National University.

Muhuri, P.K., and S.H. Preston
1991 Family composition and sex mortality differentials among children in Matlab, Bangladesh. *Population and Development Review* 17(3):415-434.

Okediji, F.O.
1975 Socio-economic status and attitudes to public health problems in the Western State: A case study of Ibadan. In J.C. Caldwell. ed., *Population Growth and Socio-economic Change in West Africa.* New York: Columbia University Press.

Orubuloye, I., and J.C. Caldwell
1975 The impact of public health services on mortality: A study of mortality differentials in a rural area in Nigeria. *Population Studies* 29(2):259-272.

Simons, J.
1989 Cultural dimensions of the mother's contribution to child survival. Pp. 132-145 in J.C. Caldwell, S. Findley, P. Caldwell, J. Braid, and D. Broers-Freeman, eds., *What We Know About Health Transition: The Cultural, Social and Behavioural Determinants of Health.* Proceedings of an International Workshop, May 1989, Health Transition Centre, Australian National University, Canberra, 2 vols.

Sushama, P.N.
1990 Social context of health behaviour in Kerala. Pp. 777-787 in J.C. Caldwell, S. Findley, P. Caldwell, J. Braid, and D. Broers-Freeman, eds., *What We Know About Health Transition: The Cultural, Social and Behavioural Determinants of Health*. Proceedings of an International Workshop, May 1989, Health Transition Centre, Australian National University, Canberra, 2 vols.

Whyte, S.R., and P.W. Kariuki
1991 Malnutrition and gender relations in western Kenya. *Health Transition Review* 1(2):171-188.